# Children with Developmental Disabilities

# Children with Developmental Disabilities
## a training guide for parents, teachers and caregivers

# S. Venkatesan

**Sage Publications**
**New Delhi/Thousand Oaks/London**

**For the kids, my kids—who made this endeavour possible ...**

First published in 2004 by

**Sage Publications India Pvt Ltd**
B-42, Panchsheel Enclave
New Delhi 110 017

**Sage Publications Inc**
2455 Teller Road
Thousand Oaks, California 91320

**Sage Publications Ltd**
1 Oliver's Yard, 55 City Road
London EC1Y 1SP

Published by Tejeshwar Singh for Sage Publications India Pvt Ltd, typeset by S.R. Enterprises, New Delhi in 10/12.5 Zapf Ellipt BT and printed at Chaman Enterprises, New Delhi.

**Library of Congress Cataloging-in-Publication Data**

Venkatesan, S.

    Children with developmental disabilities: a training guide for parents, teachers and caregivers/
S. Venkatesan
      p.  cm.
    Includes bibliographical references and index.
    1. Developmentally disabled children—Care. I. Title.

RJ135. V465           618.92—dc21          2003          2003010926

**ISBN:** 0-7619-9775-X (US-Pb)        81-7829-259-9 (India-Pb)

**Sage Production Team:** Ankush Saikia, Rajib Chatterjee, Rahul Sharma and Santosh Rawat

Illustrations by L. Nanda Kumar

# Contents

# List of Tables

# List of Figures

# List of Illustrations

# List of Abbreviations

| | |
|---|---|
| AAG | Activity Assistance Guide |
| ACPC-DD | Activity Checklist for Preschool Children with Developmental Disabilities |
| AD | Autistic Disorder |
| ADA | American Disabilities Act |
| ADHD | Attention Deficit Hyperactivity Disorder |
| ADIP | Assistance for Disabled Persons |
| ALIMCO | Artificial Limb Manufacturing Corporation |
| AsD | Aspergers' Disorder |
| AYJNIHH | Ali Yavur Jung National Institute for Hearing Handicapped |
| | |
| BASIC-MR | Behaviour Assessment Scales for Indian Children with Mental Retardation |
| | |
| C | Communication Domain under ACPC-DD |
| CAg | Coefficient of Agreement |
| CAT | Computerized Axial Tomography |
| CBR | Community-based Rehabilitation |
| CDD | Childhood Disintegrative Disorder |
| Cg | Cognitive Domain under ACPC-DD |
| CHC | Community Health Centre |
| CP | Cerebral Palsy |
| CRRC | Composite Regional Rehabilitation Centre |
| CSF | Cerebrospinal Fluid |
| | |
| Db | Decibels |
| DD | Developmental Delays |
| DDRC | District Disability Rehabilitation Centre |
| DQ | Developmental Quotient |
| DRC | District Rehabilitation Centre |
| DSM | Diagnostic and Statistical Manual |
| DST | Developmental Screening Test |
| DWCRA | Development of Women and Children in Rural Areas |
| | |
| EEG | Electroencephalography |

FM           Fine Motor Domain under ACPC-DD

GM           Gross Motor Domain under ACPC-DD
GOI          Government of India

ICD          International Classification of Diseases
ICDS         Integrated Child Development Scheme
ICIAP        International Classification of Impairments, Activity and Participation
ICIDH        International Classification of Impairments, Disabilities and Handicaps
ICMR         Indian Council for Medical Research
ICSSR        Indian Council for Social Science Research
IPH          Institute for Physically Handicapped
IQ           Intelligence Quotient
IRDP         Integrated Rural Development Programme
ISIC         Indian Spinal Injury Centre

JEE          Joint Entrance Examination

KR-20        Kuder Richardson-20

MCD          Motor Co-ordination Disorder
MDPS         Madras (Minnesota) Developmental Programming System
MPRWs        Multipurpose Rehabilitation Workers
MRI          Magnetic Resonance Imaging
MSJE         Ministry of Social Justice and Empowerment

NAB          National Association for the Blind
NASEOH       National Society of Equal Opportunities for the Handicapped
NCERT        National Council on Educational Research and Training
NGO          Non-governmental Organization
NICDR        National Information Centre on Disability and Rehabilitation
NIHH         National Institute for the Hearing Handicapped
NHFDC        National Handicapped Finance Corporation
NIMH         National Institute for the Mentally Handicapped
NIOH         National Institute for Orthopedically Handicapped
NIPCCD       National Institute for Public Co-operation and Child Development
NIRTAR       National Institute of Rehabilitation, Training and Research
NIVH         National Institute for Visually Handicapped
NOS          National Open School

| NPRPD | National Programme for Rehabilitation of Persons with Disabilities |
| NSSO | National Sample Survey Organization |
| | |
| P | Play Domain under ACPC-DD |
| PA | Preacademic Domain under ACPC-DD |
| PDD | Pervasive Developmental Disorder |
| PET | Positron Emission Tomography |
| PHC | Primary Health Centre |
| | |
| RCI | Rehabilitation Council of India |
| RD | Retts' Disorder |
| RRTC | Regional Rehabilitation Training Centre |
| | |
| S | Sensory Domain under ACPC-DD |
| SDS | Service Delivery Systems |
| SHS | Self-help Skills Domain under ACPC-DD |
| SQ | Social Quotient |
| SSD | Specific Speech Delays |
| | |
| TRYSEM | Training of Rural Youth for Self-employment |
| | |
| UGC | University Grants Commission |
| | |
| VRC | Vocational Rehabilitation Centre |
| VRWs | Village Rehabilitation Workers |
| VSMS | Vineland Social Maturity Scale |

# Preface

Different professionals carry out the assessment of individuals with developmental disabilities with different aims and purposes. A lot of time has been invested on the development and standardization of assessment tools for diagnosing developmentally disabled persons. This is the essence of most normative tests of intelligence, developmental schedules and/or adaptive behaviour scales available in our country. Today hard diagnostic questions about persons with developmental disabilities are not so much a preoccupation with professionals in the field as are questions related to programme planning, training and rehabilitation of these individuals. Therefore, it is apt to explore new avenues that facilitate assessment for programme planning, training and rehabilitation of persons with developmental disabilities. A preliminary start in this direction was the development and standardization of 'Behaviour Assessment Scale for Indian Children with Mental Retardation' (BASIC-MR) (Peshawaria and Venkatesan, 1992a). This Scale is proving to be popular and useful for special teachers of children with mental handicaps for planning individualized training programmes in school settings. But a major limitation of this scale, as well as with other similar scales available in the country, is that it caters to the needs of older children. There is no standardized tool for using with children of a lower age, i.e., infants, toddlers and preschoolers. Most items in the existing scales are predominantly tilted towards older children, adolescents and adults with disabilities. This present work is exclusively intended for preschoolers, toddlers and infants with developmental disabilities. The book has six chapters spread over three sections:

(1) Introduction on Developmental Disabilities
(2) Development and Standardization of ACPC-DD
(3) Assistance Guide for Training on ACPC-DD

The three chapters in Section A cover a wide range of impairments, disabilities and handicaps commonly seen in young children. This overview is meant to enable beginning students and parents of children with developmental disabilities to appreciate their manifestations, prevalence and characteristics. The importance of home-based training programmes and the steps in carrying out such programmes are also delineated. An agenda for carrying out problem-behaviour management programmes is also included for those children who exhibit negative behaviour during skill training programmes.

Section B deals with the development and standardization of an 'Activity Checklist for Preschool Children with Developmental Disabilities' (ACPC-DD). All teaching objectives and items included in the ACPC-DD are purported for teaching children below six years of age. The items are empirically validated and located along a hierarchical scale of developmental difficulty. They are worded in behavioural terms so that trainers can readily start working on the given goals for initiating changes in behaviour in their children. An elaborate glossary is enclosed at the end with a broad scheme and context under which target items are to be taught to infants, toddlers and preschoolers with developmental disabilities.

Section C is an 'Activity Assistance Guide' (AAG) for care-givers on ACPC-DD. A practical, 'ready-to-use' or 'do-it-yourself' advisor-type of approach has been endeavoured in writing this for trainers or care-givers of children with developmental disabilities. A portion of this section is also devoted towards sensitize readers on contemporary trends, problems and issues relating to rights, immunities and privileges of persons with disabilities in India.

There is a pressing need for this advisor since many trainers are groping for concrete suggestions from professionals not only on what to train these children, but also how to train within their own homes. This book is intended to serve that purpose. The contemporary scene of early developmental disabilities in India cuts a pathetic image. Professionals invest a greater portion of their expertize on making obvious diagnoses of children with developmental disabilities by way of expensive and unnecessary radiological investigations (like CAT scans, PET scans, MRIs, X-rays, etc.). Diagnosis-making or labelling becomes the dead end of the tunnel for many parents of children with developmental disabilities. The crucial questions are 'What happens after that?' 'How do I deal with this special child now?' 'What do I teach him now?' 'How do I programme an effective home-based training programme for my child who has an early developmental disability?' The present scale endeavours to answer some of these queries and prepare the ground for practitioners to deal effectively with the training of these children.

The completion of this work, which was undertaken a decade ago, has run through difficult terrain. The customary contrivance and compulsion of authors to catalogue several names in gratitude for their contributions to the preparation of a book is herein refrained. As it were, the completion of this work has vanquished all those designs seeking to obtrude the smooth flow of this endeavour over the past seven years. However, of course, acknowledgement remains due only for the members of my immediate family (an inescapable and most lovable institutional contraption), but for whose unfailing emotional support, probably, this work would never have been completed ... er ... so late!

**S. Venkatesan**

# SECTION A

Introduction on Developmental Disabilities

# CHAPTER 1

# INTRODUCTION

*This chapter attempts to provide an informative overview on the possible types/sub-types of psychological disorders, disabilities, impairments or handicaps usually encountered in infants, toddlers and preschoolers. No claim has been made to this overview being intensive or exhaustive. It is only meant as an eye-opener for students and parents of children with disabilities.*

A variety of life situations, including the aging process, manifest themselves as impairments. We often use the term impairments, disabilities and/or handicaps interchangeably; hence incorrectly. To begin with, parents need to be clear about these terms as the terms themselves profoundly influence their opinions and attitudes towards their own children with such problems.

## Impairments, Disabilities and Handicaps

Impairments are generally not recognized until they interfere in the performance of daily activities by an individual. *Impairment* is any visible structural/anatomical loss of physical or sense organs in an individual. The loss of a little finger is an *impairment*. *Disability*, usually a consequence of impairment, is the functional inability of an individual to perform any activity in the manner or within the range considered 'normal' for any human being. It is a restriction of activities as a result of an impairment. Disability interferes in the performance of daily activities by an individual. Temporary or permanent disabilities can be caused by diseases, accidents or genetic causes, and may vary from case to case. The scale of abilities–disabilities exists, as it were, along a continuum. Thus, going back to our earlier example, a person who has lost his little finger (impairment) may not be experiencing any disability when compared to another individual who has lost his upper limbs. *Handicap* is a disadvantage resulting from, or the consequence of, impairment as well as disability. It is the manifest limitation that prevents fulfilment of the social role expected for the age, sex or cultural background of an individual (WHO, 1980). A person may lose a limb and still not face any impediments at his job. Thus, he is physically impaired but not handicapped. The concept of handicap is subjective, situational and subject to social perception. The official document to distinguish these terms is the International Classification of Impairments, Disabilities and Handicaps (ICIDH) first published by the World Health Organization (ibid.). A revision of the ICIDH is expected shortly, as a renamed instrument called the *International Classification of Impairments, Activities and Participation* (ICIAP) (WHO, 2002). This renaming is to do away with the stigma and negative connotations attached to the words 'disability' and 'handicap'. Further, the 'linear, theoretical or medical-disease' model underlying the earlier understanding of impairment-disability-handicap as a consequence of 'illness-disease' is being increasingly challenged by the alternative 'human-rights model' that advocates primacy of the individual with impairments. The term 'disability' has been replaced with 'activity', and 'handicap' with 'participation', to indicate the nature and extent of a person's involvement in life situations. The qualifiers that indicate the degree of difficulty and assistance required to overcome this difficulty (formerly called 'handicap') is now referred to as 'restriction in participation'. In this new classification, a list of environmental/contextual factors commonly impacting on participation are delineated.

> **Impairment is any structural loss, disability is functional incapability and handicap is a social disadvantage experienced by a person**

## Magnitude

The magnitude of impairments, disabilities and handicaps has been estimated differently in different counties. A WHO report suggests that 5.21 pcr cent of the population of developing countries is disabled. This comes to, roughly, a colossal 50 million persons with disabilities in India. There has been no nationwide survey on the prevalence of disabilities to date. Most epidemiological reports are part of specific disease-morbidity statistics, results of disability detection camps, profiles of case distributions seen at Child Guidance Clinics (CGCs) across the country, etc. While such reports indirectly reflect on the magnitude of disability in our country, they cannot be assumed to give the complete and accurate picture.

> **In India 16.15 million people are affected with one or the other of the four major types of disabilities**

The first sample survey covering specific pockets in India estimated that 16.15 million people in the country are affected with one or the other of the four major disabilities, viz., visual, hearing, locomotor and/or mental handicaps (NSSO, 1991a, 1991b). The National Sample Survey Organization (NSSO) (47th round) had its own criteria for defining/identifying various disabilities. For example, it defined a person with visual disability as one with no light perception, and also those with light perception, but who could not count the fingers of a hand correctly (even with the aid of glasses) from a distance of three metres in broad daylight. Hearing disability was defined as a persons inability to hear properly, or a person being able to hear shouted words only when the speaker was sitting directly in front. Obviously, these definitions are subjective. Table 1.1 lists the estimated prevalence of disabilities per thousand persons according to the NSSO (1991a). Even though one appreciates the diligence of field investigators who undertook such a massive exercise across the country, their medical competence in accurately diagnosing impairments and disabilities is doubted by fastidious social scientists. Nevertheless, the figure of 1.9 per cent as given by the NSSO continues to be the official benchmark for comparison of disability-prevalence statistics with other countries like China (5 per cent), Pakistan (4.9 per cent), Philippines (4.4 per cent), Nepal (5 per cent), etc. A census estimate is always a more comprehensive statistic than sample surveys. Interestingly, the first census in India in 1871 included questions not only on physical disability but also on intellectual disablity! The practice was discontinued in 1931. Thereafter, during The International Year of the Disabled (1981), an attempt was made to collect information on disabled persons under the census, but a correct estimate could not be given. This was discontinued again 1991. It is heartening to note that the 2001 Census in India has included the disability count as an ingredient in the national agenda.

**Table 1.1**

**Prevalence of Disabilities (per thousand population) as per NSSO (1991a)**

| Type of Disability | Rural | Urban | Overall |
|---|---|---|---|
| All handicaps | 19.75 | 15.75 | 19.95 |
| Locomotor disability | 10.74 | 9.62 | |
| Visual disability | 5.25 | 3.02 | |
| Hearing disability | 4.67 | 3.39 | |
| Speech disability | 2.73 | 2.37 | |
| Developmental disability | 31.00 | 29.00 | |

(14.56 million persons, or 1.9 per cent of the general population, in India is disabled.)

## Types of Handicaps

Handicaps in human beings classified according to their site of occurrence include:

1. Physical/locomotor handicaps
2. Visual handicaps
3. Hearing handicaps
4. Mental handicaps
5. Learning handicaps
6. Multiple handicaps

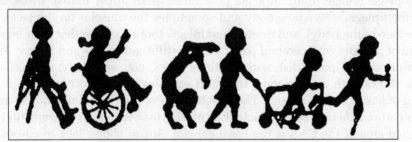

**Illustration 1.1  Types of Handicaps**

### 1. Physical/Locomotor Handicaps

Physical/locomotor handicaps occur due to impairment of the limbs or extremities. It involves an inability to execute distinctive activities associated with moving the self or other objects from one place to another. The inability results from an affliction of the muscular-skeletal and/or nervous system. The cause of physical/locomotor handicap may be congenital or developmental (cerebral palsy or phocomelias), acquired or infective (tuberculosis of the spine, chronic osteomyelitis or leprosy), traumatic (amputations, sports injuries or accidents), metabolic (rickets, vitamin B12 deficiency or gout), degenerative (motor neuron disease, multiple sclerosis or Parkinson's disease), etc.

Locomotion impairments are also classified according to where they occur, such as, cerebral (cerebro-vascular accidents), spinal (traumatic paraplegia), nerve lesions (peripheral nerve injury), muscular lesions (muscular dystrophy), skeletal (fractures and dislocations), etc. For the purpose of government benefits and concessions, persons with locomotor handicaps are graded under various severity levels, viz., mild (less than 40 per cent), moderate (40 to 74 per cent), severe (75 to 99 per cent) and profound (100 per cent). Some commonly seen types of physical/locomotor handicaps are:

**Cerebral Palsy:** Cerebral palsy is a non-progressive neurological disorder of muscle co-ordination and control. It usually manifests itself at birth and continues to disable the individual throughout life. The damage does not directly affect the muscles of the extremities or the nerves connecting to the spinal cord. Rather, it is the brain's ability to control or co-ordinate those muscles that is affected.

> **Case Vignette**
> Vishal, a five-year-old, was brought in with complaints of an inability to stand or walk, weakness of the hands in grasping objects and poorly articulated speech; all this despite an improved comprehension of single-step instructions. He could communicate his wants through gestures. Someone suggested that the child could be 'a case of polio' (sic)—which he was obviously not! Vishal's problems related to motor development and co-ordination and were part of the symptoms of cerebral palsy.

The various types of cerebral palsy classified according to the affected part of the body are: monoplegia (single limb), diplegia (legs rather than upper limbs), triplegia (any three limbs); quadriplegia (the whole body and sometimes the muscles on the face), hemiplegia (only one side of the body), and double-hemiplegia (both hands rather than legs). The muscular tone of persons with cerebral palsy may be stiff/rigid or low and floppy. Another classification of cerebral palsy distinguishes three types, viz., spasticity, athetosis and ataxia. *Spasticity* shows high muscle tone, tight/stiff muscles with rigid type of movements and scissoring of hands or legs is seen. The affected area of the central nervous system (CNS) is the motor cortex. *Athetosis* shows fluctuating muscle tone with jerky movements of the limbs. The affected area of the CNS is the basal ganglia. *Ataxia* shows lack of co-ordination and balance in gait, and muscle tone is low. The affected area of the CNS is the cerebellum. A majority of children with cerebral palsy have oral and dental problems like difficulties in swallowing, sucking, biting, drooling, chewing, dental caries and malformed teeth. They may also show contractures and deformities. Around 60 per cent of children with cerebral palsy have low levels of intelligence. Not all children with cerebral palsy are mentally handicapped or vice versa. Parents must be wary of a tendency among professionals to over-diagnose co-morbidity of these twin conditions without making appropriate allowances for the masking effect of one on the other. Such underestimation of a child's potential can jeopardize their remediation planning programmes.

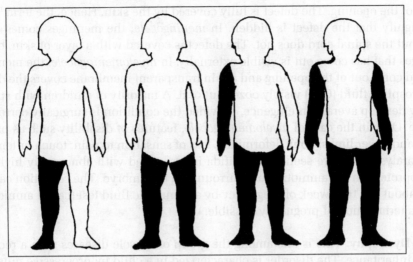

**Illustration 1.2  Types of Cerebral Palsy**

**Amputation:** Loss of limbs (either partly or wholly) may occur due to trauma, accident or disease. Some common causes of amputation are gangrene, leprosy, malignant tumors (osteosarcoma) or some congenital disease (phocomelias). Lower limb amputations are generally more common than upper limb amputations. Amputations below the knee are the most common form of physical impairment.

**Deformities and Contractures:** A deformity is an abnormal position that is not passively correctable. It is assumed by a part of the body as a result of some disease or injury. Additional factors such as muscular weakness, imbalance, gravity, faulty posture or walking patterns, limb length discrepancy, etc., can aggravate deformities of persons with physical handicaps. Some lower limb deformities occur at the foot or ankle, or as scissoring of the legs, flexion contractures of hip and knee, *genu recurvatum, equinus deformity,* etc. Trunk deformities can be in the form of scoliosis (lateral deviation of the backbone), kyphosis (hunchback or sharply localized forward angulation of the spine resulting in the appearance of a lump), kyphoscoliosis (abnormal curvature of the spine both forward and sideways), lordosis (inward curvature of the spine). Foot deformities may include club foot (*tali pes*), flat foot (*pes planus*), claw foot (*pes cavus*), etc.

**Spina Bifida:** Within the first week of conception of a child, the neural tube is closed as basic prerequisite for normal development of the spinal cord in the foetus. In some instances when the neural tube fails to close due to a virus infection or some harmful agents, it leads to a serious congenital disorder called spina bifida. Thus, the newborn baby has part of the spinal cord and its coverings exposed through a gap in the backbone. There are three types of spina bifida, viz., spina bifida occulta, meningocele and myelomeningocele. In all these conditions, the posterior arches of the vertebrae are not fused.

In *spina bifida occulta*, the spinal cord and meninges (the three connective tissue membranes that line the skull and vertebral canal and enclose the brain and spinal cord) do not come out of the opening. The defect is fully covered by the skin. Hence, the term 'occulta' is used to signify that the defect is hidden. In *meningocele*, the meninges comes out of the opening, but the spinal cord does not. The defect is covered with a layer of skin, but the sac of meninges that has come out is visible externally. In *myelomeningocele*, the meninges and spinal cord come out of the opening and a thin transparent membrane covers the defect, and the cerebrospinal fluid (CSF) visibly oozes out of it. A majority of children with spina bifida eventually develop average intelligence, provided the condition is surgically corrected at an early stage. Only in the case of *myelomeningocele*, features of disability such as paralysis of the trunk and lower limbs, bony deformities, loss of sensation to pain, touch or temperature, bladder paralysis, etc., are seen. Spina bifida is associated with abnormally high levels of 'alpha fetoprotein' in the amniotic fluid surrounding the embryo. The condition can be diagnosed by about the 16th week of pregnancy by an amniotic fluid test (called amniocentesis), and makes termination of pregnancy possible.

**Muscular Dystrophy:** This is one among the group of muscle diseases with a recognizable pattern of inheritance. The disorder is characterized in a child by progressive muscle weakness after an initial phase of normal motor development till about three years. Usually, the lower limbs get affected before the upper limbs. The weakness progresses from the muscles of the ankle joint to the muscles of the hand, face and neck. The muscles around the pelvic girdle and shoulder girdle are more affected, leading to a typical manner of getting up from the floor which is called *Gower's Sign*. The calf muscles show false enlargement (pseudo-hypertrophy) owing to the deposit of fatty materials in place of degenerated muscle tissues. The confirmation of diagnosis is based on electromyography (EMG) and muscle biopsy. There are many types of muscular dystrophy based on the age of onset, distribution of weakness, progression of the disease and mode of inheritance. The most common form is 'duchenne dystrophy' that is inherited as a sex-linked recessive character and nearly always seen only in boys. The respiratory and cardiac muscles get terminally affected leading to death. Most of these cases show normal or below-average levels of intelligence, but seldom features of mental retardation.

**Post-polio Residual Paralysis:** Poliomyelitis is the result of an infectious neuro-tropic virus disease affecting the anterior horn cells in the brain stem and spinal cord of the CNS from the fecal matter of infected persons. Therefore, the disease is most common where sanitation conditions are poor. Epidemics occur in unhygienic conditions where individuals have not acquired immunity to the disease during infancy. The symptoms usually occur within 7 to 12 days after infection. In most cases paralysis does not occur. In *abortive poliomyelitis*, only the throat and intestines are infected, and the symptoms are stomach upsets and influenza. In *non-paralytic poliomyelitis*, these symptoms are accompanied by muscle stiffness, particularly in the neck and back. *Paralytic poliomyelitis* is much less common. The mild symptoms at the beginning are soon followed by weakness and the eventual paralysis of muscles. In *bulbar poliomyelitis*, the muscles of the respiratory system are infected and breathing is affected.

## 2. Visual Handicaps

*Visual handicaps* occur owing to total absence of sight or visual acuity not exceeding 6/60 or 20/200 (Snellen chart) in the better eye with correcting lens and/or limitation of field of vision subtending an angle of 20° or worse. Persons with *low vision* have impairment of visual functioning even after treatment or standard refractive correction. They may use or are potentially capable of using vision for planning or executing tasks with appropriate assistive devices. Some common eye diseases are cataract, glaucoma, corneal ulcer, optic atrophy, xeropthalmia, nystagmus, tracoma, astigmatism, short-sightedness (myopia), long-sightedness (hypermetropia), etc.

## 3. Hearing Handicaps

Hearing handicaps are where the sense of hearing in individuals is not adequately developed for the ordinary activities of life. They do not hear/understand sound at all, even with amplified speech. By definition, there must be a loss of hearing of 60 decibels (dB) or more in the better ear for conversational range of frequencies. There are various severity levels (in terms of dB) for classification of hearing impairments based on audiological evaluations of the better ear (Table 1.2).

| Table 1.2 Severity Levels in Hearing Loss | |
| --- | --- |
| *Hearing Level (in dB)* | *Severity of Hearing Loss* |
| 0–25 | Normal |
| 26–40 | Mild |
| 41–55 | Moderate |
| 56–70 | Moderately severe |
| 70–90 | Severe |
| 91+ | Profound |

The types of hearing loss are also distinguished on the basis of the site of the lesion, such as, conductive-hearing loss, sensori-neural hearing loss, mixed hearing loss, central auditory disorder and retro-cochlear pathology. *Conductive-hearing loss* occurs when transmission of sound is interrupted in the outer or middle ear. The usual cause of conductive-hearing loss in children is middle ear infection (such as otitis media), and, in adults, it is due to osteosclerosis. *Sensori-neural hearing loss* occurs when the hair-cells of the cochlea or the acoustic nerves are damaged. This loss of hearing through bone conduction is more or less permanent, and can be due to the side effects of drugs (including antibiotics), infections (such as meningitis or rubella), syphilis or anoxia at birth, aging, etc. A *mixed hearing loss* involves a combination of sensori and conductive hearing loss with damage to the air and bone conduction pathways, even though latter may the be better of the two. *Central auditory disorder* originates from lesions in the central auditory system with damage to the auditory nerve rather than the external and/or middle ear. A *retro-cochlear pathology* involves damage to the nerve fibers along ascending auditory pathways from the internal auditory meatus to the cortex. Parents should be conversant with the hearing responses of infants so that any abnormality is detected early (Table 1.3). Hearing loss is suspected to occur when infants fail to respond to loud or soft sounds, fail to follow commands not accompanied by gestures, stop babbling after six to eight months or have speech, articulation or voice problems, etc.

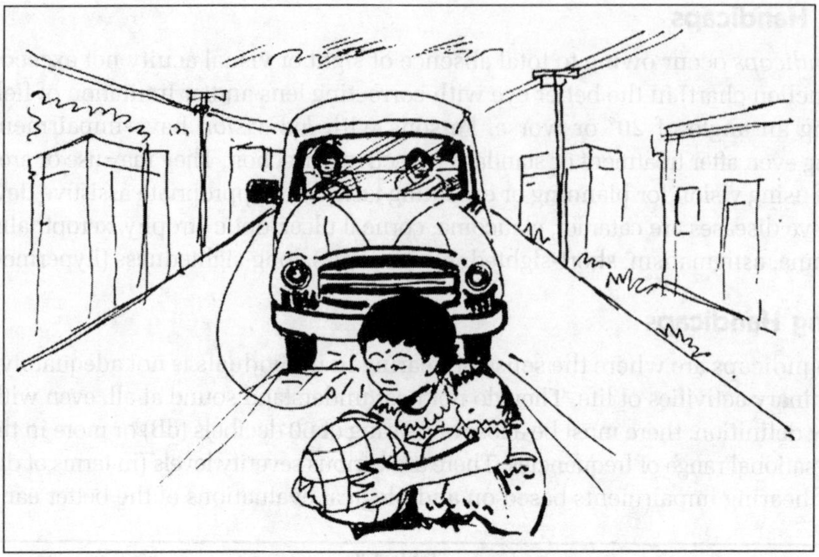

**Illustration 1.3  Hearing Handicap**

**Table 1.3**
**Normal Hearing Responses in Preschool Children**

| Age Range | Behaviour Responses |
|---|---|
| 0–3 months | Infant awakens to loud sounds, alarms or claps even while sleeping. |
| 3–6 months | Recognizes mother's voice and stops crying, smiles when spoken to by mother. |
| 6–9 months | Localizes the source of sounds. |
| 9–18 months | Comprehends words like 'no!', follows simple commands like 'come-go!', 'sit-smile-stand!', 'give-take!', etc. |
| 18 months+ | Follows simple/single step instructions like 'get me that box!' |

## 4. Mental Handicaps

Mental handicap (or mental retardation) is identified as a significantly sub-average level of intellectual functioning associated with deficits in adaptive behaviour and manifests itself during the developmental period (Grossman, 1972). In a more recent definition, mental retardation is defined as a disability characterized by significant limitations both in intellectual functioning and in adaptive behaviour as expressed in conceptual, social and practical adaptive skills. This disability originates before the age of 18 (AAMD, 2002).

The five assumptions essential to the application of this definition are:

1. Limitations in present functioning must be considered within the context of the community environments typical of the individual's age peers and culture.
2. Valid assessment considers cultural and linguistic diversity as well as differences in communication, sensory, motor and communication factors.
3. Within an individual, limitations often coexist with strengths.
4. An important purpose of describing limitations is to develop a profile of needed supports.

5. With appropriate personalized supports over a sustained period, the life functioning of the person with mental retardation will generally improve.

Mental retardation is not something that you have, like blue eyes or a bad heart. Nor is it something that you are, like short or thin. It is not a medical disorder, nor a mental disorder. Mental retardation is a particular state of functioning that begins in childhood, and is characterized by limitation in both intelligence and adaptive skills. It reflects a 'fit' between the capabilities of individuals and the structure and expectations of their environment. The definition of mental retardation has undergone revisions at least over ten times since 1908 based on new information, changes in clinical pratice or breakthroughs in scientific research.

The core element in classification of individuals with mental retardation is their level of intelligence (calculated as IQ or 'intelligence quotient') and their ability to adapt to demands of daily living (calculated as SQ or 'social quotient'). In infants and preschoolers, IQ is more pertinently referred to as DQ (or 'developmental quotient'), which is a lower extension of the same construct. Unlike IQ, the DQ of young children is subject to great instability and variations owing to either differential rates of growth or experience.

The IQ of a person is calculated as a percentage quotient against his/her chronological age. Thus the IQ of a 10-year-old with equal mental age of 10 years will be 100. A 10-year-old with a mental age of 11 years will get an IQ of 110. A child of 10 years with a mental age of five years will have an IQ of 50. In sum, any person who has an intellectual capacity of less than 70 per cent of his physical age can be called mentally retarded (Table 1.4).

**Table 1.4**
**Classification of Mental Retardation (MR)**

| Severity Levels | Range of IQ |
| --- | --- |
| Mild MR | 50–70 |
| Moderate MR | 35–49 |
| Severe MR | 20–34 |
| Profound MR | Below 20 |

Persons with mental handicaps show typical features of slowness in mental development from birth or before the end of their developmental period (which is considered to be 18 years). Other features of mental retardation are listed under Table 1.5 to enable readers to easily identify such persons in their surroundings.

## Mental retardation is not mental illness

Mental retardation is not to be confused with mental illness, even though in laymans' terms they are used interchangeably. Mental retardation is a condition or disability with its onset usually at birth or during childhood/adolescence. It has to do with low levels of intelligence in a person to think rationally, act purposely or solve problems effectively in their lives. Mental illness is a disease. It can occur at any time in a person's life. It involves disease symptoms like talking to oneself or laughing for no reason self, crying spells, hearing voices in the absence of any known source of such sounds, sleeplessness, irrelevant or incoherent speech, etc. Mental retardation requires habilitation of a person on skills identified as deficits, whereas mental illness requires rehabilitation of learnt skills that are lost due to the disease process. A further clarification on differences between disabilities and disorders will be given in the later pages.

---

**Table 1.5**

**Typical Features of Mental Retardation**

Does the child/person show:

1. Slow rates of development since birth in all areas?
2. Discrepancy between physical and mental age?
3. Poor school/academic performance with repeated failures at school?
4. Dependence on others for carrying out day-to-day activities like dressing, bathing, etc.
5. Appearance of being dull, and being slow in understanding, memory, attention-concentration, thinking, problem-solving, decision making, etc.
6. History of delay in all developmental milestones?
7. Difficulties in expression/control of feeling/emotions?
8. Disturbances in communication skills (expressive/receptive)?
9. Difficulties in managing money, lack of time skills for his age?
10. Incompetence in performing vocational activities or lack of social skills for his age?
11. Associated features like behaviour problems, fits, sensory handicaps, etc.

[If you answer 'yes' to more than five of the above questions, then the child/person in question may be mentally retarded.]

---

## 5. Learning Handicaps

Learning handicaps (also called *learning disorders* or *academic-skills disorders*) are invisible handicaps. Children with this handicap appear to have average or even above-average intelligence. They have had normal exposure to school or academic training. They show no apparent physical or sensory handicaps by way of hearing loss, visual impairment, mental illness and/ or mental retardation. There is no evidence of any organic pathology, psychological disease or disorder. They may even show sparks of overt intellect in many facets of daily life. Yet, these children show an intriguing slowness or incapacity in dealing with one or more of subjects like reading, writing, spelling or arithmetic.

**Case Vignette**

Vinayaka, an eight-year-old pupil of the second standard, was brought in with complaints of poor academic performance. According to his parents, he appeared fairly intelligent and behaved his age in all areas of life. He could ride a bicycle, speak fluently, play games with his peers, use the computer to browse the Internet and play games, etc. However, his greatest dislike and weakness was mathematics. He showed great difficulty in carrying out simple calculations involving addition, subtraction, multiplication and/or divisions, in negotiating numerals greater than 100 and so on. For example, he would write 107 as 1007, or read 204 as 24. He could not write numbers beyond one hundred on dictation, write before numerals to a specific number, add up the prices of small items from a neighbourhood store, etc.

The child with a learning handicap shows a curious discrepancy between his tested intellectual abilities and their expected educational levels. For example, a 10-year-old child with matching mental age and expected school-level performance of the fifth grade may actually show reading levels of the first grade. For any given child, a learning handicap may occur in isolation in one area of school performance (such as reading, spelling or arithmetic), or in a cluster of mixed variety (reflected as generalized scholastic backwardness). Learning disorders are diagnosed when the child's academic achievement in individually administered, standardized tests in reading, mathematics or written expression is substantially below that expected for the child's age, schooling and level of intelligence. The learning problems significantly interfere with academic achievement or activities of daily living that require reading, and mathematical or writing skills. A diagnosis of learning disorder is generally avoided if the difficulties can be explained by sensory deficits (such as hearing or visual impairments). Learning disorders persist into adulthood. The identification of learning disorders is necessarily a diagnosis by exclusion (Table 1.6).

| Table 1.6 | |
| :-- | :-- |
| Diagnostic Criteria for Learning Disorders | |
| No. | Inclusion/Exclusion Criteria |
| 1. | Child must have average or above-average levels of intelligence. |
| 2. | Global/generalized delays in developmental milestones (as in mental retardation) is not seen. |
| 3. | Delays seen only in one or odd areas (usually speech and language) of development. |
| 4. | There is always sufficient quality or quantity of exposure to school/academic training. |
| 5. | No apparent cultural, social or economic deprivation in the child. |
| 6. | No evidence of mental illness, organic brain pathology, manifest sensory handicaps. |
| 7. | In spite of ruling out all the above, wherein a child reflects an academic performance of at least two grades or more lower than his expected levels of academic performance, there arises possibility of considering a diagnosis of learning disorder. |

## 6. Multiple Handicaps

Multiple handicaps refer to conditions where the child has two or more disabilities concurrently. For example, a child that has visual impairment along with primary mental retardation. Dual or multiplicity of handicaps a single person is more frequently encountered in clinical practices than can be imagined. In case a child has a dual diagnosis, the helper should be conversant about both the conditions independently, as also their mutually interactive effects, for the proper planning or implementation of training programmes.

> **Multiple handicap is the co-existence of two or more disabilities in an individual**

## Disabilities and Disorders

Impairment, disability and handicap are further distinguished from disorder, disease or illness. Disorders represent the co-existance of syndromes with a clinical course. Disease represents a professional understanding of pathophysiological process constituting certain signs or symptoms in conjunction with their aetiology and pathology. Illness refers to parent/family recognition, labelling and experience of these processes as abnormal or as a departure from wellbeing. Illnesses can affect individuals, both physically as well as mentally. Mental illnesses or psychological disorders are often confused for mental disabilities or handicaps. Mental retardation is not mental illness, though sometimes they may co-exist.

Disabilities are relatively permanent conditions, whereas illnesses are not necessarily so. There is usually a normal pre-morbid history predating psychological disorders/illnesses. Intervention for disabilities usually involve habilitation programmes, whereby fresh learning has to be initiated on several living skills. This is the basis for making a distinction between habilitation and rehabilitation programmes. More appropriately, psychological illnesses require rehabilitation whereby learnt skills that have been lost are retrained. Handicaps require habilitation. Illness is generally treated completely or successfully if identified/diagnosed early in the life of an individual. Some common psychological disorders in children confused for/ as existing along with a primary disability are given below. Parents must be conversant with these conditions since some of them may be present in their preschool children, if not as primary disorders, at least as associated features of a primary disorder.

1. Pervasive developmental disorders
2. Attention deficit and disruptive disorders
3. Communication disorders
4. Motor skills disorders
5. Feeding or eating disorders
6. Elimination disorders
7. Emotional disorders
8. Epilepsy or convulsion disorders

## 1. Pervasive Developmental Disorders

Pervasive developmental disorders (PDDs) are characterized by severe and ubiquitous impairment in *several* areas of a child's development, including reciprocal social and communication skills. PDD is distinguished from mental retardation, wherein impairments occur in *all areas* of a child's development. The general intellectual/developmental level of children with PDD, or their history of early development milestones, will be typically age appropriate. In a few cases, a degree of mental retardation may be evidenced, usually as a consequence and not as a cause of PDD. Therefore, the normal history of early developmental milestones predating the onset of PDD is a critical element in their final diagnosis. Terms like 'childhood psychosis or schizophrenia' were once used to designate these children. There is now enough evidence to suggest that PDD is distinct from these conditions. However, a few of these children may eventually develop adolescent/adult schizophrenia.

> **Case Vignette**
>
> Vipin, a six-year-old child, was brought in with complaints of behaviour disturbances characterized by lack of sleep, an erratic appetite, alternating crying-laughing spells without apparent reason, talking to himself, etc. These symptoms used to persist for three to five months before decreasing by themselves to some extent. After a gap of a few months there would be an exacerbation of these symptoms. When these symptoms decreased, Vipin showed a better propensity to learn new behaviours. When the symptoms reappeared, his learned skills would regress. Any amount of disciplining procedures would not help when the symptoms increased. A course of medication prescribed by the psychiatrist helped to some extent. Vipin's is a typical case of PDD. There are five major sub-types of PDD.

**Autistic Disorder:** Autistic disorder (AD) usually shows an onset during infancy or early childhood (below three years). Unlike mental retardation, children with AD show an early developmental history of near normal sensori-motor and/or even language milestones followed by typical qualitative abnormalities in reciprocal social interactions and patterns of communication, and by restricted, stereotyped and repetitive interests and activities. Abnormal pattern of social interaction, language and restricted or repetitive behaviours are, so to speak, the elemental triadic properties of autism (Table 1.7).

**Table 1.7**
**Clinical Features of Autistic Disorders**

| No. | Clinical Features |
|---|---|
| 1. | Difficulty in interacting and playing with other children. |
| 2. | Acts as if deaf and does not react to speech or noises. |
| 3. | Strong resistance to learning new behaviours or new skills. |
| 4. | Lack of fear about realistic dangers; may play with fire for example. |
| 5. | Resists changes in routine—a slight change may produce disproportionate anxiety. |
| 6. | Prefers to indicate wants by gestures and speech may or may not be present. |
| 7. | Laughs or giggles for no appropriate reason. |
| 8. | Not cuddly as a baby. |
| 9. | Marked physical over-activity. |
| 10. | No eye-to-eye contact; persistently looks past or turns away from persons. |
| 11. | Unusual attachment for inanimate objects like soap case, plastic, paper, etc. |
| 12. | Spins objects, especially round ones. |
| 13. | Repetitive and sustained odd play, such as rattling stones in a can. |
| 14. | Stand-offish manner—treats persons as objects rather than as persons. |

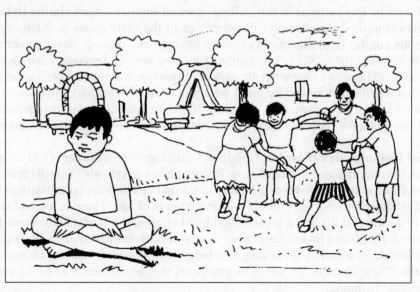

**Illustration 1.4  Autistic Disorder**

Impairment in *social interaction* manifests itself as an inadequate appreciation of social-emotional cues, a lack of response to other people's emotions, deficient pro-social contacts, poor modulation of social contexts, deficient use of social signals, weak integration of social, emotional and communicative behaviour and lack of social-emotional reciprocity. Qualitative impairment in *language* manifests itself as a lack of social usage of language skills, impairment in make-believe and social-imitative play, deficient eye contact, poor synchrony or lack of reciprocity in conversational interchange, poor flexibility in language expression and relative lack of creativity and fantasy in thought processes, lack of emotional response to other people's verbal/non-verbal overtures and a lack of associative aids, gestures, variations/modulation in spoken communication.

Autism is also characterized by restricted, repetitive and stereotyped patterns of behaviour, interests and activities. This manifests itself as a tendency to impose rigidity and routine on a wide range of aspects of daily functions, including play patterns. There is behavioural insistence on the sameness of certain activities, rituals or routines of a non-functional nature, over-attachment to inanimate objects, a stereotyped preoccupation with interests and motor activities, and a resistance to change. Along with these core features, there may be disturbances in sleep or appetite, fears/phobias, self-injurious behaviour, temper tantrums and aggression. All levels of IQ occur in autism. Distinguish autism as a primary developmental disorder in some children and/or against few autistic features seen in association with some other primary condition like hearing impairments, learning handicap, severe-profound mental retardation, etc. Note that an occasional finger flick or a rare occasion of muttering to oneself, withdrawn social mood or disinterest in play does not necessarily mean a child should be labelled as 'autistic'! Such over-generalization and faulty observation leading to misdiagnosis can cause havoc in the lives of individuals.

**Retts' Disorder:** Retts' disorder (RD) lies in close proximity to ADs in children, and is often confused with it. The patterns or difficulties in social interaction are similar in both conditions. There is normal psychomotor development in the early phase of infancy/childhood, and there are similar impairments of expressive/receptive language development. However the similarities end there; RD is invariably diagnosed only in females, whereas ADs occur more in males. RD shows a characteristic pattern of head-growth retardation, loss of previously acquired hand skills (evidenced by hand wringing or hand washing), appearance of poorly co-ordinated gait/trunk movements and only transient loss of social engagement early in course of this disorder. Normal social interactions sometimes develop spontaneously later.

**Childhood Disintegrative Disorder:** Childhood disintegrative disorder (CDD) is also called Heller's syndrome, dementia infantilis or disintegrative psychosis. The diagnosis is made only when there is at least a two-year history of normal developmental milestones before the onset of this disorder, and the child is within 10 years of age. There is a significant loss of previously acquired skills and a greater likelihood of mental retardation towards the end of this course. A significant loss of previously acquired skills occurs in areas like expressive or receptive language, social skills or adaptive behaviour, bowel or bladder control, play and motor skills. These changes are not to be attributed to schizophrenia, head injuries or some known organic pathology.

**Aspergers' Disorder:** Aspergers' disorder (AsD) shares several features with autistic disorders. There is marked impairment in multiple non-verbal behaviours such as eye-to-eye gaze, facial expression, body posture and gestures to regulate social interaction. Children with this disorder show a failure to develop peer relationships appropriate to their developmental level. They lack spontaneous sharing or interests, achievements or enjoyments with others. There is general lack of social or emotional reciprocity. A crucial difference between AsD and AD lies in the fact that there are no delays in language development. There is no clinically significant delay in cognitive development of age-appropriate self-help skills, adaptive behaviour and curiosity about the environment in childhood, either before or after the onset of this disorder. The core criteria for AsD is listed under Table 1.8.

**Table 1.8**
**Core Criteria for Aspergers' Disorder**

| No. | Core Features |
| --- | --- |
| 1. | Severe impairment in reciprocal social interaction: |
|  | (a) lack of interest and/or inability to interact with peers |
|  | (b) lack of appreciation of social cues |
|  | (c) socially and emotionally inappropriate behaviour |
| 2. | All absorbing narrow interest: |
|  | (a) at the exclusion of other activities |
|  | (b) repetitive adherence to the same range of activities |
|  | (c) more rote than meaning |
| 3. | Imposition of routines and interests: |
|  | (a) on self, in all aspects of life |
|  | (b) on others |
| 4. | Speech and language problems: |
|  | (a) superficially perfect language expression |
|  | (b) formal, pedantic language |
|  | (c) odd prosody, peculiar voice characteristics |
|  | (d) impairment of comprehension including misinterpretation of literal/implied meanings |
| 5. | Non-verbal communication problems: |
|  | (a) limited use of gestures |
|  | (b) clumsy/gauche body language |
|  | (c) limited facial expressions |
|  | (d) inappropriate expressions |
|  | (e) peculiar, stiff gaze |
| 6. | Motor clumsiness: |
|  | (a) poor performance on neuro-developmental examination |

**Early Onset Schizophrenic Disorder:** Although schizophrenia is primarily an adult psychological disorder, some early writers describe its occurrence in children. The concept of childhood psychoses led to terms like autistic disorders and, eventually, PDDs. The early literature as we know it today may actually be descriptive of what we now call PDDs. A distinct category of childhood schizophrenia is still justified by some authors against disintegrative, autistic and/or PDDs. Childhood schizophrenia is characterized by an early onset, presence of positive or active behaviour symptoms like hallucinations, delusions and bizarre or disorganized thinking. Negative symptoms consist of paucity of speech, decreased pro-social behaviour, avolition, apathy and flat affect. Additionally, there are serious disturbances in sleep and appetite. Most children with PDDs require a supplementary course of medicines, especially if there are noticeable disturbances in their sleep and/or appetite. Otherwise, behaviour therapies and non-drug interventions suffice fairly during the rehabilitation processes of these children. An accurate and expert diagnosis at the hands of specialists is recommended before putting the label of PDD on young children.

## 2. Attention Deficit and Disruptive Disorders

The two categories of psychological disorders that come under this category are:

**Attention Deficit Hyperactivity Disorders**: ADHD (earlier called 'hyperkinetic') disorders have an early onset, either in childhood (below five years) or early adolescence. It is typically characterized by a short attention span, over-activity and impulsivity. The manifest behavioural patterns often reflect in reckless/impulsive or accident-prone actions. Individuals with this disorder often find themselves in disciplinary trouble due to their unthinking rather than a deliberately defiant breach of rules. They appear to be socially uninhibited, often lack social reserve or caution and are generally unpopular with their peers. Parents experience immense stress in routine management of children with ADHD in home settings.

All levels of IQ occur in ADHD. It is vital to distinguish ADHD as a primary disorder and/ or against few of these features seen in association with some other primary conditions like hearing impairment, learning handicap, severe/profound mental retardation, etc. There are instances wherein a restless child seen briefly in a clinic (presumably tired after a long journey)

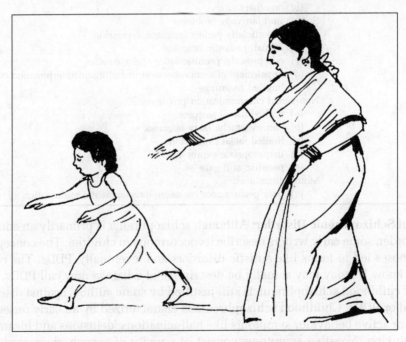

**Illustration 1.5  Attention Deficit Hyperactivity Disorder**

has been hastily diagnosed with ADHD and even put on strong anti-psychotic or stimulant medication!

> ### Case Vignette
> Vimal is a six-year-old. Since two or three years his parents observed that Vimal has become excessively over-active. He does not sit in one place for more than a few minutes or complete any given activity. He is always restless and unstable. His parents weren't able to predict what Vimal would end up doing next. Someone had to continually monitor him all the time for fear that he would disturb somebody or something. At times, his mother was so vexed with his antics that she ruefully wondered if she had 'ever killed a monkey in her previous birth'—as a punishment for which the Gods had given her such a child.

> **Short attention span, impulsivity and over-activity are core triadic features of ADHD**

**Behavioural Problems and Conduct Disorders:** Behavioural problems are actions that are harmful either to the child himself or to others who are around. They interfere in the learning/teaching process, are age inappropriate or socially deviant and are a cause of immense strain for care-givers. Some examples of problem behaviour are hitting others, screaming, stamping of feet, rolling on the floor, pulling objects from others, biting oneself, etc.

> ### Case Vignette
> Vikram, a five-year-old child, was brought in with complaints of behaviour problems like shouting, temper tantrums, biting himself, hitting others, throwing things, etc., since a period of six months. These problem behaviours started insidiously. He began by crying for every small thing that was denied by his parents, who then started to yield to most of his demands. When they refused him something, he would shout at the top of his voice, fall on the floor and throw a tantrum. Such behaviours increased in front of guests at home. Initially his parents continued to give in to most of his demands for fear of him misbehaving in front of the guests. His parents tried all sorts of techniques to change Vikram's problem behaviour. They scolded him, threatened him, advised him, compared him with other children who behaved well and even spanked him. However none of these techniques worked.

Behaviour problems and conduct disturbances exist in isolation or co-exist along with some other primary conditions like hearing impairments, learning handicap or severe/profound mental retardation. When they co-exist with other conditions, it is often mistaken as an inherent or inevitable feature of such a condition. For example, when a child with mental handicap throws things, shouts or stamps its feet, people attribute these problem behaviours to his primary condition of mental retardation. This is however not true. Problem behaviour may be viewed as learned patterns of behaviour or as a function of the contingencies/rewards received by children in their respective environments. The correction of problem behaviour needs always to be taken up in priority before implementing any remedial programme for teaching specific skills to children with disabilities. A recommended reading on this topic is Peshawaria and Venkatesan (1992b).

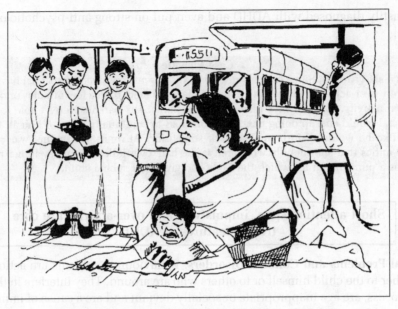

**Illustration 1.6 Behavioural Problem and Conduct Disorder**

## 3. Communication Disorders

Communication disorders manifest independently, or they co-exist with some other primary disability. In any case, they must be recognized and intervened with for their own merit. Some commonly seen communication disorders originating during early childhood are:

**Expressive Language Disorder:** Children with this disorder show expressive language abilities below their current chronological/mental age levels when assessed on standardized normative language tests. Both verbal and non-verbal (sign) language skills are markedly lower than their expected general intellectual abilities for other non-language tasks. The intelligence levels (IQ, DQ and SQ) of these children are within average levels, or sometimes even more. At times, deficient expressive language skills in children are seen as result of mental retardation, PDDs, identifiable sensory/organic neurological conditions or simply as a function of lack of exposure to explicit language tasks in early childhood. Presenting symptoms may include limited speech and vocabulary, difficulties in learning new words or word finding difficulties, telegraphic sentences, limited/simplified grammatical structures, omissions of critical parts of sentences, use of unusual word orders and slow rate of expressive language development.

This disorder is usually recognized by the time a child is five years old, although mild forms may not become apparent till early adolescence, when language becomes more complex. The outcome of this disorder is variable. About half of those affected overcome these initial difficulties without therapy and develop near-normal expressive language abilities by adolescence. Others require intensive or regular speech therapy. They show difficulty in communicating their needs, thoughts and intentions through spoken language. Their speaking vocabulary is limited, both in size and variety. They use sentences that are short, incomplete and ungrammatical. They relate stories and events in a disorganized, confused and unsophisticated manner. The non-verbal aspects of their communicative abilities, general intelligence, speech and hearing apparatus are intact. In other words, the non-verbal aspect of a child's development history is age appropriate. Only the expressive aspects of speech or spoken language are seriously underdeveloped. There should be a lag of at least two years on a standardized expressive language assessment device in order to confirm a diagnosis of this disorder.

**Mixed Receptive-Expressive Language Disorder:** A major feature of this disorder is that there is significant impairment in both expressive as well as receptive language abilities, which are much below normal chronological/mental age levels as assessed on standardized normative language tests. Both verbal and non-verbal language skills are affected to a range which is in variance from their general intellectual abilities for other non-language tasks. Therefore, the intelligence levels (IQ, DQ and SQ) of children with this disorder are well within average levels, or sometimes even more.

It is important to rule out features of mixed receptive-expressive language disorder due to mental retardation, PDDs, learning disorders, identifiable sensory/organic neurological conditions or simply as a function of lack of exposure to explicit language tasks in early childhood. The presenting symptoms include, in addition to features under expressive language disorder, receptive language deficits like difficulty in understanding words, sentences and in understanding specific types of words, pointing skills, spatial relationships, 'if-then' sentences, discrimination of sounds, symbols, storage, recall and sequencing.

This disorder has a clinically close relationship with a child's language and cultural background. This disorder is apparently aggravated by early childhood factors like restricted language use, poorly co-ordinated multiple use of language at home, play, peer and preschool settings, combined with limited social/play opportunities, excessive engagement with computer/video games, television, etc. This disorder is discernible by the time a child is four years old, or even earlier. Many children with this disorder eventually acquire normal language skills, though the outcome of this disorder is generally poor compared to only expressive language disorders. This is particularly true for certain specific types of this disorder, such as Landau–Kleffner syndrome (acquired epileptic aphasia), which occurs between three to nine years and causes brain lesions or strokes. There is evidence to believe that many children showing language disorders are likely to develop learning disorders with regular academic exposure, or during middle childhood.

A category of children with only receptive language disorder and intact expressive language is not generally recognized. This is because in normal language development, comprehension precedes expression/production. These children show behavioural features almost similar to those with expressive language disorders. However, in addition they also have problems with understanding and reception/comprehension of spoken language. They have difficulty in learning new words, particularly those with uncommon or abstract meanings. They misinterpret conversational questions or comments, leading them to make inappropriate or nonsensical remarks. They fail to understand lengthy or grammatically complex instructions, directions or explanations. These difficulties are often misunderstood by caregivers as signs of stubbornness, inattention or other behavioural problems. As with all specific developmental disorders, the exclusion criteria of not attributing these receptive-expressive language difficulties to low intelligence, sensory impairments, emotional disturbance, cultural, environmental or economic disability and lack of adequate instruction is applicable for this disorder too.

**Phonological Disorder:** The essential feature of phonological disorder (formerly called developmental articulation disorder) is a failure to use developmentally expected speech sounds that are appropriate for an individual's age and dialect. This involves errors in sound production, use, representation or organization, such as substitution, omission, distortion and/ or addition. Specific articulation problems owing to primary mental retardation, cerebral palsy, sensory (hearing) impairments, neurological conditions or environmental deprivation must be ruled out. Sound omissions are typically viewed as more serious than sound substitutions, which in turn are more severe than sound distortions. The most frequently (mis)articulated sounds are those acquired later in the developmental sequence (like l, r, s, z, th, ch). However, sometimes consonants and vowels that develop earlier may also be affected. Lisping is also a common phonological disorder.

**Stuttering:** Stuttering is a disturbance in normal fluency and time patterning of speech that is inappropriate for an individual's age. Frequent repetitions or prolongation of sounds or syllables characterizes speech. There may be associated interjections, broken words (pauses within a word), audible or silent blocking (filled or unfilled pauses in speech), circumlocutions (word substitutions to avoid problematic words), words produced with excess of physical tension and monosyllabic whole word repetitions. These disturbances interfere with the academic, social and occupational functioning of an individual. Stuttering occurs more or less in different situations or life areas of an individual, and is often aggravated with subjective distress or anxiety. Stuttering is often absent during reading, singing or talking to inanimate objects or pets. Children with stuttering often develop avoidance behaviour when faced with situations where they have encountered difficulties in the past in their oral presentations. They might also develop secondary behaviour features like accompanied motor movements (eye blinks, tics, tremors of the lips or face, jerking of the head, breathing movements, fist clenching, etc.). Stuttering should be distinguished from normal non-fluencies, particularly in toddlers and young children. However, whole word or phrase repetitions, incomplete phrases, interjections, unfilled pauses and parenthetical remarks are common but transient features in the speech of some children. They should not be confused with stuttering.

## 4. Motor Skills Disorders

Developmental co-ordination disorder is a major form of impairment in this area. It manifests itself as a failure to co-ordinate routine or age-appropriate motor activities like walking, crawling, buttoning clothes, somersaulting, sitting, tying shoe laces, using scissors, assembling blocks, building models, throwing/catching a ball, standing or walking, handwriting, etc. These difficulties are seen despite average or above average general intellectual abilities in the child. In other words, primary conditions like mental retardation, ADDs, cerebral palsy, muscular dystrophy, PDDs, sensory impairments, neurological conditions or allied conditions of environmental deprivation cannot explain these difficulties. Only a history of delay in motor development is evidenced.

Distinction should be made between writing disorder and motor-skills co-ordination disorder. There are other names for this condition like choreiform syndrome, congenital maladroitness, psychomotor syndrome, developmental apraxia or dyspraxia, congenital clumsiness, developmental agnosia, developmental dyspraxia-dysgnosia, clumsy child syndrome, specific developmental disorder of motor functions and so on. The main symptom of this disorder is poor motor co-ordination. This is seen as difficulties in fine and/or gross motor functions, activities and routines. The motor skills may be clumsy rather than globally impaired. The co-ordination problems manifest in motor skill disorders are listed in Table 1.9.

**Table 1.9**
**Typical Co-ordination Problems in Motor Skills Disorders**

| No. | Type of Problem | Behavioural Features |
|-----|-----------------|----------------------|
| 1. | Dyspraxia | Inability to produce correctly sequenced, co-ordinated motor movements when presented with a demonstration/oral request. |
| 2. | Synkinesia or muscle overflow | Manifests as unintended muscle movements. Mirror movements like finger twitching on the opposite hand when the child is asked to perform a finger opposition task. Facial grimaces when asked to make hand movements. |
| 3. | Hypotonus | Characterized by flaccid or sleepy quality of the child's facial expression or general muscle tone. |
| 4. | Hypertonus | Characterized by high levels of muscle tone, with an inability to finish drawing a line at a given point and overshooting it, or throwing a ball too hard/inaccurately over short distances. |
| 5. | Tremors | Marked by irregular unsteadiness in muscular movements, mostly in tasks requiring walking and/or drawing. |
| 6. | Impersistance | Inability to maintain or sustain various body postures for reasonable periods of time. The task involves how long the child can remain standing without movement when instructed to, for instance, 'stick out your tongue!' or to become a 'statue'. |
| 7. | Asymmetry | Describes motor behaviours that affect only one side of the body. If the child executes motor movements more fluidly on one side than on the other, it might indicate an asymmetry. |

The developmental history of these cases show delays in motor milestones (such as neck holding, turning over, crawling, creeping, sitting, standing, walking and so on). Their motor-co-ordination problems are evident in simple gross muscular activities like running, balancing, throwing and kicking, or fine muscular activities like fastening laces, sewing, buttoning, unbuttoning, stitching, tracing or writing. These difficulties must not be due to avoidance or lack of opportunities for performing these activities. As with all specific developmental disorders, the exclusion criteria of not attributing these motor problems to low intelligence, sensory impairments, emotional disturbance, cultural, environmental or economic disability and lack of adequate instruction is relevant herein too. The diagnosis is not to be confused with such difficulties seen in other neurological conditions like cerebral palsy or lesions, mental retardation, PDDs, etc. It is not infrequent to encounter toddlers in restricted tenements who are denied opportunities for outdoor play coming up with complaints of poor motor/

muscle co-ordination. Caregivers are strongly advised to involve such children in regular outdoor play to save them from the misdiagnosis of motor skills disorder.

## 5. Feeding or Eating Disorders

Feeding or eating disorders are characterized by persistent disturbances in feeding and eating during infancy or early childhood. An area of intense concern for the mothers of toddlers is the feeding/eating behaviours of these children. Most mothers carry a long list of complaints regarding their children's eating habits. The sub-types of this disorder are:

**Pica:** An essential feature of pica is the persistent eating of non-edible or non-nutritive substances for a period of at least a month. The items ingested vary with the child's age. Common items that are ingested are plaster, paint, insects, leaves, hair, cloth, thread, sand, pebbles, animal or bird droppings, clay and soil. There is no aversion to food. The behaviour is inappropriate for the child's age and culturally sanctioned practices. It is important to distinguish pica from behaviour problems in some children with PDDs, ADD and/or mental retardation who cannot discriminate between edible and non-edible substances. Pica in infants can lead to several medical complications like lead poisoning from ingesting paint or paint-soaked plaster, mechanical bowel problems, intestinal obstruction as a result of hair-ball tumors, intestinal perforations or infections, etc.

**Rumination Disorders:** Rumination, regurgitation and re-chewing of ingested food are fairly frequent during the first month of an infant's life. However, after the first month, rumination disorders are diagnosed if partially digested food is brought into the mouth without apparent nausea, retching, disgust or associated gastro-intestinal disorders. The food is either brought out or, more frequently, chewed and reswallowed. These symptoms are not due to any gastro-intestinal or other general medical condition, nor due to eating disorders like anorexia nervosa and bulimia nervosa, primary mental retardation, PDDs, etc. Infants with this disorder display a characteristic position of straining and arching with the head held back, and making sucking movements with their tongues to give the impression of gaining satisfaction from the activity. Infants display irritability and hunger between episodes of regurgitation. Malnutrition, weight loss and failure to thrive are common. Associated psychological problems like lack of stimulation, neglect, stressful life situations and problems in parent–child relationships are predisposing factors. Rumination disorders should be distinguished from normal vomiting owing to forced feeding.

**Psychogenic Vomiting:** Psychogenic vomiting (also called psychogenic hyperemesis gravidarum) occurs as recurrent episodes of nausea and vomiting with no organic basis to explain such symptoms. A gastro-intestinal endoscopy would reveal a normal digestive tract with no medical explanation for the recurrent episodes of vomiting.

## 6. Elimination Disorders

These are disorders of the gastro-intestinal tract precipitated by psycho-social rather than medical or organic factors. Some common sub-types included under this disorder are:

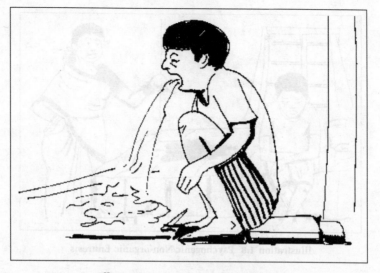

**Illustration 1.7  Psychogenic Vomiting**

**Psychogenic/Non-organic Encopresis:** The essential feature of this disorder is the repeated passing of faeces in inappropriate places (for example, in clothes or on the floor). Most often this is done involuntarily, or at times it may be intentional. For this disorder to be diagnosed, the event must occur at least once a month for at least three months, and the child must have crossed the chronological or mental age of four years. Faecal incontinence occurs due to the direct physiological effects of a substance (like laxatives) or some medical condition.

The child with faecal incontinence suffers an intense degree of subjective embarrassment, guilt or shame; the condition is often a function of the extent of ostracism, punishment or rejection on the part of others in his environment. Smearing of faeces may be deliberate or accidental resulting from the child's attempt to clean or hide them. If the child's intention is clearly established, it could be a behaviour problem or a symptom of conduct disorder. Two types of encopresis are identifiable. Primary encopresis is where the individual has never established faecal continence, and secondary encopresis is where the disturbance develops after a period of established faecal continence.

**Psychogenic/Non-organic Enuresis:** This disorder is characterized by involuntary or intentional passing of urine, by day and/or by night, which is abnormal in relation to the child's mental age and which is not a consequence of lack of bladder control, neurological disorder, epileptic attacks or structural abnormality of the urinary tract. Two types of enuresis are identifiable. Primary enuresis is where the individual has never established urinary continence, and secondary enuresis is where the disturbance develops after a period of established urinary continence. Emotional problems (birth of siblings, parental neglect, etc.) arise either as a cause or consequence of enuresis. However, enuresis is not ordinarily diagnosed in children under five years or under a mental age of four years.

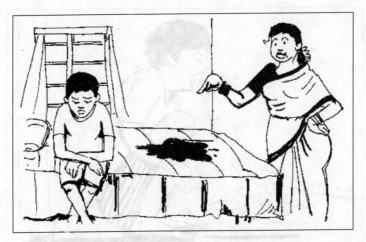

**Illustration 1.8  Psychogenic/Non-organic Enuresis**

**Case Vignette**

Vinod, a six-year-old student of the first standard, had developed severe problems with controlling his stools. He came back from school on several occassions with soiled clothes. When this started to happen regularly, his parents were alarmed. He had been fairly continent and under control till a year earlier. They consulted their paediatrician, who ruled out any physical and/or organic basis for Vinod's problem. There was no weakness or any pathology related to the anal sphincter muscles to explain his feeble control over his toilet habits.

## 7. Emotional Disorders

Emotional disorders reflect a heterogeneous group of problems in a child's social-emotional relationships with his peers and family, and outside members of society. These problems begin during the toddler phase after an initial period of normal social development. It is important to distinguish these disorders from PDDs that are characterized by a primary constitutional social incapacity/deficit that pervades all areas of functioning. Some important disorders that fall under this category are:

**Attachment Disorders of Early Infancy or Childhood**: Attachment refers to a bio-behavioural system whose goal is to co-ordinate balance between the need for safety in proximity to caregiver(s) and the tendency for exploration and autonomy during infancy and early childhood. A clearly expressed preference for a small number of care-giving adults, separation protest and wariness of strangers are fairly established between 7 to 12 months in normal infants. A key feature of this disorder is the abnormal pattern of relationship the child develops with the caregiver before the child is five years old. The child shows strongly contradictory or ambivalent social responses that are most evident during unions or partings. Such infants respond to their caregivers with an averted gaze. They may show a mixed response of approach, avoidance and resistance to comforting actions offered by caregivers. In most cases these children show interest in peer interaction, but social play is impeded with negative emotional responses. The preference of a child for selective attachment with one or the other parent is not to be mistaken for this disorder. This disorder is distinguished from PDDs on five different counts. These children show a normal capacity for social responsiveness, whereas children with PDD do not. The social responsiveness of these children remit once they are placed in social situations which are continually care giving. Their language patterns are not abnormal as in children with PDDs. Further, persistent cognitive impairments unresponsive to environmental changes are not seen in this disorder as in children with PDDs. The persistent pattern of repetitive/stereotyped behaviours, ritualistic activities or interests as occurs in PDDs are not seen in these children.

**Elective or Selective Mutism:** This disorder is characterized by emotionally determined selectivity in speaking. The child shows his language competence in some social situations or relationships, but fails to speak in others. There is social anxiety, withdrawal, sensitivity or resistance to speaking at home, with strangers and friends and at school, while paradoxically showing normal language expressions in some other situations. This pattern of behaviour is seen consistently in similar situations over time.

**Childhood Phobias:** Phobias are anxiety-evoking circumscribed situations or objects outside of an individual which are not currently dangerous. The individual understands this very well and yet is unable to confront the specific object or situation. The specific and subjective symptoms of phobia are not distinguishable from other types of anxiety. Mere contemplation of the entry of phobic situations usually generates anticipatory anxiety. The specific objects/situations of phobia may include animals (zoophobia), darkness (nyctophobia), sharp objects (acrophobia), water (hydrophobia), enclosed places (claustrophobia), disease (nosophobia), etc. Phobias in children must be distinguished from normal or age-appropriate developmental fears. For example, fear or reticence from contact with strangers, avoidance of darkness and/or furry objects is fairly common in infants transgressing into the toddler phase. They usually outgrow such fears with or even without any therapeutic interventions.

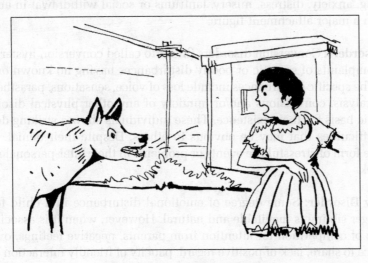

**Illustration 1.9  Childhood Phobias**

**Depressive Disorders:** The core features of adult depressive disorders are essentially same across the lifespan. The developmental level appears to influence the expression of certain mood symptoms with greater frequency than others. For example, loss of pleasure in daily activities or psychomotor retardation which is characteristic of adult depression is seldom seen in children or adolescents. There might be greater evidence of irritability and violent or destructive behaviour as a form of expressing subjective feelings in adolescents than adults with depression. Suicidal thoughts or ruminations are equally common in children and adolescents as with adults having depression. Some common depressive symptoms seen in children and adolescents with depression are sad feelings, crying without apparent reason, irritability, social withdrawal, somatic complaints, behavioural problems, etc.

Depression in children usually starts as severe problem behaviour. The behavioural disorders (usually irritability, refusal to go to school, opposition actions and so on) may be a reflection of underlying depression. In such cases, conduct disturbances resolve once the underlying depression is treated. Distinguish between depression and normal bereavement reactions, where there is clear life event involving loss through death. Consequently, there are expressions of grief, such as, crying, funerals, visitations and rituals; usually within two months of bereavement.

**Separation Disorders:** Separation from home or from major attachment figures during childhood is characterized by developmentally inappropriate anxiety which is sufficient to cause clinically significant distress. There is an unrealistic preoccupation about possible harm befalling major attachment figures or that they will leave and not return. There are worries about the occurence of some untoward event, like a child being kidnapped, lost, killed or admitted to hospital. There is a persistent refusal to go to school because of the fear of separation rather than the events in school. There is a persistent reluctance or refusal to go to sleep without being near or next to a major attachment figure at home. There are repeated nightmares about separation. There are somatic complaints like stomach ache, headache, vomiting, etc., on occasions involving separation from major attachment figures. There is excessive crying, anxiety, distress, misery, tantrums or social withdrawal in anticipation of separation from a major attachment figure.

**Conversion Disorders:** Conversion disorders (hitherto called conversion hysterias) are characterized by complaints of somatic or bodily disturbances having no known or discernable organic basis. The specific disturbances include loss of voice, sensations, parasthesias, hearing and vision, paralysis, convulsions and/or mimicry of any other physical disorder with no apparent organic basis for their existence. These individuals show a striking denial of their problems or difficulties that may be obvious to others. Despite their denial, psychogenic causation in the form of stressful life events or problems in their inter-personal relationships is not far to seek.

**Sibling Rivalry Disorder:** Some degree of emotional disturbance in a child following the birth of a younger sibling is inevitable and natural. However, when it is associated with an unusual degree of competition for attention from parents, negative feelings, overt hostility, strong reluctance to share, lack of positive regard, paucity of friendly interaction and physical

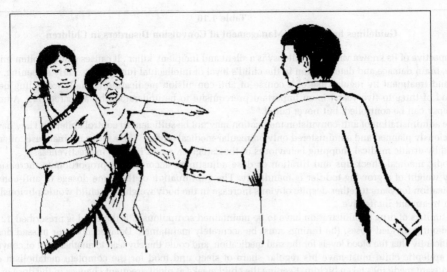

**Illustration 1.10  Separation Disorder**

trauma or maliciousness directed at the sibling, this disturbance becomes eligible for recognizing as a disorder. The emotional disturbances take the form of regressive behaviour wherein the child blindly imitates the actions of the younger sibling in a bid to gain parental approval or attention. It may co-exist with several refusals, opposition or demanding behaviour, clinging, temper tantrums, etc.

## 8. Epilepsy or Convulsion Disorders

Convulsion disorders reflect the neurological status of an individual. The clinical presentation of epilepsy depends upon its causes, anatomical lesion within the brain, pattern of spread of epileptic discharges, age of onset and a host of other factors. Several types of epilepsy can be recognized. There are 'simple' types with slight jerking or deviation of the eyes, fluttering of eyelids, oral/facial movements, isolated muscle spasms and the like. There are also more 'complex' seizures with extensive jerking movements of the upper and lower limbs, tongue bites, unconsciousness, frothing, incontinence and so on. In young infants and toddlers, there are certain types of epilepsy which are not easily detected by outward observations. There is, for example, a category of seizures called 'infantile spasms' (West's Syndrome) wherein between four to eight months of age clusters of bodily jerks occur in the form of 'salaams' intermittently. Another category called 'febrile convulsions' that occur between 3 to 60 months is invariably associated with a rise in body temperature and high fever. An undetected type of epilepsy is 'absences' (pyknolepsy), which is characterized by alteration of consciousness lasting for not more than a few seconds. The child appears to be simply staring into space or lost in his own world. There may be transient cessation of ongoing activity, which may be resumed after the brief episode. A few absences may graduate into more serious forms of epilepsy in later life.

---

**Table 1.10**

**Guidelines for Effective Management of Convulsion Disorders in Children**

1. Irrespective of its known varieties, epilepsy is a silent and incipient 'killer'. It causes gradual, often imperceptible, brain damage and deterioration in the child's level of intellectual functioning. Early screening, diagnosis and treatment by regular use of a course of anti-convulsion medication (usually extending beyond a period of three to five years) is an important prerequisite to be understood by all caregivers. Admittedly, epilepsy can be controlled, but never cured.

2. Mere administration of anti-convulsion medication may not be sufficient to control epilepsy. They have to be judiciously planned and administered only on regular medical advice. Their indiscriminate use, often aggravated by erratic medical shopping behaviours of the caregiver, result in their ineffectiveness.

3. Periodic medical check-ups and titration or dose adjustment according to proportionate increase in the body weight of a growing toddler is mandatory. The continuation of the same dosage of anti-convulsion medication for years together despite obvious increase in the body weight of a child would obviously make such treatment ineffective.

4. The timings of drug administration have to be maintained scrupulously. If the child is prescribed 12-hourly or 8-hourly divided doses, the timings must be accurately maintained. Delayed doses or missed doses can significantly alter the blood levels for the said medication, and could thereby lead to another bout of convulsions.

5. The epileptic child must have his regular share of sleep and food for the complete metabolism of anti-convulsant medicines taken by him. Keeping the child awake at night, frequent changes in the dose or regime of administered medicines, frequent shifts in seeking advice from prescribing medical practitioners, improper titration of drug dosage, stopping medicine or drug abstinence (either on one's own or on the 'friendly' advice of others), etc., are some factors contributing to repeat occurrence of fits in their children.

6. Periodic serum-level estimations of anti-convulsant medication for a given child must be carried out on medical advice to verify if the absorption levels are matching the administered dose.

7. Concurrent and periodic serum-haemoglobin-level estimates are required in patients with epilepsy. A reduction in the quantity of the oxygen-carrier pigment (haemoglobin) in the blood can lead to anemia. Iron-deficiency anaemia results from a lack of iron, which is necessary for the production of haemoglobin. There are several causes, as well as types, of anaemia. In any case, the presence of anaemia can render ineffective the effect of anti-convulsants in patients with epilepsy unless they are concurrently treated.

8. Many infants and young children run the risk of fits associated with an increase in body temperature. These type of fits are called febrile convulsions. Even though febrile convulsions are not as harmful as non-febrile ones, parents must take all precautions to ensure that the body temperature of the child does not shoot beyond risky levels. Administration of anti-pyretics, use of ice packs and other measures to bring down body temperature must be immediately followed if such cases occur.

---

Many forms of sub-clinical epilepsy are also known to exist. They are not outwardly visible at all. In some cases, they are inferred only on electro-encephalography (EEG) record in the form of spiked waves. A word on first aid for fits will not be out of place here. Many persons react spontaneously to the sight of fits in someone by holding them tightly or inserting metallic objects between their teeth. Making them sniff onions, dirty footwear or gagging is frequently used as first aid by people in public places. All these well-intentioned responses are *not* required, and are unconnected with cessation of the ongoing attack. The patient may be turned sideways to allow frothing saliva to drip outside his or her mouth. Clearing the crowd around the epileptic patient may provide enough ventilation. The patient's clothes may be loosened, and he or she may be referred to a medical practitioner after cessation of the attack. Recurrent attacks of fits without intermittent regaining of consciousness (called *status epilepticus*) can prove fatal at times. Consultation with a physician is recommended for all cases of epilepsy. Patients with epilepsy should avoid activities like driving, swimming, working on heights and near fires, etc. Table 1.10 lists some useful guidelines for the management of convulsion disorders.

There is also a form of epilepsy that is termed as psychological/functional fits, characterized by the features described above, and yet different from them since they do not have any organic basis. Such types of epilepsy show a profile of normal EEG records, CAT scan and other neurological investigations. These fits are precipitated by psychological factors such as seeking the attention of others or trying to escape the burden of some unwanted consequences by the child.

## Interventions in Planning Programmes for Children with Disabilities: The Role of Diagnosis

Diagnostic hunting by parents of preschool children affected with DDs is more frequent than imagined. It was the intention of the author in this chapter to orient parents on possible varieties of diagnostic conditions that could possibly affect children in this age group. Even though several conditions are explained under appropriate headings by outlining specific features or characteristics of each disorder/disability, they do not necessarily reflect cases as seen in actual clinical practice. It is rare to see actual cases of children who mimic classic textbook descriptions of signs and symptoms of disorders/disabilities. In actuality, several disabilities/disorders co-exist at various levels or within different degrees. For example, a child with a learning disorder may simultaneously show associated emotional disorders, behaviour problems as well as convulsion disorders. An intelligent diagnosis must take into account such overlapping layers and also take appropriate decisions about a primary condition against other associated features in any given child with a disorder, disability and/or handicap.

The accurate diagnosis of a disorder, disability and/or handicap in a child is an important prelude to planning the right programme for intervention or rehabilitation. The diagnostic label affixed on a given child lends both target as well as direction for future remediation programmes. An incorrect diagnosis can put caregivers in a vicious cycle of going round and round without seeking any intervention for the good of the child. Meanwhile precious time may have been lost. Diagnostic labels also have their limitations. It is seen that some parents are always into the cycle of searching for the right diagnosis that describes their child. They run from pillar to post seeking medical opinions on their child. So long as their search for diagnostic confirmation is on, there is no end to it, nor is there any realistic beginning for appropriate remediation/rehabilitation programmes to be commenced for their child. The acceptance of a correct and accurate diagnosis heralds the beginning of a positive acceptance about the status of their child.

Another great peril in diagnosis-making exercises is that parents tend to search and tag any or all features onto a child who has been 'diagnosed' with a particular label. For example, when a child is 'diagnosed' with an autistic disorder, parents some invariably search for even those features that may remotely appear to have some semblance with that disorder in their child. Again, one should not hastily conclude an isolated feature of some disorder to be sufficient evidence for diagnosis of those conditions themselves. A peer rejected hearing-impaired preschool child indulging in solitary play or talking to himself does not at once qualify to be branded as having an autistic disorder or CDD, as another child with an inability to squat or jump across small obstacles does not qualify as a spastic! It is both easy as well as hazardous to wreck the mental strength of an uninformed parents by faulty diagnosis of their children's conditions. It should be kept in mind that it consumes enormous effort and time to rebuild shattered confidence or set right parents' misinformed knowledge and attitudes through appropriate guidance/counselling.

### Case Vignette

Payal, who was four years old, was brought in with complaints of not being responsive to verbal instructions given by caregivers. She appeared inconsistent in her responses to people calling her name, and commands or instructions to perform certain actions. She would occasionally utter some words but they were not imitative. Her paternal grandfather, who was the head of their joint family, frequently defended her delays in development as nothing to be worried about as he had seen several children who started speaking or walking very late in childhood only to catch up with other children later. Payal's parents put-off her first medical consultation till she was over five years old, when their family doctor strongly recommended an expert opinion. Consultations were made with neurologists, paediatricians, homeopathic/ayurvedic specialists and so on. A variety of disorders like mental retardation, hearing loss, autistic disorder and Retts' Syndrome were considered. A skull X-ray, EEG, audiology screening, CT scan, MRI, several rounds of blood, urine and stool tests and the like were carried out. Someone started the child on a course of brain tonics to presumably increase (what they suspected to be) her low intelligence! Yet another doctor was eager to start Payal on a course of anticonvulsant medication as a preventive measure in case she had some kind of subclinical epilepsy! At the end of all these arduous exercises, Payal's parents were still in the dark about the final diagnosis of their child.

# CHAPTER 2

# HOME-BASED SKILL TRAINING PROGRAMMES

*The correct diagnosis and early identification of a child with developmental disability is the first step towards their effective management. An intervention programme started early can remedy or even prevent several serious and deleterious consequences. It can limit the effects of the primary handicap, and also prevent occurrence of secondary handicaps in these children.*

All prospective parents look forward to a normal baby free from flaws, blemishes and deformities. The birth of a baby with developmental disability (DD) causes serious and complex psycho-social problems in parent–child bonding. Parents undergo a variety of psychological reactions like shock, doubt, shame, guilt and denial or ambivalence before achieving any semblance of acceptance eventually. Both informed as well as uninformed parents cannot escape feelings of anxiety, consternation and despair when a child is born with a handicap. Mothers, more so than fathers, are reported to react with strong feelings of hurt, helplessness, resentment, disappointment and a sense of inadequacy when they come to know that they have given birth to a child who has a disability. However, one must be wary of sweeping interpretations. Being deeply hurt and wishing that the baby did not have the problem does not constitute rejection. Trying to find out the cause of the disability does not mean doubt, guilt or ambivalence. Parents rarely reject their children, much less abandon them.

Parents differ in the type or intensity of emotional reactions. Some feel hurt, helplessness, resentment, disappointment and/or a sense of inadequacy on knowing that they have given birth to a child who has a disability. The common areas of parental concern regarding children with handicaps is reported to range across topics including the child's appearance, desirability or the possibility of an immediate surgery that could be a 'cure-all' for their problems, anxieties as to whether the child can speak at all and feed and look after himself or herself. There may be additional apprehensions about possible reactions from the spouse or siblings in due course of time. Will the spouse accept the child? Will the siblings take care of the child as it grows up? Will other family members or relatives acknowledge the child as they would do any other normal child? Will the next child also be handicapped?

Parent queries or reactions to the birth of a child with an impairment is actually a unique individual response. While some parents may not easily or quickly reconcile to the fact that their child is different, the majority of them learn to accept the grim reality. Sometimes parents require supportive guidance/counselling from professionals and social support from family, friends and relatives, etc. Already besieged and beleaguered by a sense of guilt at having given birth to an imperfect child, caregivers may face tremendous pressure from fellow parents guiding them to seek consultations from everyone in sight. Thus some parents easily fall into this trap and embark on an endless search for the correct diagnosis and/or cure for their child. It is important that caregivers realistically appraise their own and their child's condition before coming to terms with it. This is a crucial prerequisite for the success of any home training programme that one wishes to undertake for children with disabilities. The earlier chapter would have given readers an overview of the disorders/disabilities commonly seen in preschool children.

## Perils of Diagnostic Labelling

Even though rehabilitation professionals can be of great help to parents in explaining the diagnostic condition of their child, at times they render great disservice too. Misleading labels, hasty diagnosis, repeated testing, elaborate and unwarranted investigations and other such allied pressure-provoking practices also heighten the emotional turmoil of parents already burdened with the need for accepting their child. Nevertheless, one must take diagnostic labels for what they are worth in order to understand the real position of the child. One must guard against the tendency to attach more significance than such labels are meant to carry in the rehabilitation sector.

**We label jars, not people!**

Diagnostic labels are just a lamppost for parents groping in the dark about their child's condition. At the same time, they are not to be viewed as definitive judgements on the fate of a child. It must be clearly understood that many of the conditions described in previous chapters are fairly reversible given early measures, particularly for *children at risk*. There is a great difference between *children at risk* and those who have a confirmed disability. This difference is to be identified early and intervened appropriately for the optimum betterment of infants, toddlers and preschool children.

## Training Programmes for Children with Disabilities

Parent-professional interaction for habilitation of children with DDs usually commences with diagnostic labelling. Attempting to identify the child's diagnostic condition cannot however be the end of the exercise. Even though many contemporary medical practitioners indulge in elaborate diagnostic gymnastics by routing gullible parents through several radiological investigations, biochemical tests, genetic assays and so on, these exercises should not end at just labelling the child. What is more important is the process that should take place thereafter. Preschool children with DDs require intensive multi-sensory stimulation programmes along with preventive genetic-counselling for prospective mothers. School-aged children with disabilities require day care facilities, community-based training programmes, and rarely, custodial care centres. Adults with disabilities require pre-vocational training, vocational training and placement under sheltered workshops or open employment surroundings. One of the most powerful avenues to reach children with disabilities is by extending home-based training programmes between professionals to parents and caregivers.

## Parent-professional Collaboration

Parent-professional collaboration is crucial for the success of any home training programme in children with disabilities. In the earlier days, professionals were used to working alone and not involving parents in the rehabilitation process. Parents were also wont to perceive the professional as an active service-provider and themselves as mere service-recipients. The rehabilitation professional would take all decisions for, or on behalf of, the child with a disability. Parents had to passively embrace them without any questions. Parents were viewed as beseeching help and the professional as the all-knowing, providing everything for the help-seeking caregivers. It is high time these attitudinal fixations are transformed in contemporary parents if they seek progress in home training programmes for their children with disabilities. Rehabilitation professionals are not panaceas for all problems faced by parents of children with DDs. They are human beings with their own faults and foibles that may interfere in the optimization of the rehabilitation process. Some attitudinal blocks seen in professionals are listed in Table 2.1. These psychological snags must be overcome to get closer to bettering home training programmes of parents for their children with disabilities. Simultaneously, parents also need to introspect and correct themselves on certain attitudinal impediments, if any, against professionals as listed in Table 2.2.

An ideal situation necessitates mutual matching and optimization of the relative strength in professionals and parents of children with disabilities. Parents have a greater investment in their children, both in terms of time and emotions. They have valuable information about their child's behaviour, interests, likes and dislikes, temperament, abilities, etc. They share a greater physical and psychological proximity with the disabled child. They spend more time with the child as compared to professionals, who can afford only a meagre hour or so on any given child with a disability. On their side, professionals bring with them a fund of technical knowledge and information that can supplement, lend direction and provide a scientific basis for home training programmes.

---

**Table 2.1**

**Attitudinal Blocks in Rehabilitation Professionals**

Rehabilitation professionals need to ponder over these myths and correct themselves in the interest of reposing greater confidence on parents/caregivers and optimizing success in home-based training programmes for children with disabilities:

1. Parents are the root cause of DDs in their children.
2. Parents always need help from professionals in handling or managing the day-to-day problems of children with DDs.
3. Parents are problematic, and suffer from psychological problems themselves since they are stressed/burdened with rearing a child with a handicap.
4. Parents cannot decide for or on behalf of themselves or their children with handicaps. Professionals need to make decisions for them and direct them explicitly on various issues related to rearing their children with disabilities.
5. Since professionals are more qualified and know more about disabilities than parents, it is expected that caregivers follow instructions about home management.
6. Since professionals are 'service-providers' and parents 'service-receivers', the latter are expected to go to the former rather than vice versa.
7. Since professionals are bogged down with excess work, parents must learn to adjust to their schedule in the interest of receiving services for their children with handicaps.

**Table 2.2**
**Attitudinal Blocks in Parents and Caregivers**

Parents and caregivers also need to ponder over these myths and correct themselves in the interest of their interactions with rehabilitation professionals and for optimizing home training programmes for their children with disabilities:

1. Professionals need to know everything about disabilities and impairments.
2. Professionals do not often agree between themselves on the diagnosis and/or treatment strategies for children with developmental disabilities.
3. Professionals are pedantic and use a lot of jargon and technical language that is seldom understood by laypersons and parents of children with handicaps.
4. Professionals blame parents and induce in them a sense of guilt or incompetence in their handling of children with handicaps.
5. Professionals are not as emotionally involved as parents in the training or rehabilitation process of children with disabilities.
6. Most professionals are materialistic and concerned about earning money rather than being service-oriented towards the disabled.
7. Professionals are not always ready to sacrifice in order to work with less fortunate people like persons with disabilities.

## Preparations before Starting a Home-training Programme

Knowledge about diagnostic conditions and psychological acceptance of behaviour assets/deficits in a child is an initial preparation from the parents' side before starting a home training programme. There are some other preparations (given in Table 2.3) in terms of materials and time required before undertaking home training programmes. Where should the programme be carried out? Who will take charge of the programme? Mothers in our country are expected, by convention, custom and culture, to take this role of the specialized caregiver. While fathers may conveniently absolve themselves of their home training responsibilities under some pretext, this excuse is no longer tenable in the case of children with DDs. Parents (as also grandparents, siblings and extended family members) share combined responsibility for the extra demands of child care required in home training programmes.

**Table 2.3**
**What Must You Do before Starting a Home-training Programme?**

- Collect as much correct information about the diagnostic condition of your child or about any associated conditions (if any).
- Get an idea of the intellectual/social adaptive level of functioning of your child.
- Find out just how much can be expected out of your child. Obviously, normal schooling may be ruled out for the majority of severe-profound categories of DDs.
- Observe your own feelings and expectations about your child and distinguish them from wishful thoughts or feelings. A discussion with professionals/experts may help you learn about yourself in relation to your child who has a handicap.
- An ideal situation would require co-ordination and co-operation of all members of the family in every stage of planning and implementation of the home training programmes.
- Remember that your spouse and the other members in your family may not be expectedly at the same level of psychological acceptance about your child's condition. Some may be accepting while others may be overcritical, sceptical or even reject the child. Accept the fact that it takes all sorts of people to make this world.
- While there may be many people around you, yet you may be alone when it comes to the actual training of your child with a disability. Even professionals are of limited help in a sense as they spend only an hour or so in actual terms per session with your child. As the primary caregiver, you have the opportunity for spending the most time in a day with your child.

In our country, the additional presence of extended/joint family members can be gainfully used for the benefit of home training programmes. However, this entails all family members being *equally oriented* on the special needs and procedures for handling these children. While additional hands/social support ease and facilitate distribution of child-care activities, there is the attendant risk of 'Too many cooks spoiling the broth.' Inconsistencies in child rearing practices have been found to be higher in poorly oriented joint/extended families than in nuclear families. This can be more disadvantageous while undertaking effective home training programmes. Ultimately it is not a matter of mere group living, but the quality of such group dynamics within the family which counts for benefit of constructive stimulation of children with disabilities.

It requires an amount of physical and psychological preparation for the individual caregiver as well as the whole family before planning and/or implementing home-based training programmes for children with DDs. Many caregivers raise excuses that they are too busy to be able to find enough time for carrying out a home training programme. But where there is inclination, there is time! What's more, it is not the *quantity* of time that matters in the training of children, it is the *quality*. For example, a mother may spend the whole day sitting idly or watching television in the company of her preschool child. This does not help the child gain anything compared to even half-an-hour that another parent spends actively with her child showing or teaching several stimulating things.

Parents and prospective trainers must watch their expectations of the training outcomes appropriately. While dealing with special children, one obviously cannot have the same expectations as in the case of training non-disabled children. One cannot expect the sky. The response to stimulation activities carried out on these children may not be as forthcoming as in normal children. For example, in teaching a child with disability to point to his name on a name call the parent may have to work for at least 50 to a 100 trials, as compared to a mere 10 or 15 trials in a normal child. If the parent is not mentally prepared for such a long and patient endeavour, he or she is likely to give up prematurely—hence proving insufficient to the needs of the child. In as much as parents are eager to adopt short cuts to better the quality of life of their children with disabilities, and some professionals are always zealous to sell their wares as the 'best' available remedy in the market, remember that there is never a 'canned programme'! Rather, any or every training programme for children with disabilities needs to be flexible enough to accommodate the individual needs of each child. In a sense, none of the techniques proposed in this book are new and untried. Many of these ideas or techniques have been used before. An effort has been made to compile them in one place for those wishing to teach preschool children with DDs. A cascade presentation for planning and implementation of skill training programmes for infants, toddlers and preschoolers with DDs in home settings is shown in Figure 2.1.

## 1. Identification and Listing of Deficit Skill Behaviours

The first step in any home training programme is to make a detailed list of the current level of skill behaviours in your child. This is not as easy a task as it appears to be. Many times, as parents, we presume to know enough about our children. We assume we can accurately list what our child can or cannot do. For example, in clinical practise, when we ask a parent as to whether the child can or cannot button its shirt, many parents perfunctorily dismiss the query with an emphatic 'No!'—only to be consequently faced with an embarrassing situation when the child performs the said activity in front of the clinician. Such a parent is often forced to make a defensive conclusion like 'Oh! He seems to be doing it fine in front of you. But he would never do this at home.' The lesson to be learnt by adult caregivers is that their children may be actually capable of a great deal more than they would ever have seen them doing. It may be simply a question of not having given their children the opportunities to perform those things. This situation is particularly true of children with DDs, since parents unwittingly block so many opportunities for learning. This may not occur intentionally on their part. Many parents who report that their child cannot cut with a pair of scissors or strike a matchstick may be actually hiding a good intention of playing safe with their child. Or it may be a sheer attitude of over-protection towards the special child. You must be wary of such pitfalls while making initial assessments of your child's behavioural strengths and

**Figure 2.1**
**Planning and Implementation of Skill Training Programmes**

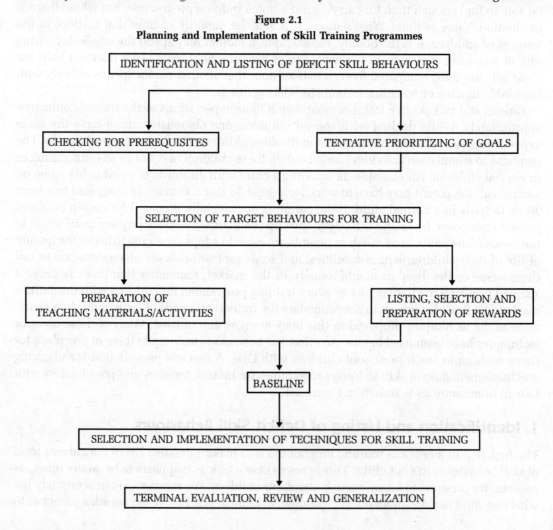

weaknesses. In sum, this initial process of observation or testing of the current level of a child's functioning is intended to profile a range of behaviours which the child can/cannot perform. This exercise becomes the basis for planning and implementation of the skill-behaviour training programme (Table 2.4).

---

**Table 2.4**

**Guidelines for Identification and Listing of Deficit Skill Behaviours**

- Observe your child's current level of skill behaviours closely in a variety of life situations.
- Keep an eye on your child's past/recent achievements over a long period, say a year or so.
- Make a list of priority needs of your child. List an exhaustive inventory of behavioural items that he or she needs to, but cannot, perform for his or her known mental/chronological age level.
- Look at your own available resources in terms of time/opportunities that can be used in home training your child.
- Go over a checklist of skill behaviours for children with DDs (such as 'ACPC–DD). ACPC–DD is an inventory of common activities of daily life in various areas like eating, dressing, toilet, play, etc. Cover as many areas/domains of behaviour listed during this initial observation (refer to Chapter 4).
- Some other checklists are also available for different age groups and severity or types of handicaps in children. For example, ACPC–DD is for infants and toddlers below six years, BASIC–MR (Peshawaria and Venkatesan, 1992a) is for school-going children with mental retardation.
- Go through each and every item in these checklists to verify whether your child can or cannot perform the mentioned activity under the set of circumstances described therein.
- Many items in these checklists, though simple and mundane, may not have been ever tried with your child. It may simply be a case of lack of opportunity for training on some of these items.
- If you are in doubt about any particular item/group of items in the checklists, there is no harm in trying it out with your child before deciding whether he or she can or cannot perform them.
- A single random check on an activity/item is insufficient. At times, children refuse to perform a particular item when asked to. This does not mean that he or she cannot perform that item. It may not be a skill deficit, just that he or she does not want to do it owing to behaviour problems. In such a case, they need to be tackled in different ways.
- An ideal way to determine, identify and list skills that are present/absent in your child is to have about a week or fortnights' time marked exclusively for observation.
- Be careful not to mix your expectations of performance of a specific behaviour in your child with his or her actual achievements. Do not also allow your affection for him or her to colour or distract your observations about what or how much he or she can actually perform during a given behaviour.
- A frequent mistake parents commit when observing their child's behavioural assets/deficits is to teach or preach in the process. For example, while observing whether a child can recite the days of the week, parents inadvertently prompt or cue as he hesitates or falters. This tendency must be resisted in order to make an objective/accurate identification of whether your child can/cannot perform a given item.
- If the child commits some mistake during the course of your observation, do not at once correct or scold him. Remember that you are only trying to discover where or how much he can do of the observed activity. You are trying to determine where or how he is going wrong, so that you can use this information to correct him later.

---

## 2. Goal Setting

Goal setting here refers to objectives or targets for teaching children with DDs. Any skill training programme requires clear and precise goals to lend meaning as well as direction to parents' efforts. There are three types of goals required for home training of children with DDs.

(a) Life goals
(b) Long-term goals or annual goals
(c) Short-term goals or teaching objectives

> **Case Vignette**
>
> Vikrant is a 20-year-old diagnosed with below-average intelligence (a slow learner). His mental age was estimated by a clinical psychologist to be around 12 years. His father is keen to see Vikrant get through his matriculation examinations. Vikrant has been moved across many schools. He has home-tutors for algebra, calculus, science, history and two languages. The parents are terribly frustrated that Vikrant could not get through his high school examinations despite appearing for them at least five times. Of late Vikrant is observed to have become grouchy, ill-tempered and occasionally violent too. He evades academic work, and is becoming unmanageable for his aged parents.

## Types of Goals

**Life Goals:** There can be many reasons for Vikrant's problems. It could be the lack of appreciation of his intellectual potential or the well intended but exaggerated expectations of his aged parents or something else too. Nevertheless, what is required is a primary acceptance of Vikrant's current level of intellectual functioning and establishing a life goal accordingly. Children with DDs have special skills and competencies. They cannot be equated with their non-disabled normal age peers, nor can they be expected to accomplish in their lives what others of their age accomplish. Nevertheless, this does not mean that these children are totally useless, nor that they are permanent liabilities to their families or society; it only means that they are differently-abled. It is for us to identify their differential abilities at the early stages, provide enough opportunities and instructions and guide them to achieve optimally according to their individual capacities. Thus they can be surely enabled to achieve a lot, both for themselves as well as for others around them. In this context, it becomes imperative to draw up life goals for children, especially as they grow older. During the preschool years, it may be still too early to draw up life goals or shrink the educational expectations of parents. However, parents need to train themselves to approach the whole issue with an open mind.

**Long-term Goals:** Long-term goals are necessary in home training programmes for preschool children. Long-term goals are statements expressing provisional expectations of caregivers about their child over the next quarter of a year. A three-month expectation regime is pragmatic since your child may even show spontaneous development/growth of skills over longer periods. One would then not be able to ascertain whether the given developmental changes are due to the efforts of your stimulation programme carried out at home.

**Short-term Goals:** Based on the broadly set group of long-term goals, one has to work out a specific set of short-term goals or behaviour objectives for teaching within a short range of time (Table 2.5). A long-term goal for Vikrant could be to teach him how to handle money. This could include teaching him that money has exchange/tender value, that money is to be preserved, to identify the values of coins/currency, to add or transact money, etc. Each of these specific behaviours to be trained/achieved is a short-term goal. Refer to the 'sample inventory of identified deficit skill behaviours' for an illustrative distinction between long-term goals and short-term goals (Table 2.6).

---

**Table 2.5**

**Guidelines for Selection of Short-term Goals**

- Short-term goals are statements of behaviours targeted to be taught or achieved by your child within short periods of time (usually no more than three to four weeks).
- Consider your child's age, abilities, needs, social aspects and current level of functioning in various areas before setting up specific short-term targets.
- Always select short-term teaching targets that have functional and utilitarian value for your child as well as for others around him.
- Select only those behaviour objectives that can be surely achieved by your child within a limited time frame of three to four weeks.
- Never establish objectives that are more difficult to achieve when your child is unable to perform on behaviours preceding it. Each behaviour objective invariably carries along with it certain prerequisites. In other words, your child must have achieved these prerequisites if he is to learn its attended behaviour. For more details on prerequisites, refer to the next section.
- Choose behaviour objectives that will help mainstream or move your child closer to his normal age peers.
- Select only about three to four teaching objectives at a time even though you may readily have a longer list to work upon in due course. Having too many teaching objectives at the same time may distract/dilute your focus while training.

---

**Table 2.6**

**Sample Inventory of Identified Deficit-skill Behaviours**

| | |
|---|---|
| Name of child: | Anoop Kumar |
| Chronological age: | 7 years |
| Mental age: | 4 years |
| Clinical diagnosis: | Mild mental retardation |

List of deficit skill behaviours observed under various domains over a two-week observation period carried out by parents in home settings.

**Motor**
- Cannot maintain balance while walking along a straight line.
- Cannot jump at same place with both feet off the ground.

**Communication**
- Cannot carry out two related set of commands.

**Play**
- Cannot blow out a candle.
- Cannot throw a ball in a specified direction.

**Self-help skills**
- Cannot unbutton his own clothing.

**Cognitive**
- Cannot match two primary colours.
- Cannot sort out objects of different sizes.

**Pre-academics**
- Cannot copy out a circle.
- Cannot relate time to clocks or watches.
- Cannot rote count up to five.

## 3. Checking on Prerequisites

Every teaching objective invariably carries along with it certain prerequisites. In other words, your child must have achieved certain preconditions before learning the next attendant behaviour. For example, no child will learn to walk before he learns to sit or stand. Similarly, no child learns to sit before learning to hold the neck steady. These are gross examples of prerequisites. Similar prerequisites exist for almost all behaviour objectives. A sample of some such prerequisites are given in Table 2.7. The guidelines for recognition of prerequisites are given in Table 2.8.

**Table 2.7**

**Sample List of Short-term Goals and Related Prerequisites**

| Teaching Objectives | Related Behavioural Prerequisites |
|---|---|
| Motor | |
| Picks objects using thumb and forefinger | Retains objects in palm |
| Sits on own or with support | Holds head steady |
| Kicks a ball in a definite direction | Kicks a ball in any direction |
| Communication | |
| Indicates body parts | Pointing skills |
| Follows simple commands | Listening skills |
| Self help | |
| Buttoning/unbuttoning of clothes | Fine finger grasp and eye-hand co-ordination |
| Puts on elastic shorts | Removes elastic pants/shorts |
| Cognitive | |
| Names colours | Matches/sorts/identifies colours |
| Identifies values of coins | Reads numbers |
| Discriminates between day and night | Differentiates between darkness and light |
| Play | |
| Skips using a rope | Jumps with both feet off the ground |
| Hops | Jumps alternatively using both feet |

**Table 2.8**

**Guidelines for Checking on Prerequisites before Selection of Short-term Goals**

- Perform the given teaching objective yourself to get a feel of the various skill components required for the activity.
- Break the teaching activity into small parts or steps as explained under the section on task analysis/task slicing.
- Observe your child performing the same teaching activity a couple of times in order to determine how he performs it.
- Observe (don't teach or correct straight away) the level of assistance your child requires to perform the target activity.
- If your child does not show the prerequisites for the given activity consider changing or revising the objective to a preceding simpler step.

## 4. Selection/Prioritizing Teaching Objectives

Based on the abovementioned steps, you are now ready with a list of specific behaviour objectives or teaching targets for your preschool child. The next step involves arrangement

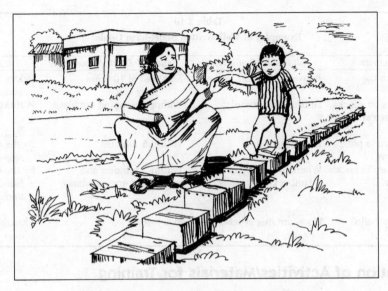

**Illustration 2.1 Maintains Balance in Walking**

of the selected behaviour objectives into a hierarchy. Select only a small list of teaching targets. Prioritize which among the selected teaching targets you would like to focus on for their achievement in the shortest possible time.

## 5. Writing Down Teaching Objectives

It is always advantageous to put down the listed and prioritized teaching targets for your child on a piece of paper rather than just committing them to memory. The advantages of this are listed in Table 2.9. How does one write down training objectives? Any teaching objective comprises four components:

- Clearly observable and measurable behaviour activity.
- Situations or conditions under which the said behaviour activity is to be performed.
- Amount or level of expected performance.
- Date deadlines for teaching or achieving the said training objective.

A few examples of well-written teaching objectives are given in Table 2.10.

---

**Table 2.9**
**Advantages of Recording Short-term Goals**

- Recording will tell you objectively where your child stands *vis-à-vis* the selected teaching objective.
- It will be a good reference point later when you want to compare any gains or losses between various teaching objectives chosen for your child. It will help you determine whether your child has made progress at the end of your teaching programme of about three or four weeks.
- You can also compare relative gains or losses between various teaching objectives chosen for your child. Did he or she gain more under motor activities than self-help skills or cognitive domains? Did he or she lose any previously learnt skills or activities during the current teaching programme?

---

**Table 2.10**
**Examples of Well Written Short-term Goals**

| Behavioural Activity | Situations/Conditions | Expected Performance Level | Deadline |
|---|---|---|---|
| Vina will match the colour red | Between 'red' and 'yellow' | Eight out of 10 times | Before 75 practice sessions |
| Vinod will pass on snacks to all children at the table | During lunch time | Without dropping crumbs | Within three sessions |
| Vishal will learn to put away his toys | After play time | Within 5 minutes | By the end of seven sessions |
| Vishnu will learn to buckle his sandals | When given his pair of unbuckled sandals | Within 3 minutes and without any assistance | By the end of seven half-an-hour teaching sessions |
| Vinitra will say 'hello' | Upon arriving at school | Every day | Through practice over 15 days |

## 6. Preparation of Activities/Materials for Training

Every skill training programme entails not only selection and prioritizing of specific teaching objectives and/or writing them down in clearly observable and measurable terms for your child, but also the preparation of relevant teaching materials or activities. Parents often assume that they have to buy costly toys or exotic play materials for their children. Of course, toys and play materials have a facilitator role in teaching children even as they entertain them. But, on many occasions, and with a little ingenuity, one can use familiar household articles or routine items as materials for teaching preschool children.

Colour and size discrimination can be taught using buttons of various colours and sizes. Old greeting cards can be cut into various shapes for teaching of shape sorting. The use of lock and key, squeezing soft clothes or sponge, picking up strewn playing cards or gem clips from the floor, using a pair of scissors and such other activities can prove to be simple but routine exercises for building eye-hand co-ordination. Old magazines or newspapers can be used for scribbling activities, finger/palm painting, leaf or block/thread painting, practising brush strokes, etc. Oral exercises can be set for children by incorporating activities like balloon blowing, playing with wind instruments (flute or mouth organ), blowing candles, soap bubbles, whistles, etc.

As far as possible, the teaching aids/materials used should be close to the real world. Your child has difficulty in generalizing what he learns in one situation to other similar situations. A child who has learnt to point to vegetables in pictures may not necessarily be able to point to real vegetables. He may be required to be taught all over again. Similarly, a child who has been taught to rote count up to 100 need not necessarily be able to count and hand over 10 tomatoes from the fridge. Therefore, teach your child as close to the real world as possible in order to avoid duplication of efforts and facilitate easy transfer of learning.

## 7. Listing, Selection and Preparation of Rewards

Rewards constitute an important agent for teaching/learning in preschool children with DDs (Table 2.11). Rewards act as incentives for children to learn, as well to perform what they have learnt. Normal children experience rewards in abundance in their daily lives since they have a large repertoire of skills or behaviours to demonstrate before others. Children with DDs do not have as many skills to show to others. Moreover, others are not usually as impressed spontaneously by these children as they are with the talents or presentations of normal children. Therefore, these children require specially focused reward-training schemes built into the context of their larger skill behaviour-training programmes.

---

**Table 2.11**
**What are Rewards?**

Consider these examples:

- Shashi recites a rhyme. Guests clap their hands.
- Mohan buttons his shirt himself. His father pats him on the back.
- Sita mops the floor. Her mother gives her a sweet.
- Varsha purchases vegetables from the market. Her father gives her a rupee.

A reward is a positive event that happens after a behaviour. It is pleasurable and makes the person want to behave similarly again and again.

---

In the examples in Table 2.11, a behaviour occurs. There is something that happens immediately after that behaviour. The person who receives it likes that 'something'. That 'something' is a reward. *A reward is a positive event that happens after a behaviour. It is pleasurable and makes that person want to behave similarly again and again*. Whether we are aware of it or not, we are all motivated by rewards or incentives. The nature, types (Table 2.12) or amount of the rewards that motivate each one of us differ. Nevertheless, every behaviour is influenced by the rewards that they get for us.

---

**Table 2.12**
**Types of Rewards**

| Type of Reward | Examples |
|---|---|
| Primary rewards | Eatables (either solid or liquid) like bananas, sweets, toffees, soft drinks, food, etc. |
| Material rewards | Things like kites, cycles, bangles, ribbons, marbles, toys, etc. |
| Social rewards | Verbal praises or actions depicting appreciation. |
| Activity rewards | Activities like riding a cycle, playing with a toy or on the swing, going for a ride on a scooter, etc. |
| Privileges | Special status positions like being made leader of a group, monitor of the class, etc. |
| Tokens | Tokens are reward items which have no inherent values. Yet they are desired because some value has been assigned to them. For example, stamps, stars in a book, marks in a test, etc. |

---

It is one thing to know the value or types of rewards that work in children, and it is quite another thing to use them effectively in achieving behaviour remediation of children. In a study, parents were asked to list all those things, events or items that they used as rewards for their children. The responses were diverse. Some said they gave eatables like bananas, colas, biscuits and so on, while others gave a list of activities like watching television, listening to music, going out on a car ride and so on. However, a surprising result of the study was the fact that while parents prioritize expensive items like primary and material rewards as having reinforcement value, they do not appear to realize the potential of easily available and

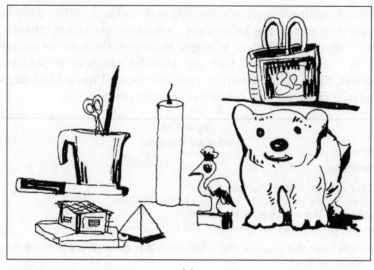

(a)

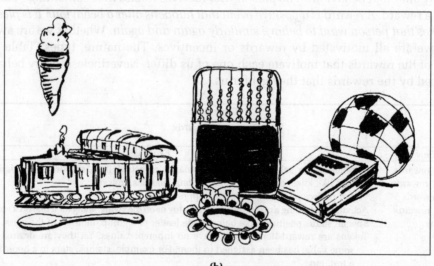

(b)

**Illustration 2.2 Types of Rewards**

inexpensive acts like praising, patting and allied social rewards in changing the behaviour of young children with disabilities (Venkatesan et al., 1996).

In actuality, it may not be that parents do not use social rewards with their children. It may only be that they do not realize their reward potential or value. Thus, there is a need for parents to be educated, not only on the selection/identification of rewards (Table 2.13), but also on the procedures for their effective use (Table 2.14) while teaching children with DDs.

**Table 2.13**

**Selection of Rewards**

Select carefully rewards that work with your child. What may be liked as a reward by one child may not be valued by another. How do you select an appropriate reward for your child?

- Ask your child directly.
- Observe him in various situations to understand his likes and dislikes.
- Use a reward checklist that contains an inventory of things or events commonly liked by children.
- Make a reward history. Recollect all those things or events your child demands and feels happy when receiving them.
- Select rewards which are easily accessible and dispensable.
- Use reward-sampling techniques. Place a variety of items in front of your child to see what he prefers frequently. His preferences will give you an idea about his reward choices.
- Never use a single reward over and over again else your child is bound to get bored or satiated. A frequent change of rewards is necessary in their use for training.

**Table 2.14**

**Dispensing Rewards**

The following rules are to be observed while dispensing rewards:

- Always reward only skill behaviours.
- Never reward problem behaviours.
- Reward clearly. Tell your child each time you reward him. He must understand why he is receiving a reward, or not receiving a reward for non-performance of certain behaviours.
- Reward consistently. Reward each and every time the target skill behaviour occurs in your child. Only then will he gradually understand the linkage between the presentation of behaviour and consequent reward experience.
- Reward immediately. There should be no delay in presentation of rewards for desirable or skill behaviours. The greater the time lag between the occurrence of a behaviour and the presentation of reward, the more the chance of your child not relating the behaviour with the reward experience.
- Reward in right quantity. There is no objective measure of how much to reward your child for a given behaviour. But rewards earned should definitely match the behaviours shown.
- It is preferable to reward in small quantities so as to keep up the interest of your child.
- Always combine social rewards with primary rewards. Social rewards are inexpensive and easy to dispense. Saying 'good!' to your child does not cost as much as buying chocolates or sweets. Surprisingly, it has been seen in research studies that most parents do not realize the potency of social rewards as much as they keep buying costly gifts or presents.
- Choose intrinsic rewards over external rewards. Even though you may start a training programme by using external rewards, your aim should be to lead the child towards working on things or activities for their own intrinsic value. Therefore, plan in advance to gradually lead your child to work for intrinsic rewards rather than for rewards from the outside world.
- Fading of rewards: the procedure of gradually tapering off costly material or primary rewards for inexpensive or easily dispensable social or intrinsic rewards is called fading.
- Change rewards sensibly. Do not give the same reward over and over again to your child. There is a danger of his or her getting bored, and the said item or activity will lose its reward potency. So keep changing the type of rewards from time to time to keep up their value in the eyes of your child.

# 8. Baseline

Baseline is a measure of targeted teaching objectives before implementation of appropriate training techniques for your child. It is important to maintain notes on your child's current level of behavioural functioning with respect to your chosen teaching objective. If your teach-ing objective is, say, to train him to join two dots to make a straight line, begin by keeping a sample note of his current level of performance. Note down how well or how poorly he performs the chosen objective. The current level of performance for any given activity may be broadly graded along a five-point rating scale (Table 2.15). Most of your teaching objec-tives vis-à-vis your child's current level of performance can be graded along this five-point continuum. In other words, what you are trying to discover during baseline is the amount/level of assistance your child currently requires to perform the chosen behavioural objective. Note that this inference cannot be based on a single observation. Try observing your child performing the given behavioural objective a couple of times before concluding decisively about the level of assistance required.

**Table 2.15**
**Grading Current Level of Performance**

| Category | Description |
| --- | --- |
| Totally dependent (TD) | When the child cannot perform the given behaviour. |
| Physical prompts (PP) | When the child requires physical assistance to perform the given behaviour. |
| Verbal prompts (VP) | When the child needs verbal instructions to perform the given behaviour. |
| Clueing/Cueing (C) | When the child requires some cues/clues to perform the given behaviour. |
| Independent (I) | When the child can perform the said behaviour on his own and requires no assistance. |

## 9. Selection/Implementation of Training Techniques

There are many behavioural techniques available for parents wishing to undertake home-based skill training programmes for preschool children with DDs. The following descrip-tions are a mere overview on training techniques for their use in home settings. However, the precise procedures for teaching target skill activities are further enunciated in the later chap-ters in greater detail.

### Task Analysis

All preschool children learn easily through small steps. This is one of the greatest secrets of teaching. Instead of teaching an activity as a whole, it is recommended you break it into separate small or simple steps to achieve the entire behavioural objective. Task analysis is simply a procedure of teaching in small and simple steps. This procedure is especially useful in teaching activities related to sensori-motor, self-help skills or play domains. Different chil-dren require different levels of assistance before being started on a teaching objective. In some ways, task analysis involves discovering the correct level or amount of assistance re-quired to teach your child a behavioural objective. The number or sequence of steps that can lead to any given behavioural objective cannot be fixed. It is tailor-made according to indi-vidual cases. Some children may require just three steps to reach a given behavioural objec-tive, while others may require more or less number of steps to achieve the same objective. Note that each step in task analysis is sequentially linked from one to another leading towards the behavioural objective. Sometimes a given child may not progress along the exact same sequence as another child. He or she may skip some step/s or may require an addition of some other step/s. A sample illustration of task analysis for an identified behavioural objective is given in Table 2.16.

---

**Task analysis involves slicing or dividing a teaching objective into small and simple steps**

---

**Table 2.16**
**A Sample Illustration of Task Analysis**

Behavioural objective: Pulling elastic shorts up on one's own
Steps:

1. Pulls elastic shorts up from the thighs.
2. Pulls elastic shorts up from the knees.
3. Pulls elastic shorts up from below the knees.
4. Pulls elastic shorts up from the ankles.
5. Sits and inserts one leg after another into shorts before pulling shorts up to the hip.

---

## Shaping

Shaping involves giving rewards in successive steps as subsets of behaviour approximated correctly towards a teaching objective. Select a target behaviour that you intend to teach. Select a set of powerful rewards which work well with your child and which may be used during training. Slice the target behavioural objective into several small steps as per task-analytic procedures. Take the last step or slice of the chosen behavioural objective and link it with the chosen rewards. Proceed to reward your child each and every time he performs the last slice of the behavioural objective. Once the child achieves the last slice of the behaviour, proceed to reward the next slice of behaviour. Remember not to reward the lower slice once the child has learnt to perform on higher steps. A sample illustration on shaping for an identified behavioural objective is given in Table 2.17.

---

**Shaping involves rewarding successive approximations of sliced behaviours towards a teaching objective**

---

## Prompting

Prompting is a procedure of giving active assistance, guidance, instructions and help when your child learns a specific target behaviour. The current level of performance for any given activity can be broadly graded along a five-point rating scale, viz., totally dependent, physical prompts, verbal prompts, cueing and independent, respectively. Prompting is viewed as a method of teaching. A child who is totally dependent on a given behavioural objective initially requires physical prompts or manual assistance in teaching techniques. For example, hold your child's hands and assist him in pointing to his nose for indication of body parts. Always associate physical guidance with a running commentary of verbal instructions on whatever you are doing. This facilitates clarity of expression of intent and purpose. Gradually use more verbal prompts even as you decrease physical prompts. Later, use only verbal and/or non-verbal cues before fading them too eventually. Some additional guidelines for using prompts while teaching preschool children are given in Table 2.19.

---

**Table 2.17**
**A Sample Illustration of Shaping**

Behavioural objective: Eye-to-eye contact training
Steps:

1. Provide a primary reward every time the child responds to any sound stimulus.
2. Provide a primary reward only when the child localizes the sound stimulus.
3. Provide a primary reward only when the child turns to your voice, even though it may be fleeting.
4. Provide a primary reward when the child passes at least a fleeting glance towards your face.
5. Provide a primary reward only when the child sustains his or her glance for 3 to 5 seconds towards your face.

---

**Table 2.18**
**Guidelines to be Used while Prompting**

- Always secure your child's attention before you provide him with prompts.
- Provide the prompts before the occurrence of the target behaviour.
- Be brief while providing verbal prompts.
- Select prompts that are easily understood by your child.
- Combine use of prompts along with other techniques for teaching skill behaviours like shaping, chaining, modelling, etc.
- Fade prompts in a sequential order beginning from physical prompts to verbal prompts to clueing, respectively.

---

**Table 2.19**
**A Sample Illustration on Prompting**

Behavioural objective: Throwing the ball in any direction
Steps:

- Place a ball in the palms of your child's hands and cover it with your hands completely.
- Assist your child in throwing the ball up in the air.
- Provide verbal instructions continuously about the ongoing activity.
- Gradually decrease your physical assistance and increase your verbal instructions each time the ball is thrown into the air.
- Much later, and after enough practice trials, decrease the verbal instructions too.
- Ask your child more and more to release the ball using his or her own hands even as you provide only some hints or cues.
- Pat or praise your child each time an attempt is made by him or her to release the ball.

## Chaining

We have understood that children learn better in small or simple steps rather than when the teaching objective is presented as a whole. The process of dividing or slicing each teaching objective into smaller steps was explained as task analysis. Further, in the same procedure, if we incorporate a scheme of sequential steps of slices of behaviour that lead to the whole behavioural objective, it is called chaining. Guidelines for the use of chaining is given in Table 2.20, and a sample of this technique is given in Table 2.21.

---

**Table 2.20**

**Additional Guidelines on the Use of Chaining**

- Delineate each step in the chain to be followed for reaching the target behaviour.
- If the behavioural objective has been sliced into six steps, begin by teaching the link between step one and step two alone. Then proceed to link the first two steps with the third step and so on.
- Make use of rewards at the end of each step in the chain.
- Move to the next step in the chain only after your child has learnt the preceding step sufficiently well.
- There are two approaches in the use of chaining techniques. You can either start at the first step or proceed to the last step of the slices towards the behavioural objective (forward chaining). Alternatively, you can also start from the last step and proceed on to the first step of the slices towards the behavioural objective (backward chaining).

---

## Modelling or Imitation

Children learn a lot by imitation. They imitate the behaviour of persons they consider important and are impressed by. It may be their favourite teacher, parent, film star, friend, etc. Imitation is a powerful tool for teaching children by means of demonstration. Don't confuse modelling with comparison. No one likes to be compared with others, more so if the comparison is based on weaknesses. Avoid comparisons. Rather, use modelling as a means to demonstrate what your child is required to do and how.

Ensure your child's attention on every detail of the model. Provide a running commentary on the activity being performed in front of your child. The model should be appropriate for the age or sex of your child. If a complex series of activities are to be taught, it is advisable to

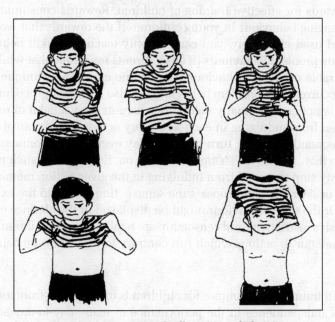

**Illustration 2.3  A Sample Illustration of Chaining**

Table 2.21

A Sample Illustration of Chaining

Behavioural objective: Taking off a pullover, shirt, *banian* or vest
Steps:

| | |
|---|---|
| 1. | Pulls off vest covering his head. |
| 1+2. | Pulls off vest covering his face. |
| 1+2+3. | Pulls off vest from about his shoulders. |
| 1+2+3+4. | Removes one hand from vest upto shoulder. |
| 1+2+3+4+5. | Removes second hand from vest upto shoulder. |
| 1+2+3+4+5+6. | Rolls up and pulls off vest around armpits. |

slice it into smaller steps and demonstrate each part separately. Ensure your child's performance at the end of demonstrating each step or sequence of behaviours. Reward the child adequately and appropriately upon every correct or nearly correct imitation of the target behaviour. Make sure that the model itself is free from flaws or imperfections. Otherwise the learner will imbibe the same errors in his learning too. Many children learn quickly by imitating the actions of their peers. They learn to clap their hands, dance to rhythm, perform physical exercises, recite rhymes, scribble with a pencil, drink with a cup/glass or just about any other imitation. Thus, parents have a powerful tool in imitation of modelling for teaching children. It can be used to teach a host of skill behaviours, or even, unfortunately, problem behaviours in children.

## Rewards Technique

We have already seen the meaning of rewards, their types, their selection and the procedures of dispensing rewards for effective training of children. Rewards constitute a very powerful technique for changing behaviour in young children. If the rewards that work for your child are identified and used effectively, you can not only teach new skill behaviours, but also reduce or eliminate problem behaviours (if any). Parents must note that while giving rewards for positive, desirable or 'good' behaviour may be one effective technique, simultaneously rewarding non-occurrence of problem behaviours is also a needed procedure for regular use with children. It is noticed that many meticulous parents have a habit of restricting or stopping their children from indulging in each and every activity. Such caregivers are found to use 'no!' more frequently at every turn of day-to-day events, with commands like 'don't do this …!', 'don't do that …!', 'no …!', 'stop …!' and so on. Even though such repeat commands may spontaneously stop the child from indulging in the given action momentarily, it will be seen that sooner or later the child repeats the same action, much to the exasperation of the chiding parent! Or the same behaviour might be displayed in the absence of the remonstrating parent. Excessive restrictions and censorship are retaliated to by children with more intensive negative behaviour or actions which run contrary to what they are being told not to do.

## Fading

The aim of all skill training programmes for children is to lead them from total dependence to a relative state of independence in the performance of many day-to-day activities. In brief, parents are to identify the behavioural potential of their children and lead them towards gradually optimizing the same to the maximum possible extent. In the process, we are providing various levels of assistance. However, the various levels of assistance and/or teaching techniques discussed so far are merely means to an end. The end is, of course, independence of your child in performance of all skills. Always remember the ultimate goal is to lead your child from dependence to independence. At the earliest opportunity, set your child free. Fade physical prompts or assistance into verbal prompts or instructions. Fade verbal prompts into cues or hints. Eliminate cues and thereby set your child moving towards independence. The process of gradual decrease in active assistance towards active or independent performance by your child when performing specific teaching objectives is called fading. Fading is not the end of any teaching activity. Plan a schedule for fading various levels of assistance well ahead of time. It should be carried out gradually and imperceptibly. An abrupt fading of assistance may cause your child to regress to previous levels of dependence.

## Generalization

Many times children learn certain specific skill behaviours in one setting. Then they might be required to perform them in some other different but related setting. For example, a child learns to greet a teacher in the classroom. Then the child extends the same greeting skills to guests who come home. A child may learn to recognize a colour (red) in a two-choice puzzle teaching situation. Then he has to extend the same recognition of colour (red) to all objects in his surroundings (such as a red post box, red flower, red sari, red *bindi* and so on). Children with DDs show severe problems in generalization. A child taught to point at vegetables in picture books need not necessarily recognize them when real vegetables are placed before him. He may have to be taught all over again. Therefore, it is apt to undertake the initial teaching of target behaviours in as natural a situation as possible. Rather than investing time and resources unnecessarily in model teaching and then arranging to transfer them to natural settings, it is economical to go in for teaching them in real life situations. A visit to a shop, railway station, zoo or a sanctuary has more direct learning for the child than a picture book/flash card depicting the same.

## 8. Terminal Evaluation, Review and Generalization

After a period of intervention by way of skill training for a given behaviour objective over target deadlines, it would be apt to undertake a re-evaluation/review of one teaching programme. For example, if your target was to teach your child to match the colour red between the colours red and yellow correctly, eight times out of 10 through 75 sessions, proceed to undertake a review at the end of this deadline. In case your child has achieved the set objective, proceed to target afresh the next objective along its continuum. On the other hand, if your child has not achieved the set objective within the stipulated time or at the set standards of chosen criteria, you must sit back to review why your child has not achieved it. There are many possibilities to be considered during this review. Many parents assume that the fault for non-achievement of set objectives lies with their child. This is seldom true. It would be more appropriate to search for an answer in other quarters. Consider these possibilities during review/reassessment of chosen target behaviours for your child with DDs (Table 2.22).

---

**Table 2.22**

**Possible Reasons for Non-achievement of Target Behaviours**

- Chosen target behaviours for skill training were not appropriate to the level of your child's development.
- Selected target behaviours might have been either too high or too low for the level of your child.
- Your child did not possess the needed prerequisite/s for learning the chosen behaviour.
- Practice sessions were inadequate.
- Teaching techniques were inappropriate for your child/chosen target behaviour.
- Rewards following performance of target behaviours during teaching/practice sessions were inappropriate, inadequate or simply not dispensed according to their mentioned guidelines for use with children.
- Presentation of teaching activities were dull, drab and uninteresting from the viewpoint of the child.
- Teaching materials were not devised or put into use according to the needs/level of the child.
- Alternative teaching devices, strategies or activities were not experimented/tried out for teaching the given behavioural objective.
- Problem behaviours requiring urgent remediation may not have been prioritized before undertaking the teaching programme for the given objective.
- Errors in performance during teaching/learning might not have been dispassionately observed for their individualized analysis and remediation.
- The teaching objective might have required further simplification through task slicing/analysis before repeat presentation.
- Your performance expectancy levels for the chosen behaviour objective may have been too high and required retuning according to the needs/level of your child.

---

## Additional Guidelines for Training

Given below are a few more guidelines to be used (Venkatesan, 1994a) while training pre-school children with DDs in home settings. Some of these points may even be understood as common pitfalls that caregivers face, thereby leading to the failure of their home training programmes.

### Simple to Complex

Always plan and proceed to teach from simple to complex tasks. Success in simple tasks will interest and motivate your child to do more. For example, the sequence of teaching colour concept can proceed through colour matching, sorting, identification and naming, respectively.

### Familiar to Unfamiliar

Always start teaching your child from a step which he knows and then proceed to tasks that he does not know. For example, if between the tasks of throwing, catching and/or kicking a ball the child knows throwing, start teaching at that step before leading onto other steps.

### Concrete to Abstract

Most preschool children show difficulty in learning or understanding abstract concepts. You can see this difficulty in their inability to interpret fables/proverbs, finding out similarity between things, expressing the morals of stories, etc. On the other hand, it is easy for them to relate with tangibles or actual objects and events. While teaching follow direct and practical ways or illustrations rather than leaving them to your child's imagination.

## Whole to Part (General to Specific)

Always proceed to teach your child from the whole of a concept to its component parts. If you want to teach the concept of body parts, begin with the whole concept—face. Then proceed to parts of the face: eyes, ears, nose and mouth. Still later, proceed to specifics of the mouth like lips, teeth, tongue, etc.

## Recognize Differential Learning

No two children are alike. Therefore, be flexible in setting teaching objectives and planning or implementation of teaching techniques. Your approach should make allowances and accommodate differential rates of learning/performance that are frequently encountered in the real world of children.

## Avoiding Pressurized Learning

With contemporary life becoming increasingly fast paced, the expectations of most parents regarding their children are on the rise. Both parents and teachers stand guilty nowadays for placing a high premium on academic performance. Even disabled children are not spared, and are pressurized to perform beyond their capacities. While an optimum level of stimulation is appreciated, an excess can be emotionally shattering for parents as well as children. Too much comparison with other well-performing and normal peers, frequent fault finding, expressions of frustration over non-performance, etc., are symptoms of either your expectations being high or of your child's abilities being low. Evidently, there is a mismatch somewhere that needs to be rectified. In this connection, an appropriate degree of activity scheduling is advised.

## Overcoming the 'Laid-back' Attitude

While pressurized learning has a deleterious effect on the child, equally dangerous is the opposite extreme of a 'laid-back' attitude among parents. In fact, this tendency is encountered more frequently in parents of children with DDs. It may probably be the outcome of repeated failures/frustrations encountered while teaching their children. Every parent of such children runs this risk of developing an attitude of helplessness. It is a feeling that 'there is no way out of this'. Eventually, it leads to negative thinking, hopelessness, pessimism and a 'can't do' kind of attitude. Indeed, the road to teaching these children is not as smooth or rewarding as with normal children, but your right attitude has got a lot to do with what or how much your child can or will achieve in home training programmes.

## Unstructured Pace of Learning

As mentioned earlier, there are clear stages in the acquisition of various skill behaviours. Obviously, your child can be located at different steps or levels along these complicated interwoven matrix of observable skills. Unless you correctly identify the step/level at which your child is located along the continuum of skills it becomes questionable if the desired teaching objectives can ever be reached. Consequently, an inability of the child to acquire target behaviours is misinterpreted as his 'incapacity' or 'fault' rather than as miscalculated teaching procedures. Therefore, it is important to pace the learning/teaching for your child to his respective speed rather than push it forward at a prescribed momentum of an irrelevant curriculum.

## Faulty Communication of Intent and Purpose

The communicative relationship between a parent and a child is also an important dimension in the success of skill training programmes. Often, faulty networks in communication may exist within the framework of parent–child interactions, which could trigger serious problems of non-compliance during teaching in home settings. The child who is repeatedly referred to as being akin to some vagrant relative in the family will assiduously pick up such behavioural tendencies from a negative model. Sometimes, there is a disparity between intended communication and its actual interpretation by the child. For example, you may mean well in showing a particular child who is well behaved as a model for your child to emulate. However, in actuality, the use of your words could suggest a comparison that is resented by your child.

## Self-fulfilling Prophesy

Many teaching sessions between a parent and a child are jeopardized as a result of implicit and unwary comments unwittingly passed by adults. The mother who tells everyone about her child's dislike for a particular food is preparing the child to become fastidious about it. Similarly, a father who continues to say in front of his child that he is very 'reserved' and does not 'mix' with other children is indirectly teaching the child to behave in that particular way. Note that implicit and incidental learning is more deep-rooted and easily picked up by children than events or elements which are intentionally programmed to be taught to them.

## Deficient Opportunities for Learning

Most children with DDs are victims of under-stimulation and of inadequate opportunities for learning. While parents are busy providing stimulation for their non-disabled siblings, quite unintentionally, the disabled child may be well provided for, but inadequately stimulated. Many of their skill deficits are a result of not being given chances to do things on their own. A child is not given a knife to cut vegetables for fear that he may harm himself. Another teenage retarded girl is not allowed to go out shopping for fears of security. Rather, these children require ample supportive opportunities for learning.

## Desist from Looking for Quick Remedies

We have understood that mental retardation is a relatively permanent handicap and not a disease. It requires a patient, prolonged and planned training programme to identify and teach each deficit skill in the child. In as many parents wish, there is no short cut or quick remedy for rehabilitation of these persons. There are no drugs, surgeries or operations to do wonders and help the child achieve all the skills parents intend to teach. However, careful planning and meticulous implementation of skill training will yield positive results slowly but surely. Parents who have not reconciled themselves to this truth are seen seeking advice from one specialist after the other, or trying various non-scientific remedies endlessly. In the process quite a lot of money is wasted, and more than that, precious time is lost where training could have been effectively implemented.

## Avoid Physical or Corporal Punishments

In principle, almost everyone agrees on the demerits of physical punishment and advocate that it should not be used on young children. Even though extreme forms of corporal punishment on children like branding, spanking, hitting with a cane, undressing for public display, etc., are on the wane, in practice, subtle forms of physical abuse continue to take place in most homes or even preschools. The presence of a stick/scale on the table may be only a symbol of the teachers status and superiority, but it implicitly conveys wrong signals to the young learner. Small pinches, quick slaps, angry stares and disapproving frowns are commonly hurled at young children during many frustrating teaching situations by unwitting elders. Such negative experiences are bound to create an atmosphere not conducive to the child enjoying the learning activity. These incensed exchanges between a mother and a child may not be carried out intentionally. The affectionate mother wishes the child learn more effectively! She may even attempt to undo her punishments immediately with an overdose of affectionate hugging, kissing or defending her actions as justified for the good of the child. Even as one is justified for speaking in defense of children on the issue of punishments, at the same time, excess laxity in discipline is not what is being advocated here.

## Errors in Teaching and Learning

When training is undertaken in a systematic and scientific manner, children make gradual and steady progress in learning. Sometimes errors occur which then hinder the learning process. Errors show up as insufficient or incorrect responses to specific target instructions. Understand that errors can occur due to: (*a*) Insufficient training or learning in prerequisite skills to perform a given task. For example, the child who has not achieved an understanding of 'darkness'/'light' may not be ready to be taught to discriminate between 'day'/'night'. The child who does not know how to differentiate between 'more'/'less' is not prepared for the concept of 'greater than'/'lesser than'; (*b*) incorrect application of strategy in performance of an activity. For example, the rule that all plural forms will have an added 's' (such as, book-books, chair-chairs, etc.) may be misapplied to all plural forms (such as, box-boxs, sheep-sheeps, fish-fishs, etc.); and (*c*) non-compliance with the teaching or learning process.

---

**Table 2.23**
**Some Techniques/Tips for Error Correction**

- Identify and correct errors immediately. Avoid delay in error correction during teaching.
- Reward your child for non-occurrence of errors more than punishment for occurrence of errors. This procedure is called the differential rewards technique.
- Do not compel your child to perform a teaching activity when he or she is bored or tired. This will trigger more errors than learning.
- Do not teach any activity that your child perceives to be too simple or easy. Match the difficulty level of a teaching activity with the abilities of your child.
- Communicate the error to your child in clear, simple and brief terms.
- Avoid use of disparaging terms/words during communication of errors to your child.
- Use the error-correction procedures consistently.
- Avoid communicating errors of your child in front of others. The shame or discomfort associated with what others may think would disturb more than help him or her seek ways to correct them.

---

# CHAPTER 3

# PROBLEM-BEHAVIOUR MANAGEMENT PROGRAMMES

*Even as parents learn the basic principles for applying skill-behaviour training programmes in home settings, they must simultaneously be competent with strategies for problem-behaviour management too. Although there is no direct link between problem behaviours and disability, some children (whether disabled or otherwise) show a propensity towards manifesting such behaviours. Problem behaviours require intervention before any skill-training programme is started. This chapter outlines steps in the planning, development and implementation of problem-behaviour management programmes for children with DDs in home settings.*

Behaviours in children with DDs may be classified as skill behaviours and problem behaviours. *Skill behaviours* are positive behaviours that children have or need to be trained in for successful personal and social living. Examples of skill behaviours are 'indicates need to go for toilet', 'buttons own clothing', 'points to body parts', 'identifies the colour red', 'greets guests', 'recognizes values of coins', etc. The range of skill behaviours cover domains like motor activities, activities of daily living, language, reading, writing, managing money and time, domestic and community orientation, social and prevocational activities, leisure and play activities, etc. Obviously, all these categories of skill behaviours are not applicable to all ages/levels of DDs. Sensory-motor behaviours are more relevant for infants and toddlers. Community living and sex/hygiene related skills are more appropriate for older or higher functioning persons with disabilities.

Problem behaviours are negative behaviours. Not all children with DDs show problem behaviours. There is a wrong notion that disabilities inherently predispose children towards developing problem behaviours. This is not true. Nor are all so-called 'normal' children free from problem behaviours. There are and can be many children with DDs without problem behaviours. However, whenever behaviour problems are present, they constitute the most visible aspect among symptoms of DDs in children. Further, as a study shows, the most sought-after area of professional consultation by parents of disabled children is related to deficient 'communication skills' followed by 'problem behaviours in these children' (Peshawaria et al., 1990). The definition of problem behaviour encompasses five features listed in Table 3.1. Examples of problem behaviours are hitting others, screaming, stamping of feet, rolling on the floor, pulling objects from others, biting oneself, sucking of thumbs, hoarding unwanted things, banging of the head, not sitting in one place for a required length of time, etc. A comprehensive list of problem behaviours commonly reported in children with disabilities is listed in Part B of Behaviour Assessment Scales for Indian Children with Mental Retardation (BASIC-MR) (Peshawaria and Venkatesan, 1992a).

**Table 3.1**
**What is Problem Behaviour?**

Any or all behaviours in children that fulfil the following criteria are defined as problematic:

- Their presence causes great strain on parents and caregivers.
- They can be a potential source of danger for the children or people around them.
- Their behaviour may be inappropriate for their age or developmental level.
- Their behaviour may interfere with the teaching/learning of new skill behaviours or in the performance of already learned skill behaviours.
- They may be socially deviant (such as stealing, telling lies, etc.).
- Their presence interferes in the teaching/learning process of other children in group settings.

**Case Vignettes**

Radha is a five-year-old child with a mild developmental delay. Whenever she points to herself on being asked 'who is Radha?' by her mother, she is given a pat on her back. Radha likes being patted. She learns to point to herself in order to get patted by her mother.

Raju, another child with a mild developmental delay, falls on the floor and cries and shouts at the top of his voice. Raju likes chocolates. Raju's mother gives him chocolates to quiet him whenever he cries or shouts at home. Raju learns to cry or shout in order to get chocolates.

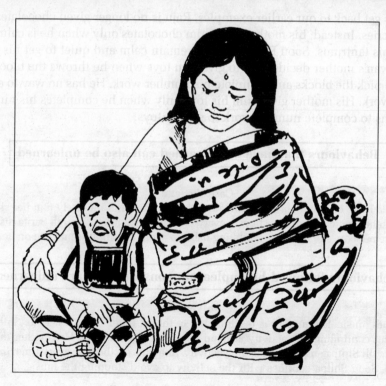

**Illustration 3.1  Case Vignette of Raju**

# How are Problem Behaviours Acquired?

From the above case vignettes, it is clear that behaviours in children are learned. Both skill behaviours and problem behaviours are also learnt. Radha learns to point to herself on hearing her name because her behaviour is followed each time by her mother's pat/praise. Raju learns to cry and throw a tantrum because his behaviour is followed each time by pleasant consequences, namely, chocolates.

| Behaviours followed by pleasant consequences are learned |
| --- |

### Case Vignette

Pawan is a six-year-old with a specific articulation disorder. Whenever his mother asks Pawan to count blocks, he throws them away. Pawan dislikes working with numbers. His mother gives him some toys to play with instead. So he learns to throw away the blocks in order to avoid the unpleasant consequences of working on something he dislikes. Thus, many behaviours are learnt by children to avoid unpleasant consequences.

| Behaviours are learnt in order to avoid unpleasant consequences |
| --- |

Now let us get back to our earlier examples. Raju is no longer given chocolates whenever he shouts or cries. Instead, his mother gives him chocolates only when he is calm and quiet. She ignores his tantrums. Soon Raju learns to remain calm and quiet to get his chocolates. Likewise, Pawan's mother decides not to give him toys when he throws the blocks. Instead, he is made to pick the blocks and complete his number work. He has no way to escape from the number work. His mother gives him his toys only when he completes his number work. Soon he learns to complete number work to get the toys.

| Behaviours that have been learned can also be unlearned |
| --- |

### Case Vignette

Sarita has a habit of biting her nails. She does this so often and intensely that her skin peels off. Her mother decides to dip her fingers every now and then into neem oil. Sarita dislikes the taste of neem. Soon, she unlearns her biting habit to avoid the unpleasant taste on her fingers.

| Behaviours followed by unpleasant consequences are unlearned |
| --- |

### Case Vignette

Shilpa loves music. Her mother is teaching her to thread beads using a needle. Shilpa has a habit of not continuing any activity at hand beyond a few minutes. Her mother decides to play music till Shilpa engages in beading activity. She puts off the tape every time Shilpa gets distracted. Soon Shilpa contines with the activity to avoid stopping the music.

| Behaviours followed by removal of pleasant consequences are unlearned |
| --- |

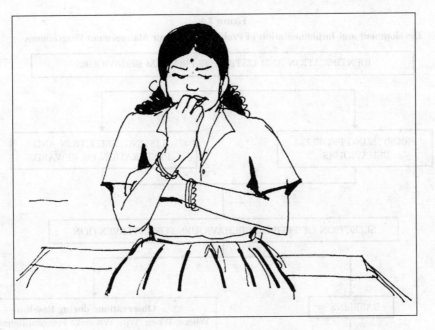

**Illustration 3.2  Case Vignette of Sarita**

To summarize, parents need to remember:

- Behaviours followed by pleasant consequences are learned.
- Behaviours are learnt to avoid unpleasant consequences.
- Behaviours learned can also be unlearned.
- Behaviours followed by unpleasant consequences are unlearned.
- Behaviours followed by removal of pleasant consequences are unlearned.

## Steps in Development and Implementation of Problem-behaviour Management Programmes

There are many techniques to teach children desirable skill behaviours or to unlearn undesirable problem behaviours. A formal and systematic programme for decreasing or eliminating problem behaviours in children with DDs must go hand-in-hand with any skill-training programme. A cascade presentation for development and implementation of problem-behaviour management programmes in children is given in Figure 3.1.

### 1. Identification of Problem Behaviours

The first step in undertaking any home-based behaviour remediation programme for management of problem behaviours is to make a detailed list of problem behaviours in your child. In case there are no problem behaviours present in your child, you may as well skip this entire exercise. It must be understood that recognition/identification of problem

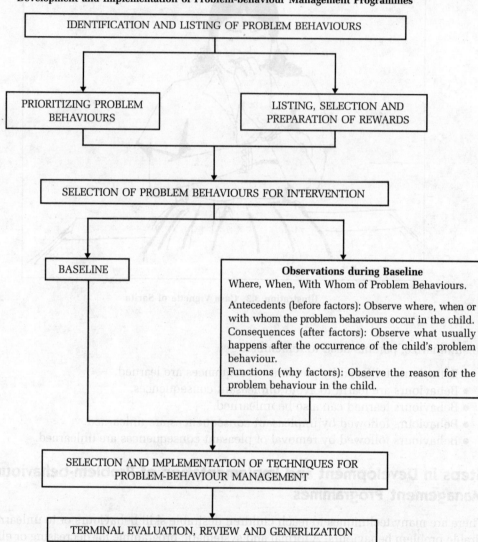

**Figure 3.1**
**Development and Implementation of Problem-behaviour Management Programmes**

IDENTIFICATION AND LISTING OF PROBLEM BEHAVIOURS

PRIORITIZING PROBLEM BEHAVIOURS

LISTING, SELECTION AND PREPARATION OF REWARDS

SELECTION OF PROBLEM BEHAVIOURS FOR INTERVENTION

BASELINE

**Observations during Baseline**
Where, When, With Whom of Problem Behaviours.

Antecedents (before factors): Observe where, when or with whom the problem behaviours occur in the child.
Consequences (after factors): Observe what usually happens after the occurrence of the child's problem behaviour.
Functions (why factors): Observe the reason for the problem behaviour in the child.

SELECTION AND IMPLEMENTATION OF TECHNIQUES FOR PROBLEM-BEHAVIOUR MANAGEMENT

TERMINAL EVALUATION, REVIEW AND GENERLIZATION

behaviours in a given child is a matter of interpersonal differences. A specific behaviour recognized as problematic by the child's mother may not be recognized as a problem at all by the father, grandfather or teacher. In a relevant study, it was found that teachers' perception and prioritizing of problem behaviours in a group of children with disabilities (Peshawaria et al., 1990) was entirely in variance from those of their parents. For example, whereas teachers reported not sitting in one place as the foremost problem behaviour in these children, parents rated not obeying commands as the major problem in the same group of children with disabilities.

Problem behaviours can be person- or situation-specific too. A problem behaviour which occurs in school may not occur at home, and vice versa.

---

**Table 3.2**

**Guidelines for Listing Behaviour Problems**

- Observe your child's problem behaviours in a variety of situations.
- Take note of reports of others about certain behaviour problems in your child.
- Use a ready-made and standardized problem-behaviour checklist, such as BASIC-MR (Peshawaria and Venkatesan, 1992a), to help identify and make an inventory of problem-behaviours in your child.
- In the beginning, the list of problem behaviours can necessarily be exhaustive, or even over-inclusive.

---

## 2. Statement of Problem Behaviours

After identification of problem behaviours in your child, the next step involves writing them down in clear observable and measurable terms. It is not appropriate to note that your child is 'naughty' or 'mischievous'. These terms may mean different things to different people. For some, 'mischievous' may mean that the child is restless, for others it may mean that the child messes the house or breaks things. Therefore, make the list of problem behaviours in an objective way. If you are using Part-B of BASIC-MR (Peshawaria and Venkatesan, 1992a) the problem behaviours are already listed therein in an observable and measurable way. This step of writing down problem behaviours in clear observable and measurable terms enables parents to be objective and clear about the specific targets they want their child to achieve. It avoids confusion and ambiguity regarding the proposed problem-behaviour management programme you are about to undertake in your home settings.

| Sample List of Problem Behaviours | |
|---|---|
| *Correct Statements* | *Incorrect Statements* |
| Ajay hits other | Arun gets angry |
| Rohan throws things | Bhavana is sad |
| Renuka bangs objects | |
| Sona bites nails | |
| Ajit pinches others | |

## 3. Selecting and Prioritizing Problem Behaviours

You may initially list many problem behaviours in your child. But, obviously, you cannot plan a management programme for all behaviours at the same time. Select only one or two problem behaviours for immediate remediation. Some guidelines for selecting and prioritizing problem behaviours are:

- Choose only one or two problem behaviours for remediation at a time.
- Choose problem behaviours that are easy to handle first. Later, as you gain confidence in handling some problem behaviours, you may select others for intervention.
- Choose problem behaviours that pose a danger to your child or to others in his surroundings.
- Choose problem behaviours that interfere in your day-to-day teaching activities.

- Choose problem behaviours for management only after ascertaining their frequency, duration and severity of occurrence.
- Choose problem behaviours whose remediation will enable the child to mingle with other children and enter the mainstream.

## 4. Identification of Rewards

Please go through the section on 'Rewards' in Chapter 2 for the meaning, procedures on identification, selection and use of rewards with your child. The same principles enunciated under skill-behaviour training programme hold good for problem-behaviour management programme too. Nevertheless, you must keep ready a list of identified rewards that work for your child so that they are readily dispensed when the occasion arises during the problem-behaviour management programme. The list of identified rewards for any given child must be what is actually pleasurable or liked by the child and not what you think is suitable.

## 5. Recording Baseline of Problem Behaviours

Just as baseline measures were suggested before undertaking of skill training programmes, it is necessary to measure your child's current severity of problem behaviours. A measure of problem behaviours in your child as they exist currently is referred to as recording baseline. There are many reasons to justify this exercise.

- It helps decide if a specific problem behaviour is indeed serious enough to warrant intervention.
- It helps you to know whether any changes have taken place at all in the problem behaviours of your child at the end of the problem-behaviour management programme.
- It is also an objective way of communicating to others that the implementation of the problem-behaviour management programme has been beneficial.
- In case of failures in any problem-behaviour management programme, the baseline measures will indicate the reasons thereof.

Baseline recording of currently observed problem behaviours in your child should be done for a minimum of three to four sessions. This can be done in two ways:

(a) **Event Recording** is a measure of how many times the selected problem behaviour occurs under specific conditions. Examples:
    Radha cries three times in an hour.
    Ravi spits six times in half-an-hour.
    Guru throws things six times in two hours.

(b) **Duration Recording** is a measure of how long the selected problem behaviour occurs under specific conditions. Examples:
    Vaibhav sucks his thumb for half-an-hour on average over a three-hour session.
    Ramu rocks his body on an average for 40 minutes in four one-hour sessions at home.

## 6. Functional Analysis of Problem Behaviours

In a related study, parents were asked to list what they considered were the possible causes of problem behaviours in their children. The list is reproduced with it's three headings, viz., child-centred, parent-centred and environmental-centred causes (Table 3.3). It was found that many parents locate the cause of problem behaviours in their children, or in their own parenting styles/attitudes, or in some limitations in their environment. While some of their perceptions on the causes of problem behaviours were apparently correct, others were erroneous (Venkatesan and Vepuri, 1993a). It is important for parents to self-correct faulty perceptions of causes since they can come in the way of effective home management of problem behaviours in their children. Before you continue any further, it is recommended that you take the twin questionnaires on parental knowledge and opinion on causes and management of problem-behaviours in children (Tables 3.4a and 3.4b).

Behaviour problems are not an exclusive property of children with DDs nor is it due to their primary condition per se. If this were true, then non-retarded children would never show any behaviour problems at all. Nor are all behaviour problems a result of some psychological illness. The notion that it is natural for children to misbehave is not tenable. Equally wrong is the expectation that behaviour problems in children get resolved on their own as they grow older. In fact, the presence of behaviour problems in older children is much more burdensome. Remember that as your child gets older and physically stronger, you grow comparatively weak! It will become a difficult proposition to counter his or her physical strength with your increased age. Therefore, planning/implementation of behaviour management programmes at the earliest is most advisable.

Although some parents invoke supernatural causes for problem behaviours in their children, the belief should not come in the way of taking concrete steps to remedy them. Expecting clearance of the influence of a supposedly evil star or the child's fate may delay the behavioural remediation programme. By that time, your child would have 'learned' a given problem behaviour so well that it will be more difficult for him or her to unlearn it in a short time. It is common to ascribe bad moods as the culprit for problem behaviours in children. The concept of 'mood' is subjective, non-observable and non-measurable. Is it 'bad mood' that

---

**Table 3.3**

**Parental Report on Perceived Causes of Problem Behaviours**

Child-centred Causes
- Primary condition of the child
- Psychological illness
- Psychological/physical trauma
- Natural for children to misbehave
- Mood fluctuations
- Deliberate and intentional actions
- Skill deficits
- Perceived discriminations by children
- Attention seeking
- Heredity

Parent-centred Causes
- Poor parenting
- Magico-religious influences

Environmental-centred Causes
- Boredom/under-stimulation
- Poor models

**Table 3.4a**

**Short Questionnaire on Knowledge and Opinion of Parents on Causes of Problem Behaviours in Children**

(Part A)

Attempt to answer these questions to check your knowledge and opinion on causes of problem behaviours in children. Answer all questions in terms of either 'Agree' or 'Disagree'.

|  | Agree | Disagree |
|---|---|---|
| 1. Behaviour problems in children and ill-tempered or badly behaved children are all a question of parents' fate. | ☐ | ☐ |
| 2. It is quite natural for children to misbehave. | ☐ | ☐ |
| 3. Children outgrow their behaviour problems as they grow older. | ☐ | ☐ |
| 4. The root cause of all behaviour problems in children lie in faulty or deficient parenting skills. | ☐ | ☐ |
| 5. Children with developmental disabilities show on an average a greater number of behaviour problems than do same aged non-disabled children. | ☐ | ☐ |
| 6. The developmental disability in a child may itself be a cause of behaviour problems. | ☐ | ☐ |
| 7. Behaviour problems in children may also depend on their moods. | ☐ | ☐ |
| 8. Bad moods can lead to problem behaviours even in well-behaved children. | ☐ | ☐ |
| 9. Behaviour problems in children may be inherited from parents who are temperamentally aggressive or who show ill-tempered behaviour themselves. | ☐ | ☐ |
| 10. Behaviour problems in children may be intentional or deliberate actions in order to trouble elders or parents. | ☐ | ☐ |
| 11. Children may sometimes behave badly under the negative influence of evil stars. | ☐ | ☐ |
| 12. The cause of behaviour problems cannot be always ascertained. Sometimes a child may misbehave for no reason at all. | ☐ | ☐ |

**Table 3.4b**

**Short Questionnaire on Knowledge and Opinion of Parents on Management of Problem Behaviours in Children**

(Part B)

Attempt to answer these questions to check your knowledge on management techniques for problem behaviours in children. Answer all questions either as 'Agree' or 'Disagree'.

|  | Agree | Disagree |
|---|---|---|
| 13. A good technique to overcome behaviour problems in children is to give into whatever they demand. | ☐ | ☐ |
| 14. When a child indulges in some problem behaviour, parents can try diverting his or her attention to something that is neutral. | ☐ | ☐ |
| 15. Spanking or hitting is the most powerful deterrent for severe behaviour problems in children. | ☐ | ☐ |
| 16. What spanking or hitting cannot achieve can be achieved in children with loving and friendly advice. | ☐ | ☐ |
| 17. Another technique to manage problem behaviours in children is to laugh away the child's misbehaviour as though it is a joke. Soon the child will learn to forget repeating such actions. | ☐ | ☐ |
| 18. When none of the techniques to manage a problem behaviour works, the best thing is to just wait for the child to mend his or her problematic ways. Sometimes patience and forbearance on the part of the parents has paid good dividends. | ☐ | ☐ |
| 19. At times, it is advisable for parents to show 'well-behaved' children as models for the problem child to learn or imitate good behaviour from. | ☐ | ☐ |
| 20. Sometimes parents can use techniques like cursing, shouting or reprimanding as means to instil fear in their child so that he or she does not repeat the misbehaviour again and again. | ☐ | ☐ |

'causes' a 'bad behaviour', or is it 'bad behaviour' that makes one ascribe it to a 'bad mood'? The concept of 'mood' is a circular logic that is at once a non-testable hypothesis! Thus, in 'questionnaire-part A' (Table 3.4a), all statements are *false*. If your answer to any question was 'true' (or 'agree'), you need to make amends and correct them before proceeding to implement a behaviour remediation programme. The best way to understand behaviour problems in your child is to analyse each problem behaviour by undertaking a procedure called behaviour/functional analysis. This involves splitting each behaviour into three components:

*(a)* **Antecedent (before) Aspects:** This refers to what happens immediately before the chosen problem behaviour. Observe your child during all those situations or at all those times when he manifests the chosen behaviour problem. Look out for when, where, with whom, why or how many times he shows the chosen problem behaviour.

*(b)* **Behaviour (during) Aspects:** This refers to what happens at the time of occurrence of the chosen problem behaviour. In other words, observe how many times or how long your child shows the given behaviour. You have already done this during your baseline recording.

*(c)* **Consequence (after) Aspects:** This refers to what happens after the occurrence of the chosen problem behaviour. How do people in the child's environment respond to the problem behaviour? What effect does the problem behaviour have on others around? How does your child benefit by indulging in the said problem behaviour? In the same study mentioned earlier, parents were asked to report what usually happened or what management strategies they used to cope with problem behaviours in their children (Venkatesan and Vepuri, 1993a). Their listed techniques are delineated in Table 3.5.

---

**Table 3.5**

**Parental Reports on Perceived Techniques for Management of Problem Behaviours**

1. Reward the problem behaviour.
2. Yield to the demands of the child.
3. Change environment in favour of the child.
4. Resign or wait for the child to mend his or her ways.
5. Divert the child's attention to something else.
6. Coax, cajole, love or advise.
7. Clueless about what to do.
8. Compare the child to other children who behave well.
9. Laugh away the child's misbehaviour as a joke.
10. Curse, shout, scold or reprimand the child.
11. Threaten the child verbally.
12. Physically abuse or hit the child.
13. Physically restrain or time out.

---

It is seen from Table 3.5 that parents show ambivalence ranging from extreme indulgence (yielding to all the demands of the child) to extreme punitiveness (physically abusing or hitting the child). There is also vacillation or indecision about not knowing 'what to do' when a problem behaviour occurs in the child. Therefore, it is necessary for parents to appreciate the 'real' factors that lead to problem behaviours in their children. Thus, in 'questionnaire-part

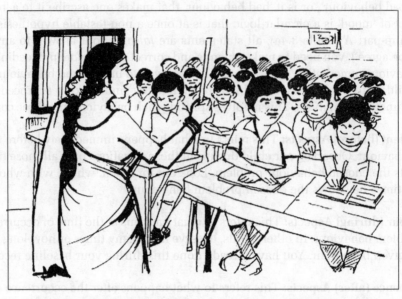

**Illustration 3.3  Classroom Scene: Teacher with a Stick**

B' (Table 3.4b), all the statements are *false*. If your answer to any question was 'true' (or 'agree'), you need to make amends again and correct them before proceeding to seriously implement the problem-behaviour remediation programme. From the psychological point of view, it is understood that there are five major factors to explain the occurrence of problem behaviours in children:

**(a) Attention:** All of us love to be at the centre of attention. Most problem behaviours in children may be attempts to attract attention from others. A child who bangs his head against a wall may be doing so to be picked up by his mother. Sometimes, there is negative attention-seeking behaviour. A child puts a slipper in his or her mouth just to receive a scolding or reprimand. It may seem surprising to hear that a child would want to receive a scolding. But, from the child's point of view, he or she is at least getting the attention of an elder who has otherwise ignored him or her. A child who keeps tugging at his mother's sari while she is busy talking to her friend in the market is attempting to seek negative attention. The child knows that out of the 10 times she is pestered, the mother would respond at least once by responding 'Hold on, dear! Let me finish talking to auntie.' Whenever you discover that a particular problem behaviour increases every time you pay attention to the child, then you may safely conclude that it is nothing but attention-seeking behaviour.

**(b) Self-stimulation:** It is aptly said that 'an empty mind is the devil's workshop'. This summarizes a factor that influences problem behaviours in children. When children do not have sufficient activity stimulation, they indulge in a variety of problem behaviours. Most self-stimulating behaviours of children are placed under this category. The severely handicapped child who has the pernicious habit of poking his eyes may be doing so only for the light flashes he experiences in his eyes with every poke. When children do not have a structured timetable of activities, they may resort to problem behaviours. Sometimes, self-stimulation appears when children find the given teaching activities not up to their expected level of stimulation. For example, you may think that you have kept your child engaged in beading activity. But, in the child's view, this activity is boring or monotonous. Hence, he indulges in problem behaviours. If the chosen target behaviour for a child is not age appropriate, difficulty level matched and/or graded to the needs of your child, the situation may manifest as a problem behaviour.

**(c) Skill Deficits:** Sometimes problem behaviours result from a skill deficit. The child who lacks pointing skills may bang the fridge every time he wants water. A child who does not have the social skills to ask for the ball during play with a verbal statement may snatch the ball from his peers. Another child who does not have the communication skills to ask for chocolates kept high up a shelf throws a tantrum. In these cases, the problem behaviour is a means of communicating the wishes or needs of the child.

**(d) Escape:** Some problem behaviours in children are a means of escape from the undesirable consequences of a particular behaviour. The child who throws colour pencils every time he is asked to colour diagrams is probably doing so because he does not like colouring work. The teenage girl who grumbles at her mother may be attempting to escape the burden of domestic work.

**(e) Tangible Rewards:** On many occasions, we inadvertently reward problem behaviours of a child. Of course, nobody does this intentionally. The mother who gives sweets to her crying child is probably teaching him to cry whenever he wants sweets. Whenever you notice a problem behaviour in your child, try and analyse which of the abovementioned factors could be precipitating it. Also, note that for any given problem behaviour there need not be only a single factor contributing to it.

Sometimes, a combination of these factors precipitates a given problem behaviour. A child may mouth a slipper initially because she does not discriminate between edibles and non-edibles (skill deficit factor). Later, the same behaviour may reflect an attention-seeking behaviour. The parent must be discerning enough to discover which factor or set of factors are at play in precipitation of a given problem behaviour. This is crucial because, as we shall presently see, the selection of management techniques for problem behaviours greatly depends on identified functions or factors that go into the problem behaviours.

## 7. Development and Implementation of Problem-behaviour Management Programmes

Many people have a wrong notion that techniques of behavioural management are based on specific problem behaviours. This is untrue. Rather, they are based on functions identified as underlying the targeted problem behaviours. Therefore, it is crucial that you correctly identify the utilitarian functions that benefit your child for presenting a problem behaviour. There are several techniques for management of behaviour problems in children. Note that selection of an appropriate technique for management of a problem behaviour depends on the specific functions underlying them.

**Changing the Antecedents (before Factors):** We have seen that some behaviour problems are precipitated by certain antecedents or before factors. Antecedent factors in problem behaviours can result even from faulty programme planning of skill behaviours. If you select teaching objectives that are too difficult/easy for a given child, it may lead to a teaching situation where he throws up some problem behaviours. We have seen how there can be a self-fulfilling prophecy with implicit expectations of parents getting unwittingly communicated to the child and resulting in problem behaviours. The skill training programme, schedule, materials used or even actual practice of teaching by the parent are all contributory antecedent factors in problem behaviours. Whenever you encounter an antecedent-controlled problem behaviour in your child, immediately try to discover the trigger that initiates it. Obstruct the occurrence of the trigger by changing their place, person, time or location.

> ### Case Vignettes
> Whenever Sunil settles down to study in his room, Anil interferes by snatching his books or talking with him. Their mother observes that the very act of Sunil carrying his books to his room is a sufficient trigger for his handicapped brother to go after him. In this example, there is a clear antecedent and trigger behind the occurrence of Anil's problem behaviour. Sunil is advised by his mother to lock his room before settling down to study.
>
> Ashwini is reported to throw away all the teaching material whenever her mother settles down to teach her. She finds it very difficult to commence any teaching activity. During baseline observation, it was seen that the trigger for her problem behaviour is an antecedent involving the act of spreading all the materials in front of her. The mother is recommended to take only one teaching material at a time for teaching Ashwini.

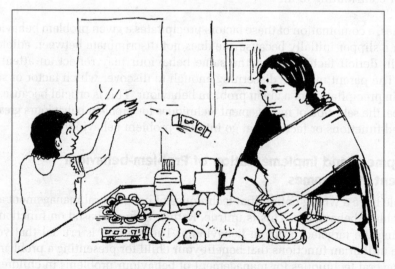

**Illustration 3.4  Case Vignette of Ashwini**

**Extinction/Ignoring:** This is the technique of first choice for use with all attention-seeking problem behaviours. When you identify that a particular problem behaviour is meant to seek the attention of others (either positive or negative), use extinction. Never pay any attention to the occurrence of such behaviours. Note that you should not provide even negative attention. Be consistent in the use of extinction procedures each and every time the attention-seeking problem behaviour occurs in your child. Never use extinction for behaviour problems that involve harming the self or others. Avoid giving lengthy sermons or lectures on how to behave well. These 'talks' or 'coaxing/cajoling' only tend to reward the child's problem behaviour. It is not so easy for parents who are accustomed to paying attention to every small peccadillo with a repeated 'No!', 'No!' to change overnight and stop paying negative attention towards the problem behaviour. Also, note that when you use extinction techniques, your child may initially show an increase of the attention-seeking problem behaviour. Nevertheless, you should be steadfast. Soon the child will realize that his behaviour is not paying the same dividends as it used to earlier.

---

**Case Vignette**

Jaya makes grunting noises every now and then in front of guests. The guests laugh at these peculiar sounds and this makes Jaya very happy. Her mother has understood that Jaya's noise making is an attention-seeking behaviour. She decides to implement extinction techniques. The guests as well as everyone at home are advised to refrain from laughing or paying any attention to her behaviour. Soon Jaya gives up making grunting noises.

---

**Time Out:** Some problem behaviours are so serious that mild techniques like extinction or changing of antecedents may not be sufficient. When the child pulls the hair of others and throws or breaks things, you cannot just wait for things to take their own course. At such times, a more active technique for use by parents is time out. Time out simply means removing your child from a rewarding situation or removing a rewarding situation from the child. No child would prefer to keep away from a rewarding experience for long. Therefore, time out can act as a powerful deterrent against violent, destructive or aggressive behaviour. There are many forms of time out. A simple procedure involves separating the child from the sphere of learning activity to the corner of the room for a specified amount of time. The child may be asked to sit heads down or with finger on lips and so on. However, this may not be sufficient for aggressive children. You may require shutting them away in a solitary place for a specified amount of time. We all would have undergone such forms of punishment during

---

**Case Vignette**

Rajiv was brought in with complaints of throwing things, hitting his sister, falling on the floor and crying for every small unfulfilled demand. Behaviour analysis revealed that his demands were met most of the time. A behavioural programme was initiated wherein his parents were instructed not to fulfil any demand if it was accompanied by his problem behaviours. Additionally, a time out technique was suggested if he became violent towards others. All the members in Rajiv's house were counselled to follow the techniques in mutual agreement. Though there was an initial increase in Rajiv's behaviour problems, thanks to the perseverance of his family in consistently using time out techniques all his problems subsided in two-weeks time.

childhood. Remember time out is not merely shutting the child in a room away from other friends or rewards. There are several rules and guidelines to be understood in the implementation of time out techniques in home settings (Table 3.6).

**Physical Restraint:** Violent and destructive behaviour in a child may not be amenable to mild forms of behaviour control. Then you have to resort to strong techniques like physical restraint. Physical restraint involves restricting the physical movements of your child for some time following the problem behaviour. Self-injurious behaviour, behaviour involving physical harm to others, hitting, slapping, etc., are amenable to physical restraint techniques. When you use this technique, make sure you vocalize a strong verbal command like 'No!' in

---

**Table 3.6**

**Guidelines for Implementation of Time Out**

- When your child indulges in a problem behaviour for which you have decided to use this technique, tell him clearly why he is going for time out. The child must know the reason for time out. Many parents assume that the child will understand on his or her own. This is not true. The time out could be for one thing and the child could have misunderstood it for something else.
- Be brief in your communication with your child. This is not the time for long lectures or sermons. Remember not to talk to your child when he or she is in the time out area.
- Place the child in the time out area only for a brief time. The child should not be shut in it for hours together. At the same time, he or she should not be set free even when continuing to cry, wail or shout in the time out area. The moment your child stops crying, you may release him or her. Again, you must clearly state the reason for the child being released.
- Sometimes children come out of the time out area and begin to shout or cry again, insisting why they were given time out. In such cases, there is no other option but to send the child into the time out area again with clear instructions that he or she can come out only when the misbehaviour ceases.
- Use of the time out technique will initially show a rise in problem behaviours, but do not get alarmed. This means you are using the technique correctly. After repeated pairing and use of time out each and every time with the problem behaviour, the child will learn that there is no other option than to comply.
- If you are using a time out room, make sure that it does not have any danger spots like exposed wires or other things that could harm your child. In a moment of emotional agitation, the isolated child may end up doing something rashly.
- Do not lose your temper while implementing the time out technique. Remain as calm as possible and provide matter-of-fact instructions before or after the time out.
- Do not pity, sympathize or discuss on time out experience after the child has come out of the room. The child should not be given any special treatment like being asked whether he or she wants some water or was frightened, etc.
- Time out is a more effective technique with children who are outgoing and who prefer being with people. Children who are withdrawn may actually enjoy time out. Be careful to judge the nature of your child accordingly before you plan to implement time out techniques.
- Be consistent in the use of time out. There is no point in using time out once in a while for targeting problem behaviours. The link between the behaviour problem and time out will not get established if this technique is used inconsistently.
- Note that time out only teaches your child what *not* to do. It does not teach what he or she should do. Therefore, use time out in combination with other behaviour management techniques.
- You will need to prepare yourself and other members in your family sufficiently before implementing time out techniques. Even if one member of the family sympathizes with the child or contravenes the rules of time out, the whole technique will fail.

accompaniment to the restraint you apply on your child. Apply physical restraint only for very brief time. No other physical contact should be made or verbal instructions given during implementation of physical restraint.

**Restitution/Over-correction:** The use of this technique not only decreases occurrence of problem behaviours in your child, but it also gives him a chance to learn alternate skill behaviours. If your child throws things all around the house, you must insist on him not only clearing the mess, but also clearing the entire area. You must be firm in implementation of restitution. There is no point in your giving instructions and the child ignoring them or you yourself clearing the mess later. This technique is useful only with children who can follow instructions. Never reward a child at the end of complying with over-correction procedures. This would mean that you are indirectly rewarding the child's problem behaviour. Do not nag, talk, lecture, sermonize or argue as you implement this technique.

**Conveying Displeasure:** This involves telling your child in clear and explicit terms whenever he indulges in problem behaviour. This technique is also known as reprimand. Reprimand is not merely telling your child how not to behave; it also means telling your child how he is expected to behave. Reprimands are implemented immediately following your child's problem behaviour. Be firm in your voice and looks when you use reprimands for specific problem behaviours. Remain calm and composed yourself when you use reprimands. Never reprimand a child in public. Do not keep reminding your child about reprimands given for past problem behaviours. Do not forget to convey pleasure for positive behaviours, even as you convey displeasure for negative behaviours.

**Differential Rewards:** Irrespective of the functions identified for a behaviour problem or choice of appropriate techniques for their management, you must always use the differential rewards technique. Differential rewards involve use of rewards for non-occurrence of problem behaviours. Many times we consider using strategies for reducing or eliminating problem behaviours in a child. But we seldom give thought to rewarding non-occurrence of problem behaviours. Just as it is crucial to use, say time out for assaulting behaviours, it is equally important to use rewards when your child does not manifest the same behaviours. It is apt for you to convey to the child that he or she has not shown a given problem behaviour for quite some time and hence deserves a reward. Differential rewards may be used for non-occurrence of behaviour problems during a specific period of time, or for a specified number of times. It can be simultaneously used for occurrence of alternate desirable behaviours, and so on.

**Activity Scheduling:** One of the reasons for occurrence of problem behaviours in children is lack of adequate stimulation. This is typical for most children with DDs. These children do not have enough opportunities to learn or show their limited skills. Even if they did, rewards are not sufficiently forthcoming. Therefore, appropriate scheduling of the daily timetable of activities is necessary to keep the child constructively engaged. Often when your child is engaged in training activities appropriate for his or her age/level, the scope for occurrence of problem behaviours reduces considerably.

**Case Vignette**

Varsha's therapy started with activities requiring her to point at various pet animals, vegetables, vehicles, fruits and household articles on picture cards. Every time the therapist settled down to teach her with picture cards, Varsha would look around and seem easily distracted. An intensive behavioural observation and assessment revealed that Varsha had long since acquired enough competence in picture reading. What she required were activities involving picture arrangement, sequencing pictures depicting her daily routines, arranging pictures on fables, etc. The faulty programming was immediately rectified. Her therapeutic activities were rescheduled, and her behaviour problems were no more observed during the therapy sessions.

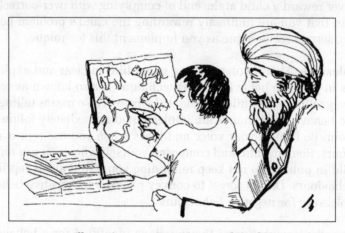

**Illustration 3.5  Case Vignette of Varsha**

**Contingency Contracting:** Contingency contracting is to be used with older children. This technique involves declaring, in clear and unambiguous terms, your intentions or expectations of a given behaviour in your child. The desired target behaviour should be identified and communicated clearly to the child. The conditions for their occurrence should also be specified. The consequences of showing or performing that behaviour should involve presentation of some reward/s to the child. For example, if *'Irfan keeps his belongings on his shelf everyday (and not throw them around the house) after returning from school continually for six days in a week, he would be rewarded with his favourite ice cream on Sunday.'* The main feature of contingency contracting is that there is an 'if' and 'then' clause attached to these contracts. The communicated sense is that 'if you do this, then you shall get that'. Obviously, it also implies that if the child does not do it he or she would not get the promised reinforcement too. There should be no concession or bargaining in this matter.

Many people misunderstand contingency contracting as an euphemism for bribing. Hence, they are against the use of this technique on moral/ethical grounds. This argument is untenable. In the first place, rewards are not bribes. Bribes are advantages or benefits offered to an individual even *before* performance of target behaviours. Further, there is a conscious understanding and prior agreement on the terms and conditions of mutual advantage between the giver and receiver. This is not the case in behavioural contracting. The rewards are never to be dispensed *before* the occurrence of the agreed target behaviours. The focus of this technique is not mutual benefit between parent and child, but rather the correction of a problem behaviour in the child.

**Token Economy:** Tokens are reward items with no inherent values. Yet they are desired since some value has been assigned to them. Example are stamps that are valuable to a philatelist, stars in a book, marks in a test, etc. Parents can even devise their own tokens like plastic coins or paper stars, which are then ascribed some tender value. The child can exchange, for example, every three such tokens for a chocolate or five tokens for a 10-minute television programme or 20 tokens for a weekend movie, and so on. Tokens can be used as immediate incentives for encouraging a desirable behaviour, or also as a fine for indulging in a problem behaviour.

> **Case Vignette**
>
> Remo has been soiling his clothes (psychogenic encopresis) at home or at school for the past six months. His mother would scold him for his lapses and end up washing his clothes for him. Upon advice of the therapist, his mother stopped doing his clothes for him. Additionally, token economy was undertaken. For each day that Remo did not soil his clothes, as per the therapists advice, he was given a 'star marking' on the calendar. For every five stars that he collected, Remo was given a toy car. There was also an understanding that for every time he soiled his clothes he would stand to lose two of the stars earned by him. Soon this twin system of reward and penalty made him give up the habit of soiling his clothes.

## 8. Terminal Evaluation

This involves terminal check-up to ascertain whether the targeted problem behaviours have indeed been reduced or eliminated completely consequent to the implementation of a behaviour management programme. Any failures, reasons thereof or difficulties are to be noted for future implications.

## Additional Guidelines for Management of Problem Behaviours in Home Settings

In Chapter 2, certain guidelines for training preschool children with DDs in home settings were given. While all of them hold relevance for caregivers even during management of problem behaviours, some more additional points (Venkatesan, 1993) are listed below:

### Disagreement among Caregivers

You have crossed an important hurdle in understanding why or how your child shows problem behaviours. You have learnt how to decide on appropriate techniques for their management. However, this does not really ensure success for your programme. The greatest challenge for parents is the implementation of a behaviour management programme. For example, a mother identifies that her child throws things to receive attention from others. She decides to use extinction. The test is the implementation of this strategy. The mother may be determined to implement the programme. But the support or agreement of other family members may not be forthcoming. Many homes share this predicament. One or two members in a family begin implementing the required or appropriate behavioural techniques. But a third person may be doing something that undermines the attempts of the first two persons. All members in a family must mutually agree on what constitutes the child's problem behaviours, what functions appear to be mediating them or which technique should be implemented for their successful remediation by all of them at all times. Also, discussions on what behaviour problems to target for remediation, how to implement the remediation programme, what is to be done for non-compliance, etc., should never take place in front of the child. Half- or ill-conceived behaviour remediation programmes rarely succeed in reducing or eliminating problem behaviours in children.

> **Case Vignette**
> Paresh was identified as having a problem behaviour of falling on the floor or throwing tantrums. Time out was decided upon to reduce this misbehaviour. His mother and father started using time out at home. However, Paresh's grandmother objected to this, insisting that the 'poor' child should not be 'tortured' thus. 'Look! He is a retarded child. Over and above that how can you have the heart to lock him in a room', she would say in front of the child. This gave Paresh support to continue with his problem behaviours.

## Disciplining is Akin to a Card Game

The business of disciplining your child is akin to a game of cards between two players. The child throws a card from his deck and you throw another. The child throws another again and you throw another again and so on. The child manifests a problem behaviour and you counter it with a technique. He musters up energies to present yet another serious problem behaviour and you should be ready with yet another stronger technique to counter it. This is called testing of limits. Usually a child may start with behaviour problems like shouting or shrieking at the top of his or her voice. If the parents do not respond, the child may proceed a step further to harm others, throw things or even harm himself or herself. It is as though the child is testing the parents' resilience to tolerate his or her behaviour problems. At some point or the other, owing to some weakness, when parents relent—that becomes the reinforcement for the problem behaviour to occur again and again.

> **Case Vignette**
> Anita began with the problem of nagging for small things again and again in the house. Her mother identified it as attention-seeking behaviour and decided to ignore it. Anita's nagging increased, but her mother continued to ignore it. Soon Anita showed another problem behaviour of shouting or crying to attract the attention of elders in the house. When even this did not fetch her rewards, she begins throwing things around and hitting others. The mother found it difficult to ignore these actions anymore.

This illustrates the various levels of problem behaviours in some children. You must be wary of such strategic levels in problem behaviours of children. You must also be adept in countering problem behaviours at each and every level. In other words, you must be prepared to implement counter-strategies for disciplining with every increase in the level of problem behaviour shown by the child. The ace must always be up your sleeve if you are to win the game of disciplining. Your firmness, determination, grit and resolve count for more than anything else in the interest of your child. All this does not also imply that the child with a problem behaviour is a strategist or schemer bent upon gaining advantages from elders in his or her surroundings. It is simply that the child has learned the benefit of indulging in some behaviours which have brought forth benefits rather than other behaviours which have not brought him or her similar advantages.

## Overcoming Guilt

Many parents suffer guilt in implementing behavioural remediation programmes on their children with DDs. Their rationale could be that the child is already handicapped. Over and above that, would one be justified in using strict measures on the child? Children do not naturally outgrow behaviour problems on their own. Rather, the problems worsen day by day. Remember the day is not far away when you lose your physical strength and your child gains more of it. Moreover, the use of all these behaviour techniques are not against your child; they are intended against your child's problem behaviours. Therefore, be assuaged that you are not against your child. You are only against the problem behaviours. Further, your child must unlearn them as quickly as possible if he or she is to make better adjustments in life. Your child may be demanding and getting things according to his or her whims at home from you. But children cannot always get their own way in this world. Sooner or later they must learn to adjust to other ways. That is the crux of behaviour management programmes.

## Effective Management Involves Correct Identification of Functions

It has been already highlighted that effective management of problem behaviours in children is based on correct identification of functions that those behaviour problems serve for a given child. Learn to deduce the correct functions/benefits behind your child's problem behaviour. Otherwise you run the risk of failing in implementation of behaviour management programmes in home settings. Broadly, the specific techniques for identified functions behind problem behaviours in children are summarized in Table 3.7. Problem behaviours mediated by factors related to skill deficits in your child need to be tackled by use of skill training techniques (refer to Chapter 2). These include shaping, chaining, modelling, prompting, etc. Problem behaviours allowing the child to escape the burden of performing certain activities are to be combated with physical compliance, contingency contracting, over-correction, etc. The problem behaviours acquired by a child owing to intended/unintended rewarding practices are to be unlearned by negating such rewards, implementation of appropriate reward-training techniques, use of differential rewards, etc. Self-stimulatory problem behaviours require activity-scheduling techniques involving control of antecedents, skill training, etc. Attention-seeking problem behaviours are best extinguished by use of ignoring, differential rewards and so on.

## Never Make False Inducements

Appeasement or attempting to do so is a common error on the part of many caregivers. A crying child is given a sweet, or is at least promised one. The kind or range of proffered promises

**Table 3.7**
**Sample List of Behavioural Techniques for Specific Identified Functions**

| Identified Functions | Suggested Behavioural Techniques |
|---|---|
| Skill deficits | Shaping, chaining, modelling, reward training, activity training, etc. |
| Escape | Physical compliance, contingency contracting, over correction, etc. |
| Reward | Reward training, differential rewards, etc. |
| Self-stimulation | Activity scheduling, antecedent controls, skill training, etc. |
| Attention | Extinction, differential rewards, etc. |

varies across parents and situations. Some promise an ice cream, others an evening out or just about anything without bothering about the implications of such false inducements. Parents justify such transient verbal appeasement as ordinary ploys used by everyone to placate disobedient children. The matter is not so simple. When a promise is made and then not honoured, there are serious long-term implications in the disciplining process with the child. The child begins to realize that elders merely promise or threaten but do not act. When a seriously frustrated mother threatens her son that he would be admitted into a hostel for his next misbehaviour, and then does not follow-up with the threat, she has exposed her own weakness in front of her child. He understands that his mother simply threatens but literally means nothing.

## Desist from Pleading, Begging or Nagging for Discipline

Sometimes caregivers wallow in nagging or begging for a disciplinary action from their child who has indulged in some misdemeanour. 'Now, you must say sorry!' some mothers are overheard pleading over and over again with a problem child. The child seems to care two hoots for such repeated pleas. Disciplining is no bargaining business between adults and children.

## Do not Care about what Others May Think

A common refrain heard from some parents is that they understand the implications of being inconsistent or lenient in the management of problem behaviours in their children, but are unable to implement behavioural techniques firmly. 'How can we ignore an attention-seeking problem behaviour when guests are around at home?' or 'How can we allow the child to cry and wail in a public place when everyone is looking at us?' Parents think that their prestige is at stake when their child misbehaves in front of strangers, and that they are left with no other option than to yield to the demands of their child. Some parents even tend to justify that being lenient 'once in a while' or giving in to the demands of their child 'at times' is not such a worse crime after all! In actuality, this defence is not tenable. A single act of giving in to the ways of the problem child even out of consistent refusals over 20 times can undo what they are seeking to achieve in the disciplining process of children with behaviour problems in home settings.

# SECTION B

## Development and Standardization of ACPC-DD

# CHAPTER 4

# ACTIVITY CHECKLIST FOR PRESCHOOL CHILDREN WITH DEVELOPMENTAL DISABILITIES

*This chapter provides an overview on assessment, elaborates assumptions underlying them and delineates various approaches and their limitations before introducing a newly developed and standardized 'Activity Checklist for Preschool Children with Developmental Disabilities' (ACPC-DD).*

At a general level, assessment involves forming impressions and making judgements about others. It carries an evaluative flavour while dealing with the whole person (Fiske and Pearson, 1970). At a technical level, psychological assessment is defined as the process of 'systematic collection, organization and interpretation of information about a person and his situations' (Sundberg and Taylor, 1962), to which is added, 'and the prediction of his behaviours in new situations' (Jones, 1970). The key element in assessment is 'the act of acquiring and analyzing information' (Hammill, 1987). The purpose of assessment varies from screening, identification, classification, placement and programming to certification and research (Thorndike and Hagen, 1977; Hawkins, 1979; Salvia and Ysseldyke, 1988; Venkatesan, 1991). Irrespective of their stated purpose, all assessments are based on certain assumptions which are vital to dealing with any heterogeneous population, such as children with developmental disabilities (DDs) (Table 4.1).

**Table 4.1**

**Assumptions Underlying Assessments of Children with DDs**

- Recognition of individual differences in measured phenomenon.
- Mandatory training is required for examiners before undertaking any assessment.
- Errors in assessment are inevitable and must be corrected wherever they occur.
- A developmental perspective is vital in interpretation of any assessment data.
- Assessment must be carried out in the context of cultural/experiential background of subjects.

## (a) Approaches to Assessment

There are various approaches to assessment depending upon the different types of decisions one has to make regarding children with DDs:

### Normative or Psychometric Approaches

This approach involves comparative evaluation of individual children with others who are supposedly like them (Witt et al., 1989). The procedure involves assessment of the typical performance of groups/sub-groups on a given variable as against a large collectively-representative sample of the general population known as 'norm/reference group'. The obtained raw scores are transformed into standard or transferred scores, such as percentiles, stanines, point scales, grade equivalents, etc., so as to enable interpretations and comparisons of individual scores to those of group scores. There are various types of normative assessments like intelligence tests, developmental schedules, adaptive behaviour scales, achievement tests, etc. Normative approaches to assessment have historically evolved in the context of the need to screen, identify, isolate and diagnose low-achieving children from others. To this effect, they help decide whether a given child is similar or different from other children of his age or class. They help labelling children as 'exceptional', 'special', 'sub-normal', etc.

The law and administration frequently require normative decisions to certify children for social/economic benefits (Mash and Terdall, 1976). Parents/caregivers also find it easy to understand normative comparisons of their children against age peers. Frequently, telling parents that their child is in the lower 5 per cent of the general population with respect to an ability makes more sense than providing individual-based performance scores (Singh, 1986). Normative research has yielded a vast body of technical/research data about behaviours in specific populations/sub-populations of children. This has in turn enabled large-scale policy decisions in several states. Although normative assessments lend themselves effectively to diagnostic decisions, they are only remotely connected to planning/programming of curriculum content for children with DDs (Becker and Engleman, 1976). They possess low ecological validity, i.e., individual examinees may not be required to perform their natural behaviours to perform successfully on these tests. Normative tests invoke artificially contrived situations and sample behaviours within specifically contrived situations. Such items have excellent diagnostic validity. But they are ineffective in guiding programme planning for children with DDs (Melin et al., 1983).

## Criterion-referenced Approaches

This approach follows recent trends in special education and rehabilitation medicine (Glaser, 1963). They are not concerned with the comparison of an individual with a norm or a standard. The point of reference is to an absolute standard within an individual rather than to a population norm (Glaser and Nitko, 1971; Popham, 1973). Criterion measures endeavour to answer specific questions, such as, does this child name the colour 'red' 8 out of 10 times successfully? In a sense, criterion approaches measure 'achievements', or learnt skills/activities in a child. The interest in this approach is to see whether the child can or cannot perform a given skill or activity (Kiernan, 1987). Since normative assessments place constraints on planning curriculum programmes for children, criterion approaches lend themselves directly to instructional needs of individual children. The term 'criterion' itself is derived from the experimental psychology of learning, wherein it refers to a 'critical level of mastery beyond which additional learning trials are not helpful'. Unlike normative measures, criterion measures do not sample behaviours, but measure actual behaviours per se. The purpose is not so much to compare individuals as to estimate individual skill levels/achievements in absolute terms, and to classify the individual as a master or non-master of a specific behaviour or skill.

## Functional/Behavioural Approaches

Children with DDs are frequently characterized by behaviours that can be viewed as the result of a powerful influence of environmental variables. The environmental influences may be highly variable and subject to unique interaction effects between the individual and his setting. Each behaviour is unique and bears a 'functional-utilitarian' relationship in its consequences for the individual. The proponents of this approach view behaviour as an objective, observable and measurable unit of action with precise functional consequences. Behaviour assessments involve measurement of purposeful behaviours in their interaction with the environment (Halpern and Fuhrer, 1984). Usually, the results of behaviour assessments are very specific and cannot be automatically generalized across different situations. The interpretation of results must be in the context of their intended uses, whether for providing compensation, eligibility in terms of services, development of individualized instructional programmes, charting prevalence or incidence of functional behaviour profiles, etc.

There is no single element that characterizes behavioural assessment (O'Leary, 1979). The earlier approaches to behaviour assessment involved specification of target behaviours intended for change, and their alteration through arrangement/rearrangement of environmental contingencies in a manner loosely conforming to operant conditioning principles (Skinner, 1953; Ullman and Krasner, 1965). The procedure involved obtaining the frequency, rate and duration of target behaviours by observing, recording and counting them. Later, with the concept of applied behaviour analysis (Baer et al., 1969), target behaviours as well as their antecedents and consequences came to be examined. In recent times, emphasis has been placed on viewing the individual as part of a larger network of interacting systems (Wahler, 1976), and on the vital role of cognition and emotions in mediating behaviour change (Karoly, 1981). These developments have changed the very quality of behaviour assessment from measurement of target behaviours to general problem-solving strategies based on ongoing functional analysis, and encompassing a greater range of independent/dependent variables (Venkatesan, 1994b; Venkatesan and Choudhury, 1995).

## Idiometric/Neuro-psychological Approaches

This approach draws its inspiration from the assessment of brain damaged persons in the field of neuro-psychology. The major theme is to identify specific areas of neuro-psychological functional assets/deficits in individuals or groups of individuals for inter-comparisons as well as for evolving tailor-made curriculum based on the unique structure, content or modes of cognitive operations (Venkatesan and Reddy, 1990, 1991, 1992).

In sum, no single approach to the assessment of children with DDs can suffice for enabling all types of decisions. Each approach measures behavioural phenomena at different levels and answers different questions to varying lengths and/or depths of the phenomena being studied. Ideally, a combination of all approaches to assessment at varying levels or depths is required to provide a complete and integrated view of the assessed individuals (Venkatesan, 1991). Wherein the intended objective is to assess children with DDs for enabling programme-planning decisions, it would be apt to combine use of a behavioural- and criterion-referenced functional approach rather than relying entirely upon normative evaluations for diagnostic decision making in these cases.

## (b) Guidelines for Test Construction

Some guidelines to be followed in the construction of standardized scales/tests for programme planning as recommended by various authorities are:

(i) The *purpose* of the test being developed and standardized *must be clearly stated*. For example, a stated purpose can be the development and standardization of an activity scale for children with DDs.

(ii) The *broad domains* of behaviour that are to be assessed *should be clearly specified*. The proposed domains in the scale must necessarily be relevant and exhaustive with regard to the target group. For example, the domains under activities for pre-school children with DDs can be sensory-motor, play, social, self-help, communication, preacademics, etc.

(iii) The *domains selected should be mutually exclusive*. If specific domains are overlapping, it may lead to ambiguity in scoring, administration and interpretation.

(iv) The *selected behavioural items should be arranged in a sequential order* of increasing difficulty. Item difficulty can be ascertained on the basis of their developmental perspective and/or task complexity. They are ascertained statistically by determining the relative frequency of percentage 'passes' in a given population. For example, the activity 'copies square' must be placed before the activity 'copies diamond' since the latter activity comes much later in children, both developmentally and owing to their task complexity.

(v) The *distance in terms of difficulty* between two or more items within a domain can also *depend on the extent of sensitivity* anticipated from the test. For example, if an assessment scale is required that is sensitive to three-month-changes in behaviours of pupils, the items must be more specific and easier to achieve within that period than if the tool is to be sensitive to annual changes for the same pupils or activities.

(vi) The performance objectives described in each item within each domain of the scale should be written in clear *observable and measurable terms*. The statements should specify the behaviour, conditions and deadline within which it has to be achieved or performed by the subject. For example, a well-written performance objective with all these properties could be 'When asked to give away two objects, Shyam gives away two objects from an array of five placed in front of him, at least four out of five times successfully by the end of a two-week teaching practice.'

(vii) Reliable procedures for *administration, scoring, recording of subject responses, use of test materials and interpretation of results* must be specified for every standardized assessment tool (Howell et al., 1979).

(viii) The sources from which items can be drawn for standardization and development of intervention-based assessment devices can be either 'objective-based' or 'instruction-based'. 'Objective-based' sources depend on what is to be taught to the subject. 'Instruction-based' sources depend on how it is taught to the subject (Mager, 1962).

The abovementioned guidelines for test construction and the standards for educational/psychological tests laid down by the American Psychological Association (APA, 1974) are rigidly adhered to during development and standardization of intervention-oriented assessment scales for children with DDs.

## (c) Critical Appraisal and Brief Overview of Behaviour Assessment Scales for Mentally Handicapped Persons in India

Over the past two decades, there has been a spurt in the development of behaviour assessment scales for mentally handicapped persons in India. This may appear to be a healthy and refreshing change from the earlier practise of unabashed and direct use of foreign scales. Earlier, behaviour assessment scales that were developed and standardized on a western population of mentally handicapped persons were directly adopted for their use with the Indian population, save for minor changes in content or form of expressions of certain test items. For example, an item such as 'eats with spoon/fork' was appropriately changed to 'eats with own hands', or another item like 'wears necktie' became 'wears *dhoti*', etc. Often, these changes were armchair adaptations, additions or adjustments to suit the needs of the individual investigator rather than being based on any empirical or ecological relevance or validation of such test items.

The 'Madras Developmental Programming System' (MDPS) (Jeyachandran and Vimala, 1983) could be credited as being probably the first 'Indianized' behaviour assessment scale for mentally handicapped persons, notwithstanding an allegation that it was initially a poor copy of 'The Minnesota Developmental Programming System' (Bock, 1975). While the scheme, structure and scoring procedures in both these scales showed striking similarities, the Indian version glaringly lacked details of standardization or validation. A comprehensively standardized and relatively robust assessment device was developed with the advent of 'Behaviour Assessment Scales for Indian Children with Mental Retardation' (BASIC-MR) (Peshawaria and Venkatesan, 1992a). This scale outscored the earlier available scales in terms of local application, reliability, validity or sensitivity estimates, glossary, objective administration, recording and scoring systems. In fact, it carried with it a separate training manual for teachers of children with mental retardation based on behavioural methods and techniques (Peshawaria and Venkatesan, 1992b). In recent times, there have been a host of behaviour assessment scales developed or standardized for use with persons having mental handicaps in our country (Table 4.2).

A cursory glance at available behaviour assessment scales for persons with mental handicaps in India shows serious shortcomings. Almost all scales are 'armchair' preparations seemingly developed for convenience of routine clinical use rather than with any professed research objective for standardized evaluation of children with DDs. There is diversity in the nature of these scales, their scoring systems, target age groups for whom they are intended and their utility in the context of rehabilitation for persons with DDs. Unfortunately, standardization details are unavailable for most of these scales, thereby questioning their reliability, validity and utility in our cultural context. The lure of informal classroom assessments is too easy and enticing for uninitiated special educators to scoff at formal, standardized and validated assessments for persons with handicaps.

But the peril of half-baked professionalism couched in such pseudo-scientific endeavours can prove to be a great disadvantage in the rehabilitation of persons with disabilities. Further, there is need for periodically revising/revalidating these scales at regular intervals to prevent obsolescence. There is also a need to develop/standardize several intervention-oriented behaviour assessment scales for specific target sub-groups, like children with severe/profound grades of DDs, those with multiple disabilities, preschool children with DDs, etc.

**Table 4.2**

**Summary of Existing Behaviour Assessment Scales for Individuals with DDs in India**

| No. | Title of Scale | Authors/Year | Age Range | Content Areas | Standardization Details |
|---|---|---|---|---|---|
| 1. | Madras Developmental Programming System (MDPS) | Jeyachandran and Vimala (2000) | 3–18 years | 360 items spread over 18 functional/behavioural domains | Assessment Kit available<br>Inter-rater agreement coefficient: 0.86<br>Test-retest reliability coefficient: 0.94<br>Cronbach's Alpha of Internal Consistency: 0.94<br>Face validity by expert opinion reported as high |
| 2. | Behaviour Assessment Scales for Indian Children with Mental Retardation (BASIC-MR) | Peshawaria and Venkatesan (1992a) | 3–18 years | Two parts, A and B. Part A has 280 items spread over seven skill behavioural domains. Part B has 75 items pertaining to problem behaviours | Materials kit, scoring and administration system, glossary, record booklets and supporting training manual are available<br>Inter-rater reliability coefficient: 0.835<br>Construct validity: 0.804 |
| 3. | NIMH Vocational Profile and Placement Checklist | Department of Vocational Training, NIMH, Secunderabad (1998) | 12 years+ | 97 items in two parts A and B. Part A has eight sections on generic skills. Part B has eight sections on Vocational Placement Rating Checklist | Standardization details not available |
| 4. | Assessment of Mentally Retarded Individuals for Grouping and Teaching | Department of Special Education, NIMH, Secunderabad (1995) | 3–14 years | 370 items spread across five checklists for levels like Pre-primary, Primary, Secondary, Pre-vocational and Vocational skills | Standardization details not available |
| 5. | Functional Assessment Tools | Research Division of the National Society of Equal Opportunities for Handicapped [NASEOH], Mumbai (1995) | 3–16 years | About 100 items spread across four levels like Pre-primary, Primary, Secondary and Pre-vocational | Standardization details not available |
| 6. | Curriculum Guidelines for Schools for Children with Mental Retardation | Jai Vakeel School for Children in need of Special Care, Mumbai (1991) | 0–12 years | About 100 items spread across four levels like Pre-nursery, Nursery, Primary, Pre-vocational and Vocational | Standardization details not available |

| | | | | |
|---|---|---|---|---|
| 7. | Vocational Training Checklist and Individualized Education Programme | Naviyothi Institute for the Mentally Retarded, New Delhi (1995) | 12 years+ | 88 items under six domains like basic work behaviour, personal, communication, functional academics, shopping skills nad domestic behaviour | Standardization details not available |
| 8. | Assessment of Vocational Readiness | Cornelius and Rukmini (1998) | 12 years+ | 50 items under eight domains assess vocational readiness | Standardization details not available |
| 9. | Workshop Observation Scale | BM Institute, Ahmedabad (1995) | 14 years+ | 63 items under six domains assess work skills of mentally handicapped adults | Standardization details not available |
| 10. | Student Profile Checklist | Tamanna Special School, New Delhi (1999) | 12 years+ | 275 items spread across 12 domains to be rated along a three-point descriptive scale | Standardization details not available |
| 11. | Proforma on Developmental Data and Academics | Shroff, Merchant, Adhikari and Kurani of Jai Vakeel School, Mumbai (1999) | 12 years+ | 392 items under nine domains to be rated along a five point rating scale | Standardization details not available |
| 12. | Assessment cum Curriculum Guidelines for Vocational Training School and Rehabilitation Centre | Kurani, Miranda, Shane and Shroff of Jai Vakeel School, Mumbai | 12 years+ | 93 items under six domains to be rated by vocational instructors | Standardization details not available |
| 13. | Problem Behaviour Checklist | Arya, Peshawaria, Naidu and Venkatesan (1990) | All ages | 75 items descriptive of commonly reported problem behaviours in persons with mental retardation | Standardization details not available |
| 14. | Upanayan: Preschool Programme for Children with Developmental Disabilities | Madhuram Narayan Centre for Early Intervention Services (1996) | Below 6 years | Five sets of 50 items, each covering activities like sensory, motor, communication, play and self-help skills | Training guidelines available on separate flash cards for individual items; standardization details not available |
| 15. | Portage Programme for Indian Preschool Children with Developmental Disabilities, Indian Adaptation | Kohli (1986) | Below 6 years | About 150 items covering activities like sensory, motor, communication, play and self-help skills | Standardization details not available |

**Table 4.3**
**Percentage of Passed Items in Sensory Domain**

| No. | Sensory Domain | 1M | 2M | 3M | 6M | 9M | 12M |
|---|---|---|---|---|---|---|---|
| 1. | Shows sucking responses to finger/nipple in mouth (1m) | 52.1 | | | | | |
| 2. | Turns head sideways when cheek is touched (1m) | 52.8 | | | | | |
| 3. | Pouts when lips are tapped slightly on surface (1m) | 53.4 | | | | | |
| 4. | Startles to loud sounds (1m) | 54.8 | | | | | |
| 5. | Blinks or closes eyes when tapped on forehead (1m) | 54.9 | | | | | |
| 6. | Closes fingers when touched in the palm (1m) | 55.1 | | | | | |
| 7. | Bends fingers forward when pressed above toe (1m) | 56.1 | | | | | |
| 8. | Bends fingers backward when pressed on toe (1m) | 58.1 | | | | | |
| 9. | Makes stepping movements when held upright (1m) | 58.5 | | | | | |
| 10. | Creeps forward when on stomach and pressed on toe (1m) | 58.9 | | | | | |
| 11. | Fixates eye on bright/colourful objects (1m) | 59.3 | | | | | |
| 12. | Turns head to source of light (1m) | 59.8 | | | | | |
| 13. | Turns head to source of sounds (1m) | 57.6 | | | | | |
| 14. | Gazes intently at own fingers (2m) | 42.5 | 62.5 | | | | |
| 15. | Visually tracks moving light (2m) | 41.5 | 75.4 | | | | |
| 16. | Notices dangling objects 6 to 8 inches away (2m) | 40.7 | 73.5 | | | | |
| 17. | Stops activity to listen to sounds of bell (2m) | 40.5 | 72.4 | | | | |
| 18. | Gazes intently at human face (3m) | | 28.4 | 56.4 | | | |
| 19. | Makes eye-to-eye contact consistently (3m) | | 29.4 | 54.3 | | | |
| 20. | Visually tracks moving objects/persons (3m) | | 24.5 | 53.7 | | | |
| 21. | Sits in protective cradle to swing (4m) | | | 25.7 | 68.7 | | |
| 22. | Regards own image in mirror (6m) | | | 23.5 | 63.7 | | |
| 23. | Splashes water when placed in tub (6m) | | | 22.7 | 61.7 | | |
| 24. | Laughs when tickled (7m) | | | | 45.7 | 83.4 | |
| 25. | Removes cloth from face that obscures vision (8m) | | | | 38.4 | 72.5 | |
| 26. | Reacts to different pleasant/unpleasant smells (8m) | | | | 32.5 | 71.6 | |
| 27. | Reacts to different tastes placed on tongue (8m) | | | | 28.4 | 69.5 | |
| 28. | Nods head in accompaniment to rhythm (8m) | | | | 24.9 | 68.9 | |
| 29. | Brings feet to mouth (8m) | | | | 24.2 | 62.6 | |
| 30. | Enjoys flexing of legs to tummy when lying on back (8m) | | | | 24.0 | 58.7 | |
| 31. | Enjoys peek-a-boo games/activities (9m) | | | | 22.7 | 57.6 | |
| 32. | Enjoys swirling motions when held at hip level (9m) | | | | 18.5 | 53.7 | |
| 33. | Shows hand preference (12m) | | | | | 8.9 | 56.8 |

| No. | Sensory Domain | 18M | 24M | 30M | 36M | 42M | 48M |
|---|---|---|---|---|---|---|---|
| 34. | Looks through viewing instruments (24m) | 23.3 | 69.7 | | | | |
| 35. | Listens through hearing devices (30m) | | 22.3 | 68.7 | | | |
| 36. | Sits on rocking horse (30m) | | 21.7 | 59.4 | | | |
| 37. | Discriminates between hot and cold (36m) | | | 24.6 | 68.2 | | |
| 38. | Sorts primary shapes (36m) | | | 22.6 | 64.8 | | |
| 39. | Identifies different tastes (36m) | | | 21.5 | 63.3 | | |
| 40. | Sorts size (36m) | | | 18.4 | 60.0 | | |
| 41. | Sorts by colours (36m) | | | 14.6 | 59.7 | | |
| 42. | Discriminates between rough and smooth on tactile rug (42m) | | | | 24.4 | 72.6 | |
| 43. | Identifies objects by touch (42m) | | | | 18.4 | 68.7 | |
| 44. | Stands in balance when in motion (48m) | | | | | 15.4 | 53.7 |
| 45. | Imitates breath holding: breathing in-out exercises (48m) | | | | | 12.9 | 52.9 |
| 46. | Walks in balance when blindfolded (48m) | | | | | 8.3 | 52.3 |
| 47. | Identifies shapes by touch (48m) | | | | | 7.9 | 51.9 |

| No. | Sensory Domain | 54M | 60M | 66M | 72M |
|---|---|---|---|---|---|
| 48. | Identifies objects from superimposed pictures (60m) | 18.3 | 50.9 | | |
| 49. | Identifies and seeks for correction of tastes in food (66m) | | 28.6 | 63.7 | |
| 50. | Discriminates between left and right (72m) | | | 22.7 | 56.9 |

**Note:** 'M' and 'm' both indicate months.
**Key for scoring:** NA: Not Applicable (0); TD: Totally Dependent (1); PP: Physical Prompt (2); VP: Verbal Prompt (3); C: Clueing (4); I: Independent (5)—see text page 113.

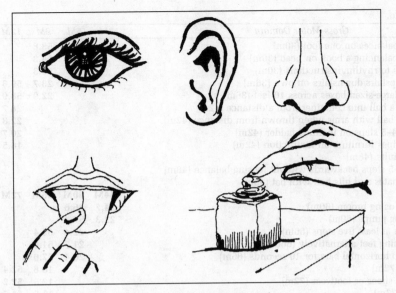

**Illustration 4.1  Sensory Domain**

| | | | | | | |
|---|---|---:|---:|---:|---:|---:|
| | **Table 4.4** | | | | | |
| | **Percentage of Passed Items in Gross Motor Domain** | | | | | |
| No. | Gross Motor Domain | 3M | 6M | 9M | 12M | 15M | 18M |
| 1. | Lifts head when lying on stomach by freeing nose off ground (3m) | 51.6 | | | | | |
| 2. | Bears weight on elbows when lying on stomach (6m) | 14.6 | 54.2 | | | | |
| 3. | Creeps forward when lying on stomach (6m) | | 38.4 | 74.5 | | | |
| 4. | Clasps both fists together and bangs at own mouth (6m) | | 32.4 | 73.3 | | | |
| 5. | Rolls over (stomach to back or vice versa) (6m) | | 31.5 | 66.4 | | | |
| 6. | Sits up with support (9m) | | 30.4 | 58.8 | | | |
| 7. | Pulls self to standing position from sitting/vice versa (9m) | | 18.7 | 57.2 | | | |
| 8. | Sits without support (9m) | | 16.5 | 54.8 | | | |
| 9. | Waves hands (9m) | | 15.4 | 53.9 | | | |
| 10. | Bounces when held by armpits in standing position (9m) | | 12.8 | 53.3 | | | |
| 11. | Crawls (12m) | | | 22.7 | 56.5 | | |
| 12. | Stands without support (12m) | | | 18.5 | 54.4 | | |
| 13. | Takes two/three independent steps before collapsing (12m) | | | 14.5 | 53.8 | | |
| 14. | Walks on own for at least 10 steps (15m) | | | | 33.7 | 63.8 | |
| 15. | Seats self without falling when placed on chair (15m) | | | | 31.4 | 59.3 | |
| 16. | Turns head down as though initiating a somersault (18m) | | | | | 22.3 | 56.8 |
| 17. | Climbs up a chair/other objects (18m) | | | | | 22.2 | 56.3 |
| 18. | Hurls ball in specified direction (18m) | | | | | 20.3 | 55.9 |

| No. | Gross Motor Domain | 18M | 24M | 30M | 36M | 42M | 48M |
|---|---|---:|---:|---:|---:|---:|---:|
| 19. | Jumps and lifts both feet off floor (24m) | 12.8 | 56.3 | | | | |
| 20. | Kicks ball in specified direction (24m) | 14.6 | 54.9 | | | | |
| 21. | Kneels on both feet (24m) | 12.6 | 53.8 | | | | |
| 22. | Runs (24m) | 12.4 | 52.9 | | | | |
| 23. | Squats (24m) | 13.6 | 51.9 | | | | |
| 24. | Jumps off one-feet height (24m) | 9.5 | 51.3 | | | | |
| 25. | Maintains balance when walking along a straight line (24m) | 2.4 | 50.6 | | | | |
| 26. | Sits cross-legged (24m) | 2.0 | 50.4 | | | | |

*Table 4.4 Contd.*

*Table 4.4 Contd.*

| No. | Gross Motor Domain | 3M | 6M | 9M | 12M | 15M | 18M |
|-----|--------------------|----|----|----|-----|-----|-----|
| 27. | Stands/balances on one foot (30m) | | 23.4 | 53.8 | | | |
| 28. | Stands balancing a book on head (30m) | | 22.4 | 54.3 | | | |
| 29. | Marches to rhythm/instructions (30m) | | 20.7 | 53.3 | | | |
| 30. | Walks upstairs/downstairs on own (36m) | | | 23.7 | 59.8 | | |
| 31. | Pushes large-sized boxes across 10 feet (36m) | | | 22.9 | 58.9 | | |
| 32. | Throws a ball into container from a distance (42m) | | | | 28.7 | 68.9 | |
| 33. | Catches ball with arms when thrown from distance (42m) | | | | 22.8 | 66.7 | |
| 34. | Climbs 4–5 steps on inclined ladder (42m) | | | | 20.7 | 63.7 | |
| 35. | Dusts/wipes furniture on instruction (42m) | | | | 18.5 | 60.4 | |
| 36. | Somersaults (48m) | | | | | 18.4 | 53.9 |
| 37. | Takes 4–5 steps backwards without loosing balance (48m) | | | | | 15.4 | 52.9 |
| 38. | Co-ordinates and hits ball with bat (48m) | | | | | 12.4 | 52.2 |

| No. | Gross Motor Domain | 54M | 60M | 66M | 72M |
|-----|--------------------|-----|-----|-----|-----|
| 39. | Sweeps using broom (60m) | 24.7 | 66.6 | | |
| 40. | Does frog jumps (60m) | 22.3 | 57.4 | | |
| 41. | Hops for at least five steps (66m) | | 22.4 | 63.4 | |
| 42. | Skips using feet alternatively (66m) | | 21.7 | 61.0 | |
| 43. | Clings to horizontal bars for 10 seconds (66m) | | 20.4 | 57.6 | |
| 44. | Swims (72m) | | | 16.8 | 52.4 |
| 45. | Polishes shoes or footwear (72m) | | | 12.5 | 52.2 |
| 46. | Skates (72m) | | | 11.5 | 51.7 |
| 47. | Bounces ball for at least 10 counts (72m) | | | 10.8 | 51.4 |
| 48. | Does sack walk (72m) | | | 9.7 | 50.4 |
| 49. | Aims and hits target 5 feet away using medium-sized ball (72m) | | | 7.5 | 50.3 |
| 50. | Clips nails (72m) | | | 7.1 | 50.2 |

**Note:** 'M' and 'm' both indicate months.

**Key for scoring:** NA: Not Applicable (0); TD: Totally Dependent (1); PP: Physical Prompt (2); VP: Verbal Prompt (3); C: Clueing (4); I: Independent (5)—see text page 113.

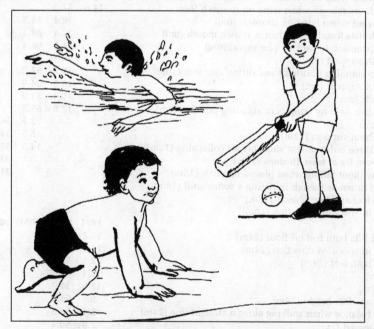

**Illustration 4.2  Sample of Gross Motor Activities**

**Table 4.5**
**Percentage of Passed Items in Fine Motor Domain**

| No. | Fine Motor Domain | 3M | 6M | 9M | 12M | 15M | 18M |
|---|---|---|---|---|---|---|---|
| 1. | Retains cube in one hand (cylindrical grasp) (6m) | 23.4 | 58.7 | | | | |
| 2. | Shows spherical grasp (6m) | 21.5 | 57.6 | | | | |
| 3. | Shows hook grasp (6m) | 18.9 | 55.6 | | | | |
| 4. | Shows opponent grasp (6m) | 17.5 | 54.3 | | | | |
| 5. | Reaches for small objects dangled in front (6m) | 26.7 | 54.7 | | | | |
| 6. | Fisting eliminated in both hands (6m) | 16.7 | 52.1 | | | | |
| 7. | Shows palmar grasp (6m) | 5.7 | 51.8 | | | | |
| 8. | Reaches out with extended arms when lying on back (9m) | | 38.7 | 54.7 | | | |
| 9. | Grasps/holds rattle or toy in palm (9m) | | 28.9 | 56.7 | | | |
| 10. | Reaches or pats image in mirror (9m) | | 18.4 | 54.9 | | | |
| 11. | Shows pincer grasp (12m) | | | 48.7 | 58.9 | | |
| 12. | Pulls away thin string or thread from face (12m) | | | 28.7 | 56.9 | | |
| 13. | Turns pages of a book singly (12m) | | | 32.8 | 56.7 | | |
| 14. | Stoops to pick up a toy (15m) | | | | 32.8 | 53.8 | |
| 15. | Puts small objects into a container (18m) | | | | | 47.5 | 56.8 |
| 16. | Inverts small bottle to obtain pea/raisin inside (18m) | | | | | 44.7 | 55.8 |

| No. | Fine Motor Domain | 18M | 24M | 30M | 36M | 42M | 48M |
|---|---|---|---|---|---|---|---|
| 17. | Opens/closes door latch (24m) | 33.7 | 63.7 | | | | |
| 18. | Unscrews lid of a bottle (30m) | | 28.7 | 75.6 | | | |
| 19. | Drops peas/pins into narrow-mouthed containers (30m) | | 23.7 | 72.5 | | | |
| 20. | Shows tripod grasp on writing instruments (30m) | | 22.7 | 64.7 | | | |
| 21. | Beads on wire/knitting needle (30m) | | 21.5 | 63.4 | | | |
| 22. | Inserts money into piggy bank (36m) | | | 42.1 | 62.1 | | |
| 23. | Inserts key into lock hole (36m) | | | 38.4 | 58.4 | | |
| 24. | Zips/unzips clothing or leather goods (36m) | | | 32.4 | 56.4 | | |
| 25. | Folds handkerchief into four (36m) | | | 31.4 | 52.7 | | |
| 26. | Screws lids of bottles (42m) | | | | 21.7 | 56.7 | |
| 27. | Walks on toes (42m) | | | | 12.7 | 53.8 | |
| 28. | Puts rubber band to strap small objects (42m) | | | | 9.4 | 52.7 | |
| 29. | Opens/closes safety pins (42m) | | | | 7.5 | 51.7 | |
| 30. | Cube assembly: level one: stacks tower at 4 cubes (42m) | | | | 6.5 | 51.3 | |
| 31. | Uses eraser (42m) | | | | 5.7 | 50.9 | |
| 32. | Pastes paper using gum/glue (42m) | | | | 5.3 | 50.4 | |
| 33. | Cube assembly: level two: makes bridges at 5 cubes (48m) | | | | | 12.6 | 56.4 |
| 34. | Uses cellotape (48m) | | | | | 10.5 | 55.4 |
| 35. | Folds paper and inserts it into envelope (48m) | | | | | 10.1 | 53.4 |

| No. | Fine Motor Domain | 54M | 60M | 66M | 72M |
|---|---|---|---|---|---|
| 36. | Uses pencil sharpener (54m) | 64.7 | | | |
| 37. | Cube assembly: level three: makes train at 5 cubes (60m) | 12.8 | 62.7 | | |
| 38. | Ties tags, slip knots or shoe laces (60m) | 10.4 | 60.7 | | |
| 39. | Operates lock and key to bolt a door (66m) | | 43.5 | 68.9 | |
| 40. | Tears paper folded into four (66m) | | 38.5 | 59.8 | |
| 41. | Fills water through a funnel into bottle (66m) | | 37.2 | 56.4 | |
| 42. | Strikes a match stick (66m) | | 32.1 | 55.4 | |
| 43. | Uses office instruments like staples, puncher and pins (66m) | | 28.4 | 53.4 | |
| 44. | Co-ordinates well in pebble play (66m) | | 25.8 | 53.8 | |
| 45. | Cube assembly: level four: makes stairs at 10 cubes (72m) | | | 24.7 | 62.4 |
| 46. | Threads a medium-sized needle (72m) | | | 43.5 | 68.9 |
| 47. | Cuts primary shapes using a pair of scissors (72m) | | | 40.4 | 64.1 |
| 48. | Wrings wet cloth by squeezing (72m) | | | 39.7 | 62.9 |
| 49. | Shows lateral grasp by holding 6 to 7 playing cards (72m) | | | 32.7 | 58.4 |
| 50. | Makes simple geometric designs on floor (*rangoli*) (72m) | | | 28.5 | 53.7 |

**Note:** 'M' and 'm' both indicate months.
**Key for scoring:** NA: Not Applicable (0); TD: Totally Dependent (1); PP: Physical Prompt (2); VP: Verbal Prompt (3); C: Clueing (4); I: Independent (5)—see text page 113.

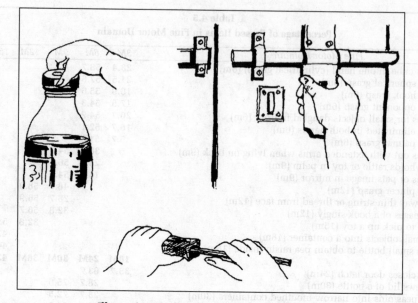

**Illustration 4.3  Sample of Fine Motor Activities**

**Table 4.6**
**Percentage of Passed Items in Communication Domain**

| No. | Communication Domain | 3M | 6M | 9M | 12M | 15M | 18M |
|---|---|---|---|---|---|---|---|
| 1. | Is calmed by voice (3m) | 78.9 | | | | | |
| 2. | Localizes source of sounds (3m) | 68.7 | | | | | |
| 3. | Responds to own name (6m) | 38.7 | 82.4 | | | | |
| 4. | Imitates babbling sounds made by others (6m) | | 42.8 | 69.7 | | | |
| 5. | Shows/extends an object when asked (9m) | | 40.8 | 66.6 | | | |
| 6. | Responds to own name by pointing to self (9m) | | 385 | 64.5 | | | |
| 7. | Comprehends simple commands that call for action (12m) | | | 42.5 | 73.5 | | |
| 8. | Uses more than three words with consistency (12m) | | | 40.2 | 72.2 | | |
| 9. | Asks for objects with vocalizing/pointing gestures (15m) | | | | 38.7 | 63.8 | |
| 10. | Vocalizes sounds of animals/machinery on request (18m) | | | | | 42.5 | 64.2 |

| No. | Communication Domain | 18M | 24M | 30M | 36M | 42M | 48M |
|---|---|---|---|---|---|---|---|
| 11. | Understands 'all gone' (24m) | 33.7 | 63.7 | | | | |
| 12. | Comprehends upto five functional commands (24m) | 30.5 | 58.4 | | | | |
| 13. | Uses 'mine' constantly (24m) | 29.5 | 56.4 | | | | |
| 14. | Understands 'yes–no' (24m) | 27.9 | 55.5 | | | | |
| 15. | Points to five body parts (30m) | | 37.5 | 58.5 | | | |
| 16. | Understands/uses 'up–down' (30m) | | 35.4 | 56.4 | | | |
| 17. | Understands/uses 'here–there' (30m) | | 32.8 | 53.8 | | | |
| 18. | Answers to 'what is this?' with the name of object (30m) | | 32.7 | 52.7 | | | |
| 19. | Names household articles (30m) | | 28.7 | 50.8 | | | |
| 20. | Says names of family members (36m) | | | 30.2 | 54.7 | | |
| 21. | Repeats rhymes/songs (36m) | | | 25.7 | 53.4 | | |
| 22. | Points to different objects when they are named (36m) | | | 22.5 | 52.8 | | |
| 23. | Differentiates between 'front–back' (36m) | | | 20.4 | 52.4 | | |

*Table 4.6 Contd.*

*Table 4.6 Contd.*

| No. | Communication Domain | 3M | 6M | 9M | 12M | 15M | 18M |
|---|---|---|---|---|---|---|---|
| 24. | Differentiates between 'inside–outside' (36m) | | | | 18.4 | 51.8 | |
| 25. | Differentiates between 'fast–slow' (36m) | | | | 15.4 | 51.4 | |
| 26. | Differentiates between 'young–old' (42m) | | | | | 24.7 | 62.4 |
| 27. | Differentiates between 'on–off' (42m) | | | | | 22.7 | 57.9 |
| 28. | Differentiates between 'good–bad' (42m) | | | | | 20.7 | 56.4 |
| 29. | Differentiates between 'near–far' (42m) | | | | | 18.4 | 53.7 |
| 30. | Tells name of five friends (42m) | | | | | 15.4 | 52.8 |
| 31. | Mimics/uses gestures during verbal communication (42m) | | | | | 12.4 | 51.7 |
| 32. | Carries out series of two related commands (42m) | | | | | 11.1 | 51.1 |
| 33. | Understands 'now–sooner–later' (48m) | | | | | 32.4 | 62.4 |
| 34. | Tells own age (48m) | | | | | 30.4 | 59.4 |
| 35. | Talks about/sings TV commercial from memory (48m) | | | | | 28.4 | 57.4 |
| 36. | Uses small courtesies like 'thank you/please' (48m) | | | | | 26.4 | 55.4 |
| 37. | Explains use of familiar objects (48m) | | | | | 25.4 | 53.4 |

| No. | Communication Domain | 54M | 60M | 66M | 72M |
|---|---|---|---|---|---|
| 38. | Relates make-believe tales (54m) | 64.7 | | | |
| 39. | Converses on telephone (60m) | 38.4 | 63.7 | | |
| 40. | Tells name of own town/village (60m) | 28.7 | 62.4 | | |
| 41. | Listens to a story (60m) | 25.7 | 60.7 | | |
| 42. | Describes action in pictures (60m) | 24.7 | 57.8 | | |
| 43. | Follows three-step instructions sequentially (60m) | 23.4 | 55.5 | | |
| 44. | Defines words in terms of use (60m) | 22.4 | 53.7 | | |
| 45. | Tells name of state and country (66m) | | | 22.4 | 62.2 |
| 46. | Gives account of short videos/TV serials (66m) | | | 20.4 | 58.4 |
| 47. | Names occupation of parents (66m) | | | 18.6 | 55.5 |
| 48. | Makes an independent query from a stranger (66m) | | | 17.6 | 53.4 |
| 49. | Points/identifies/names five different fingers (66m) | | | 15.7 | 52.7 |
| 50. | Gives complete residential address (72m) | | | 32.5 | 57.3 |

**Note:** 'M' and 'm' both indicate months.

**Key for scoring:** NA: Not Applicable (0); TD: Totally Dependent (1); PP: Physical Prompt (2); VP: Verbal Prompt (3); C: Clueing (4); I: Independent (5)—see text page 113.

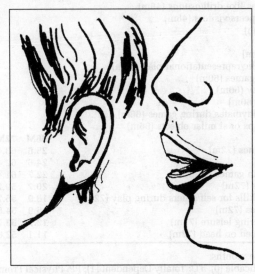

**Illustration 4.4  Sample of Communication**

**Table 4.7**
**Percentage of Passed Items in Play Domain**

| No. | Play Domain | 6M | 9M | 12M | 18M | 24M | 30M |
|---|---|---|---|---|---|---|---|
| 1. | Bangs objects (9m) | 35.8 | 62.8 | | | | |
| 2. | Plays pat-a-cake (9m) | 28.5 | 55.7 | | | | |
| 3. | Rolls ball in specific direction from sitting position (9m) | 25.4 | 53.7 | | | | |
| 4. | Regards play with shadows (12m) | | 42.5 | 64.8 | | | |
| 5. | Skips using feet alternatively (24 m) | | | | 28.6 | 56.5 | |
| 6. | Sings or dances alone to music (30m) | | | | | 28.4 | 56.6 |
| 7. | Transfers liquids from cup/glass unassisted (30m) | | | | | 26.5 | 55.5 |
| 8. | Strings four medium-sized beads (30m) | | | | | 24.5 | 54.6 |
| 9. | Imitates peers in preschool/kindergarten play (30m) | | | | | 23.3 | 52.4 |

| No. | Play Domain | 30M | 36M | 42M | 48M | 54M | 60M |
|---|---|---|---|---|---|---|---|
| 10. | Awaits turn during kindergarten play (36m) | 25.6 | 63.4 | | | | |
| 11. | Blows bubbles from soapy water (36m) | 24.3 | 62.2 | | | | |
| 12. | Slides down garden equipment (36m) | 22.2 | 61.0 | | | | |
| 13. | Swings in sitting position (36m) | 18.4 | 59.4 | | | | |
| 14. | Aims and hits large-sized objects using ball (36m) | 17.7 | 57.6 | | | | |
| 15. | Hits targets in carom board games (36m) | 15.5 | 56.3 | | | | |
| 16. | Paints impressions using different objects (42m) | | 35.7 | 58.6 | | | |
| 17. | Plays with toys/dolls (42m) | | 31.2 | 55.6 | | | |
| 18. | Blows a whistle (42m) | | 24.6 | 54.3 | | | |
| 19. | Squeezes through a tunnel (42m) | | 22.4 | 53.6 | | | |
| 20. | Scolds playmates, dolls or animals in games (42m) | | 18.6 | 52.3 | | | |
| 21. | Claps hands/sings/dances in group song (42m) | | 15.6 | 51.8 | | | |
| 22. | Imitates animals—crawls on fours, makes noises/actions (42m) | | 14.3 | 51.6 | | | |
| 23. | Shares belongings with others (42m) | | 12.3 | 51.4 | | | |
| 24. | Acts out nursery rhymes (48m) | | | 24.6 | 63.7 | | |
| 25. | Shows imitative play involving rudimentary rules with peers (48m) | | | 22.2 | 61.4 | | |
| 26. | Plays leap-frog games (48m) | | | 20.4 | 59.6 | | |
| 27. | Swings in standing position by propelling self (48m) | | | 18.6 | 57.7 | | |
| 28. | Recognizes and sets aside own play materials (48m) | | | 16.4 | 56.7 | | |
| 29. | Strikes coins on carom games to drop into pocket (48m) | | | 15.6 | 55.7 | | |
| 30. | Constructs geometrical shapes using match sticks (48m) | | | 13.7 | 54.5 | | |
| 31. | Clings onto a bar for 30 seconds (48m) | | | 12.7 | 53.4 | | |
| 32. | Imitates motor sequences like drill/*asanas* (48m) | | | 11.7 | 52.8 | | |
| 33. | Shows or offers toys to peers/visitors (48m) | | | 10.9 | 51.7 | | |
| 34. | Runs to catch peers (48m) | | | 9.7 | 51.5 | | |
| 35. | Rides a tricycle (54m) | | | | 26.7 | 63.4 | |
| 36. | Plays hide-and-seek (60m) | | | | | 24.7 | 63.3 |
| 37. | Gets involved in symbolic/representational play (60m) | | | | | 22.3 | 61.4 |
| 38. | Plays 'freeze' or 'statue' games (60m) | | | | | 20.4 | 59.8 |
| 39. | Keeps secrets during play (60m) | | | | | 18.6 | 57.7 |
| 40. | Plays blind man's bluff (60m) | | | | | 17.6 | 53.7 |
| 41. | Guides younger peers/playmates during games (66m) | | | | | 15.6 | 52.8 |
| 42. | Makes paper planes, ships or si milar objects (66m) | | | | | 12.8 | 51.8 |

| No. | Play Domain | 66M | 72M | | | | |
|---|---|---|---|---|---|---|---|
| 43. | Aims well in marble games (72m) | 25.6 | 63.4 | | | | |
| 44. | Plays hopscotch (72m) | 24.6 | 62.4 | | | | |
| 45. | Detects breach of rules in games (72m) | 22.7 | 61.4 | | | | |
| 46. | Plays simple card games (72m) | 20.7 | 59.7 | | | | |
| 47. | Maintains basic safety skills for self/others during play (72m) | 18.9 | 55.7 | | | | |
| 48. | Cheats playfully in games (72m) | 15.9 | 54.6 | | | | |
| 49. | Engages self usefully during leisure (72m) | 12.7 | 53.7 | | | | |
| 50. | Walks with books balanced on head (72m) | 11.1 | 52.6 | | | | |

**Note:** 'M' and 'm' both indicate months.
**Key for scoring:** NA: Not Applicable (0); TD: Totally Dependent (1); PP: Physical Prompt (2); VP: Verbal Prompt (3); C: Clueing (4); I: Independent (5)—see text page 113.

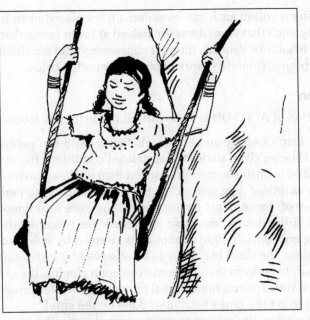

**Illustration 4.5  Sample of Play**

# (d) Activity Checklist for Preschool Children with Developmental Disabilities

The Activity Checklist for Preschool Children with Developmental Disabilities (ACPC-DD) is designed to elicit systematic and comprehensive information on current skill-behaviour levels in preschool children with developmental disabilities. The checklist is suitable for infants, toddlers and preschool children between 0 to 72 months. A teacher may find it useful even when working with non-handicapped/normal preschool children. The checklist serves as a curriculum guide, and has been field-tested primarily on a sample of preschool children with developmental handicaps (even though it includes a sub-sample of children with age-appropriate developmental levels too). Information on standardization aspects, such as reliability, validity and sensitivity of the tool, is reported below.

## Structure

The ACPC-DD consists of 400 items distributed evenly across eight behavioural domains that are relevant to the daily activities of infants, toddlers and preschool children affected with DDs, and between 0 to 72 months old. The specific number of items under each domain is intentionally fixed at 50. Special care has been taken to write every activity/item in clearly observable and measurable terms to avoid confusion in understanding or interpreting them. A separate glossary (Chapter 5) explains the content, relevance and broad implications of each item in detail for the specific conditions under which they are assessed for any given child with handicaps. An activity assistance guide (AAG) (Chapter 5) is added for this checklist to facilitate a systematic training programme for infants, toddlers and preschool children with DDs. The items within each age-level/domain are placed in an increasing order of difficulty/complexity, such that more items are passed at lower levels than at higher levels in the ACPC-DD. The reliability, validity, internal consistency and sensitivity of items included in this scale have been assiduously worked out and reported below.

## Administration

The administration of ACPC-DD is to be carried out using the following guidelines:

- Read each item carefully and assess whether a child can perform it or not upon clear instructions being given under the stipulated conditions therein.
- In case a child is unable to perform a given item on direct instruction (or is too young to do so), the examiner may give a clue to enable the child to perform the said item and mark it thereof. Some items for infants may require examiners to contrive situations under which the desired response is elicited. For example, the item 'creeps forward when lying on stomach' (9m) cannot be performed by infants on instruction from examiner. Rather, the child may have to be observed by instigating the given response.
- If a child fails to perform the said item even upon clueing, the examiner may proceed to give detailed verbal instructions (verbal prompting), or later, physical assistance (physical prompting) to get the target behaviour done by the child.
- As far as possible, the examiner must proceed upon the premise that the child can perform the said item (and not vice versa) before establishing the correct degree/level of assistance required to perform the given item.
- Examiners are advised to rely on direct observation of the child for evaluating each item, rather than on parent/caregiver interviews or reports about the child's performance.
- It is not mandatory to complete the assessment of a given child on APCC-DD within a single session. More often than not, a series of observations spread over a few sessions may be required depending on the co-operation elicited from the child. In cases where information cannot be obtained by direct observation of the child, information obtained from parents/caregivers may be supplemented. Examiners must expend all efforts to elicit the best performance of the child on each item in the checklist.
- The examiner must also make a clear distinction between a child *not knowing* to perform a given item and a child *not wanting* to perform the given item. An unwillingness on the part of a child to perform an item should not be misconstrued as the child's inability to perform the item. In such instances, a final decision on the said item should be postponed till such times as the child becomes more co-operative.
- Examiners need not administer all items for children assessed on ACPC-DD. The test administration may be stopped after five consecutive failures in a domain by a child within any age range. Usually, a child who has failed on five consecutive items within a domain is unlikely to pass any item later. Therefore, the rest of the items in that domain need not be administered and they can be scored zero. Administration should always start at a lower-age level and then proceed to higher-age levels until the child shows five consecutive failures within a specific domain (sample specimen enclosed as Annexure 1).
- Use recording sheets for scoring each child being assessed on ACPC-DD and preserve them carefully for later comparisons. The use of a separate record booklet for each child is recommended.

- Examiners must prepare a set of materials required for testing children on ACPC-DD in advance. The items must bear the same specifications as mentioned under 'Materials Required for Assessment/Training on ACPC-DD'.

## Scoring

Each child with developmental disabilities will show different levels of performance on every item on ACPC-DD. The six possible levels of performance under which each item can be scored for a given child are as follows:

**Level One: Independent (Score 5):** If a child performs a given test item without any physical or verbal assistance it is marked as independent and given a score of five. For example, on verbal instruction by the examiner to 'sit cross-legged' (Activity # 26 under Gross Motor Domain), if the child sits cross-legged without any aid or assistance he is given a score of five.

**Level Two: Clueing (Score 4):** If a child performs a given item with only some kind of verbal hints (like 'close', 'open', 'pull', 'push', etc.) and/or non-verbal clues (like pointing, shaking, nodding, etc.), it is marked as clueing and given a score of four. For example, on verbal instruction by the examiner to 'sit cross-legged' (Activity # 26 under Gross Motor Domain), if the child sits cross-legged with minimal aid or assistance, he is given a score of four.

**Level Three: Verbal Prompt (Score 3):** If a child performs a given test item with verbal assistance it is marked as a verbal prompt and given a score of three. For example, on verbal instruction by the examiner to 'sit down … fold your legs at the left knee … fold your legs at the right knee … now together' and so on (Activity # 26 under Gross Motor Domain), the child is given a score of three.

**Level Four: Physical Prompt (Score 2):** If a child performs a given test item with physical assistance it is scored as two. For example, the teacher may hold the child's legs, bring them together and fold them. Then the child is given a score of two.

**Level Five: Totally Dependent (Score 1):** If a child cannot perform a given test item despite physical/verbal assistance or clueing, it is marked as totally dependent and scored as one. For example, in spite of physical assistance, the child is unable to cross his or her legs; this fetches a score of one.

**Level Six: Not Applicable (Score 0):** In rare instances, some children may not be able to perform a listed behaviour at all owing to sensory or physical handicaps. For example, a visually-impaired child will never be able to 'read pictures'. Or a child with lower limb diplegia may not be able to walk. In such instances, it is marked as 'not applicable' and given a score of zero.

On each item of ACPC-DD, a preschool child may receive a score ranging from 0 to 5 depending on the level of assistance required to perform that given item. Enter the appropriate score obtained by the child for each item in respective columns under the profile sheet. The maximum score possible for a child on the whole ACPC-DD is $250 \times 8 = 2,000$ marks.

Add up individual raw scores in all the items secured by the child within a domain and display it on the profile sheet. The ACPC-DD is to be administered on every child on three occasions, viz., (i) *Baseline or Initial Assessment* (carried out before starting the teaching or training programme); (ii) *Quarterly Assessment* (carried out after every three months or quarter. There may be two quarterly assessments after the baseline assessment, designated as first and second assessments on the specimen scoring sheet); and (iii) *Terminal/Annual Assessment* (carried out at the end of the training programme at least once in a year, and designated as the third quarter assessment on the specimen scoring sheet).

## Discrepancies in Scores

In actual use of ACPC-DD, children may sometimes get high scores on difficult items and receive low scores on easier items. This tendency is known as intra-test scatter or intra-domain scatter. There are many reasons for the occurrence of this phenomenon (Table 4.8).

**Table 4.8**

**Reasons for Intra-test or Inter-domain Scatter on ACPC-DD**

- The child may have had a specific opportunity to learn only the difficult items listed in the checklist.
- There could be an error in test administration that requires rechecking.
- The child might have refused to perform a skill behaviour that he or she knows how to perform. In such a case, errors in scoring need to be corrected.
- The discrepancies may be due to the masking effects of associated handicaps in the child.

## (e) Development and Standardization

The ACPC-DD was tried out on a sample of 289 preschool children with various categories of DDs. The chronological ages of the sample children ranged from 2 to 120 months (Mean age: 34.82 months; Standard deviation [SD]: 18.21). The sample included 146 boys (Mean age: 35.42 months; SD: 17.24) and 143 girls (Mean age: 36.47 months; SD: 18.01). The various types of diagnostic categories covered in this sample included children with developmental delays (number of samples [N]: 94), specific receptive/expressive speech and language delays (N: 47), specific motor-co-ordination disorders (N: 12), conduct/emotional disorders (N: 29), pervasive developmental disorders (N: 18) and others (N: 89) respectively. All cases were taken from General Services of the National Institute for Mentally Handicapped (under Ministry of Social Justice and Empowerment, Government of India), Regional Centre, Patna; and/or from the Psycho-Diagnostics' Unit at the All India Institute of Speech and Hearing (under Ministry of Health and Family Welfare, Government of India), Mysore, between the years 1998 and 2001. Each case was assessed individually by a team of rehabilitation professionals including clinical psychologists, pediatricians, speech therapists, audiologists, occupational therapists, special educators, physiotherapists, etc., before affixing a final diagnostic label on the given child with a DD.

Following diagnostic assessment of an infant, toddler or preschool child with one or other type of DDs, the ACPC-DD was administered individually as per the guidelines given under administration or scoring for this checklist. All recordings for individual children were carried out and maintained scrupulously by the investigating clinical psychologist. The specific steps used in development and standardization of ACPC-DD are presented under the following heads:

**Formation of Item Pool:** The ACPC-DD is designed to elicit systematic information on current skill-behaviour levels in infants, toddlers and preschool children with DDs. The checklist construction started with the formation of a comprehensive item pool of activities related to children below the age of 72 months. A comprehensive list of 432 items was initially selected from various sources in literature for assessment of children, available intervention programmes for preschoolers in the country and abroad, etc. The specific domains included under ACPC-DD are:

- Sensory
- Gross motor
- Fine motor
- Communication
- Play
- Preacademics
- Self help
- Cognitive

During initial formation of the item pool, care was taken to see that the test items were placed in a hierarchical order of increasing performance difficulty according to the chronological ages of the children. The easier and lower chronologically-aged test items were placed at the beginning of the checklist, and the more difficult and higher-aged items were placed towards the end of the checklist. Further, it was seen that domains included in the checklist were both exhaustive and mutually exclusive. This was to eliminate repetition of test items within a domain as well as between domains. More emphasis was given on selection of items that were functional. For example, an item 'folds paper into four' seen in some developmental checklists was changed to 'folds handkerchief into four' in order to make it more functional. It was also seen whether the selected test items were 'teachable'. 'Teachability' or 'trainability' of test items is an important prerequisite for an intervention programme. Unless the assessed items can be taught to the child, the assessment becomes meaningless.

**Initial Field Try-out of Selected Items:** The initial field try-out for ACPC-DD was carried out on a select sample of 30 preschool children with developmental handicaps. The initial field trial resulted in additions, deletions, modification and restructuring of the checklist. The major type of changes that were incorporated as a result of this experience during the initial field try-out are as follows:

1. Deletions: Several test items which were non-functional, age-inappropriate or repetitive were deleted from the initial item pool. Thus, there were 28 items deleted at the end of this exercise.
2. Additions: Several test items missed out by oversight, or by intention after their use, was realized at the end of the pilot try-out. Thus, eight items and one domain (preacademics) were added at the end of this exercise.
3. Teachability: Test items were restructured or modified for want of their teachability. It was felt to be important to keep the items that showed the possibility of their being targeted for teaching. Thus, there were eight items added at the end of this exercise.
4. Behavioural Terminology: The test items were worded in observable and measurable (behavioural) terms. There is greater scope for ambiguity if an item is written as referring

to teaching 'colour concept' or 'toilet training' than specifically to, say, 'points to colour red in three-choice presentations over three out of four trials'.

5. Glossary: It is not always possible to specify the content of an item clearly in a single phrase. Often there was a need to clarify the content of an item. Therefore, a glossary was prepared to elaborate, among other things, the materials to be used to test given item/s, the number of trials or time limits required to pass that item, the procedure for assessing given items, etc.

6. Materials Kit: To avoid ambiguity or subjectivity on the part of examiners, it was found necessary to specify the nature or magnitude of materials used to assess items in the checklist. For example, the item 'jumps off a height' requires a specification on the height, the item 'throws a ball' requires specification on the size of ball to be used, 'threads a needle' requires a specification on size of the needle, etc.

**Revision of Items in Checklist:** The final form of ACPC-DD developed at the end of field trials comprised of 400 test items distributed along eight major domains. The maximum possible score for a child on any given item is five, and on the whole checklist is 2,000. This number was maintained to facilitate ease of computation and analysis of data.

**Final Field Try-out of Checklist:** The final field try-out of ACPC-DD was carried out on a sample of 289 infants, toddlers and preschool children with DDs. This sample included cases with developmental delays (DDs)(N: 94), specific speech delays (SSDs) (N: 47), specific motor-co-ordination disorder (MCDs) (N: 12), pervasive developmental disorder (PDDs) (N: 18), and others (N: 89). The 'others' category included cases of fluency disorders, eating/ elimination disorders, emotional/conduct disorders, etc. (Table 4.9).

**Table 4.9**

**Distribution of Sample Characteristics for Final Try-out**

| No. | Diagnosis | Age Levels in Years (where 'x' indicates age) | | | | | | | Total |
|---|---|---|---|---|---|---|---|---|---|
| | | $x \leq 1$ | $1 < x \leq 2$ | $2 < x \leq 3$ | $3 < x \leq 4$ | $4 < x \leq 5$ | $5 < x \leq 6$ | $6+$ | |
| 1. | DDs | 34 | 22 | 14 | 9 | 8 | 7 | – | 94 |
| 2. | SSDs | – | 7 | 21 | 16 | 3 | – | – | 47 |
| 3. | MCDs | – | 4 | 6 | 2 | – | – | – | 12 |
| 4. | PDDs | – | – | 7 | 8 | 3 | – | – | 18 |
| 5. | Others | – | – | – | 9 | 22 | 26 | 32 | 89 |
| | Total | 34 | 33 | 48 | 44 | 36 | 33 | 32 | 289 |

1. Baseline Scores: The target sample (N: 289) was individually administered ACPC-DD and the scores recorded on separate profile sheets. The baseline scores for 289 pre-school age children with DDs showed relatively high internal consistency in scores between, as well as within, domains. The highest mean scores were recorded for sensory domain (Mean: 351.69; SD: 63.4), and the lowest mean scores were recorded for preacademics (Mean: 203.49; SD: 32.4) (Table 4.10).

### Table 4.10
#### Baseline Scores on ACPC-DD for Subjects during Final Try-out

| Domain | Mean (N: 289) | SD |
|---|---|---|
| Sensory | 351.69 | 63.4 |
| Gross motor | 327.57 | 58.7 |
| Fine motor | 308.47 | 49.3 |
| Communication | 278.54 | 45.6 |
| Play | 257.46 | 43.3 |
| Self help | 227.07 | 41.5 |
| Cognitive | 214.74 | 38.7 |
| Preacademics | 203.49 | 32.4 |

2. Developmental Age Allocations for Test Items: The distribution of percentage passes under each domain of ACPC-DD shows a gradual decrease from the first to fiftieth items. Tables 4.3 through 4.7 and Tables 4.12 through 4.14 present the per cent passes for each item under the given domains. The traditional criteria of 50 per cent of children passing any given test item to determine its developmental age allocation along the age scale has been maintained (Kamat, 1967; Venkatesan, 2002a, 2002b) in development and standardization of this checklist. However, the primary focus of this percentage count was *not* to identify normative markers for items in this checklist. This cannot be so since ACPC-DD is not a normative developmental schedule. Rather, the intention was to determine the developmental hierarchy of test items in order to arrange them in sequence of complexity for planning individualized training programmes for children with DDs. The age-wise distribution of the number of items on ACPC-DD shows a relative preponderance for the >3 to ≤4 years age range (95 items; 23.8 per cent) followed by 77 items in the >5 to ≤6 years age range (19.2 per cent) and so on (Table 4.11). While the distribution of the number of test items for various domains is identical, the disparity at different clusters of age levels within preschool years is inevitable owing to differences in the domain of activities at various age levels of child development.

### Table 4.11
#### Age-wise Distribution of Number of Items on ACPC-DD

| No. | Domain | Age Levels in Years (where 'x' indicates age) | | | | | | Total |
|---|---|---|---|---|---|---|---|---|
| | | x≤1 | 1<x≤2 | 2<x≤3 | 3<x≤4 | 4<x≤5 | 5<x≤6 | |
| 1. | Sensory | 33 | 1 | 7 | 6 | 1 | 2 | 50 |
| 2. | Gross motor | 13 | 13 | 5 | 7 | 2 | 10 | 50 |
| 3. | Fine motor | 13 | 4 | 8 | 10 | 3 | 12 | 50 |
| 4. | Communication | 8 | 6 | 11 | 12 | 7 | 6 | 50 |
| 5. | Play | 4 | 1 | 10 | 19 | 6 | 10 | 50 |
| 6. | Self help | 4 | 10 | 12 | 13 | 2 | 9 | 50 |
| 7. | Cognitive | – | 3 | 12 | 10 | 11 | 14 | 50 |
| 8. | Preacademics | – | 3 | 6 | 18 | 9 | 14 | 50 |
| | Total | 75 | 41 | 71 | 95 | 41 | 77 | 400 |
| | Percentage | 18.8 | 10.2 | 17.8 | 23.8 | 10.2 | 19.2 | 100 |

**Establishment of 'Goodness' of Checklist**: The statistical measures adopted for establishing instrument goodness in this study were reliability, validity and sensitivity checks for ACPC-DD.

Reliability: Three types of reliability checks were undertaken for ACPC-DD:

1. Inter-rater reliability for ACPC-DD was attempted by taking a sub-sample of 46 children with DDs and subjecting them to repeat testing by two independent raters. The first rater was a clinical psychologist (author), and the second was post-graduate in psychology with an additional diploma in special education (mental retardation). The second rater was given a week's training on administration and scoring of ACPC-DD using didactic discussions, individual case work, personal tutoring and feedback. The Coefficient of Agreement (CAg) on 46 cases carried out independently by the two examiners came to 0.957.

2. Internal consistency estimate on Kuder Richardson-20 (KR-20) was calculated for ACPC-DD by carrying out a series of inter-item correlation within and/or between domains. The KR-20 for overall instrument and for each of the domains under ACPC-DD are given under Table 4.15. These findings confirm the homogeneity of the test item pool and the hierarchy of developmental age allocations made for items included in this checklist.

3. Two-week test-retest reliability coefficient for total scores measured on ACPC-DD within the same sample (N: 46) measured to be 0.943 (Standard error or measurement: 1.321; p: >0.05; Statistically not significant).

**Table 4.12**

**Percentage of Passed Items in Self-help Domain**

| No. | Self-help Domain | 9M | 12M | 15M | 18M | 21M | 24M |
|---|---|---|---|---|---|---|---|
| | **Eating** | | | | | | |
| 1. | Controls drooling (12m) | 26.4 | 64.7 | | | | |
| 2. | Discriminates between edibles/non-edibles (12m) | 20.2 | 56.7 | | | | |
| 3. | Drinks from cup/glass (12m) | 15.4 | 55.5 | | | | |
| 4. | Chews solid foods like biscuits (15m) | | 22.5 | 56.7 | | | |
| 5. | Finger feeds solid food (18m) | | | 18.4 | 53.7 | | |
| 6. | Unwraps candies (24m) | | | | | 18.5 | 56.3 |
| 7. | Eats seeded fruits with sufficient mastery (24m) | | | | | 22.5 | 55.8 |
| | | **24M** | **30M** | **36M** | **42M** | **66M** | **72M** |
| 8. | Retains liquids in mouth (30m) | 22.5 | 62.5 | | | | |
| 9. | Peels fruits (banana/candies) (36m) | | 23.4 | 61.7 | | | |
| 10. | Makes a fountain by releasing water from mouth (36m) | | 21.4 | 59.3 | | | |
| 11. | Picks food with own fingers to put in mouth (36m) | | 18.7 | 57.6 | | | |
| 12. | Blows (36m) | | 17.7 | 56.4 | | | |
| 13. | Mixes rice and other foods with hands (42m) | | | 21.2 | 58.7 | | |
| 14 | Sucks through a straw (42m) | | | 18.4 | 57.6 | | |
| 15. | Spits liquids (42m) | | | 17.7 | 52.4 | | |
| 16. | Swallows liquids (42m) | | | 16.6 | 51.8 | | |
| 17. | Eats with spoon (42m) | | | 15.6 | 50.7 | | |
| 18. | Follows etiquette in public eating (66m) | | | | | 52.7 | |
| 19. | Uses knife and fork (72m) | | | | | | 53.3 |

*Table 4.12 Contd.*

*Table 4.12 Contd.*

| No. | Self-help Domain | 9M | 12M | 15M | 18M | 21M | 24M |
|---|---|---|---|---|---|---|---|
| | **Dressing** | 9M | 21M | 24M | 30M | 36M | 42M |
| 20. | Removes headwear (9m) | 62.5 | | | | | |
| 21. | Takes off clothes if unbuttoned (24m) | | 28.6 | 61.4 | | | |
| 22. | Removes socks (24m) | | 25.6 | 58.7 | | | |
| 23. | Removes or puts on elastic pants/knickers (30m) | | | 26.8 | 56.4 | | |
| 24. | Unbuttons/buttons clothing (36m) | | | | 28.6 | 56.7 | |
| 25. | Takes off elastic inner/outer wear (36m) | | | | 25.7 | 55.7 | |
| | | 42M | 48M | 54M | 60M | 66M | 72M |
| 26. | Buckles shoes/sandals (48m) | 22.5 | 63.7 | | | | |
| 27. | Puts on socks (48m) | 20.4 | 59.7 | | | | |
| 28. | Buttons clothing (48m) | 18.7 | 57.8 | | | | |
| 29. | Applies facial powder/cream (48m) | 17.6 | 55.5 | | | | |
| 30. | Puts on vest/frock (48m) | 16.5 | 52.4 | | | | |
| 31. | Uses safety pins on own clothing (60m) | | | 22.4 | 62.5 | | |
| 32. | Ties simple knots/shoe laces (66m) | | | | 23.7 | 58.9 | |
| 33. | Grooms hair (66m) | | | | 22.1 | 57.6 | |
| 34. | Change clothes for laundry (72m) | | | | | 24.8 | 56.7 |
| | **Toilet** | 18M | 24M | 30M | 36M | 60M | 66M |
| 35. | Indicates toilet consistently with gestures or words (24m) | 28.3 | 56.7 | | | | |
| 36. | Seats self appropriately on toilet seat (24m) | 22.7 | 55.4 | | | | |
| 37. | Wipes hands/face with handkerchief (24m) | 18.7 | 53.7 | | | | |
| 38. | Washes hands with soap (24m) | 17.6 | 52.7 | | | | |
| 39. | Washes self if water is poured in toilet (36m) | | | 24.7 | 53.8 | | |
| 40. | Wipes/blows/cleans nose (36m) | | | 22.7 | 52.7 | | |
| 41. | Washes self in toilet (66m) | | | | | 27.6 | 63.7 |
| | **Brushing** | 18M | 24M | 30M | 36M | 60M | 66M |
| 42. | Brushes teeth (30m) | | 36.7 | 54.7 | | | |
| 43. | Cleans tongue (36m) | | | 16.7 | 54.6 | | |
| 44. | Applies paste on toothbrush (42m) | | | | 23.4 | 56.7 | |
| | **Bathing** | 42M | 48M | 54M | 60M | 66M | 72M |
| 45. | Pours water on self for bathing (48m) | 28.7 | 63.7 | | | | |
| 46. | Towels body (48m) | 22.7 | 53.7 | | | | |
| 47. | Washes face with soap and water (60m) | | | 22.4 | 56.7 | | |
| 48. | Bathes self with assistance (66m) | | | | 21.7 | *62.4* | |
| 49. | Applies soap on body (66m) | | | | 27.4 | 61.4 | |
| 50. | Bathes self unassisted (72m) | | | | | 23.3 | 53.7 |

**Note:** 'M' and 'm' both indicate months.
**Key for scoring:** NA: Not Applicable (0); TD: Totally Dependent (1); PP: Physical Prompt (2); VP: Verbal Prompt (3); C: Clueing (4); I: Independent (5)—see text page 113.

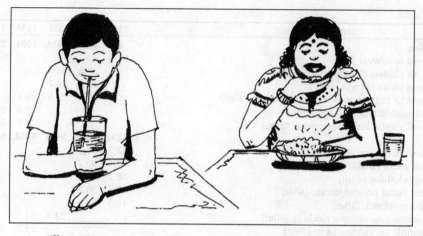

**Illustration 4.6  Sample of Eating Activities under Self-help Domain**

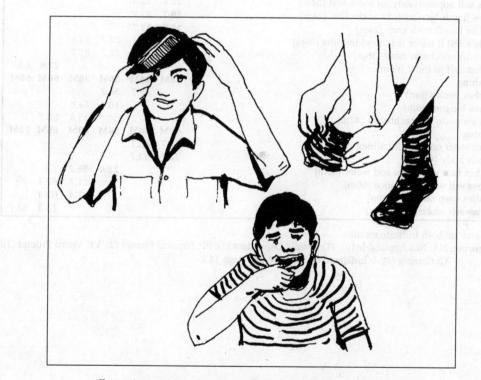

**Illustration 4.7  Sample of Dressing Activities under Self-help Domain**

**Table 4.13**
**Percentage of Passed Items in Cognitive Domain**

| No. | Cognitive Domain | 24M | 36M | 48M | 50M | 66M | 72M |
|-----|------------------|-----|-----|-----|-----|-----|-----|
| | **Clock and Time** | | | | | | |
| 1. | Differentiates between 'Darkness–light' (36m) | 33.4 | 58.3 | | | | |
| 2. | Relates time to clock (36m) | 28.7 | 55.9 | | | | |
| 3. | Differentiates between 'now–later' (36m) | 25.5 | 53.7 | | | | |
| 4. | Differentiates between 'day–night' (40m) | | 24.7 | 63.7 | | | |
| 5. | Differentiates between 'morning–evening' (44m) | | 23.7 | 58.9 | | | |
| 6. | Tells time to the hour from small hand on clock (60m) | | | 23.4 | 57.9 | | |
| 7. | Differentiates 'breakfast–lunch–dinner' (60m) | | | 21.4 | 55.8 | | |
| 8. | Differentiates 'yesterday–today–tomorrow' (72m) | | | | | 26.4 | 62.1 |
| 9. | Counts in multiples of five (72m) | | | | | 24.3 | 58.7 |
| | **Calendar** | | | | | | |
| 10. | Rote recites days of week (60m) | | | | 20.4 | 59.7 | |
| 11. | Rote recites days of week—with checks after (66m) | | | | 18.4 | 56.7 | |
| 12. | Rote recites months in year (66m) | | | | 17.4 | 55.6 | |
| 13. | Rote recites months in year—with checks after (66m) | | | | 15.7 | 53.7 | |
| 14. | Rote recites days of week—with checks before (72m) | | | | | 13.7 | 57.9 |
| 15. | Rote recites months in year—with checks before (72m) | | | | | 12.7 | 55.8 |
| 16. | Reports seasons in year (72m) | | | | | 11.5 | 54.9 |
| 17. | Identifies/names the day (72m) | | | | | 10.5 | 53.4 |
| 18. | Identifies/names specific days by reading calendar (72m) | | | | | 9.4 | 51.7 |
| | **Money** | | | | | | |
| 19. | Preserves coins/notes as money (24m) | 63.5 | | | | | |
| 20. | Sorts coins from other metallic objects (30m) | 24.7 | 63.7 | | | | |
| 21. | Knows money can buy things/has tender value (36m) | 23.3 | 61.5 | | | | |
| 22. | Discriminates between 'big–small' coins (48m) | | | 23.7 | 64.5 | | |
| 23. | Goes to neighbourhood shops for single items (48m) | | | 21.5 | 63.4 | | |
| 24. | Discriminates coins/notes (48m) | | | 19.7 | 59.7 | | |
| 25. | Can tell values of coins/notes (60m) | | | | 23.5 | 56.9 | |
| 26. | Identifies value of coins (66m) | | | | 24.6 | 59.7 | |
| 27. | Adds up coins below one rupee (72m) | | | | | 20.7 | 57.4 |
| 28. | Shops for 3 to 4 items with chits (72m) | | | | | 18.9 | 56.3 |
| | **General** | | | | | | |
| 29. | Matches two objects (24m) | 56.9 | | | | | |
| 30. | Matches objects to pictures or vice versa (24m) | 55.7 | | | | | |
| 31. | Discriminates 'more–less' in liquids (30m) | 18.6 | 57.7 | | | | |
| 32. | Understands/uses 'open–close' (36m) | 17.6 | 56.4 | | | | |
| 33. | Identifies primary colours (36m) | 16.8 | 55.1 | | | | |
| 34. | Identifies primary shapes (36m) | 15.6 | 54.7 | | | | |
| 35. | Arranges different sizes in ascending/descending order (36m) | 12.6 | 53.9 | | | | |
| 36. | Recalls at least four out of five objects that have been named (36m) | 11.5 | 52.7 | | | | |
| 37. | Discriminates sex (36m) | 10.5 | 51.4 | | | | |
| 38. | Sequences action/story pictures (48m) | | | 21.5 | 63.4 | | |
| 39. | Names/discriminates two sizes (48m) | | | 20.4 | 61.5 | | |
| 40. | Repeats rhythm claps made by examiner from behind screen (48m) | | | 19.7 | 59.7 | | |
| 41. | Compares two weights (48m) | | | 17.6 | 58.7 | | |
| 42. | Performs alternate sequencing activities (48m) | | | 16.6 | 57.6 | | |
| 43. | Differentiates between 'beautiful–ugly' (60m) | | | | 38.5 | 63.4 | |
| 44. | Identifies secondary colours (60m) | | | | 28.7 | 59.6 | |
| 45. | Defines words in terms of use (60m) | | | | 25.6 | 58.7 | |
| 46. | Performs double alternate-sequence activities (60m) | | | | 24.6 | 57.7 | |
| 47. | Differentiates between 'sooner–later' (60m) | | | | 22.2 | 56.1 | |
| 48. | Tends plants/feeds pets (60m) | | | | 20.1 | 53.9 | |
| 49. | Tells age (60m) | | | | 19.8 | 52.8 | |
| 50. | Names colours (66m) | | | | | 56.8 | |

**Note:** 'M' and 'm' both indicate months.
**Key for scoring:** NA: Not Applicable (0); TD: Totally Dependent (1); PP: Physical Prompt (2); VP: Verbal Prompt (3); C: Clueing (4); I: Independent (5)—see text page 113.

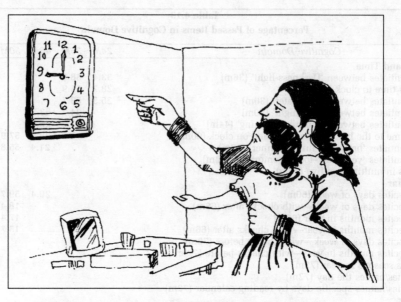

**Illustration 4.8  Clock and Time Activities under Cognitive Domain**

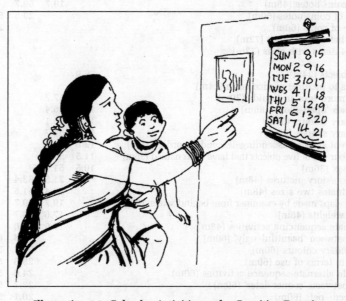

**Illustration 4.9  Calendar Activities under Cognitive Domain**

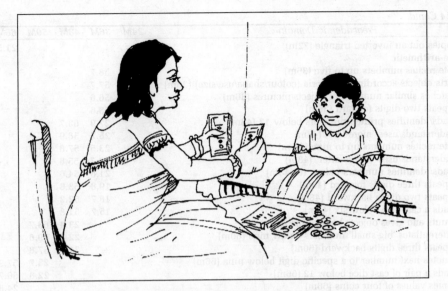

**Illustration 4.10  Money Activities under Cognitive Domain**

**Table 4.14**

**Percentage of Passed Items in Preacademic Domain**

| No. | Preacademic Domain | 24M | 36M | 48M | 50M | 66M | 72M |
|---|---|---|---|---|---|---|---|
| | **Pre-reading** | | | | | | |
| 1. | Matches similar pictures (36m) | 36.5 | 68.3 | | | | |
| 2. | Recalls at least four out of five objects shown in a picture (48m) | | 37.5 | 69.8 | | | |
| 3. | Points/identifies/reads five pictures depicting animals (48m) | | 32.4 | 67.7 | | | |
| 4. | Identifies objects from half-closed pictures (48m) | | 28.6 | 65.8 | | | |
| 5. | Reads out own name (48m) | | 22.3 | 58.3 | | | |
| 6. | Points/identifies/reads five pictures depicting vehicles (48m) | | 21.6 | 57.7 | | | |
| 7. | Points/identifies/reads five pictures depicting vegetables (48m) | | 19.6 | 56.4 | | | |
| 8. | Points/identifies/reads five pictures depicting furniture (48m) | | 17.7 | 55.4 | | | |
| 9. | Points/identifies five pictures depicting occupations (48m) | | 16.6 | 54.6 | | | |
| 10. | Identifies missing parts of a picture (60m) | | | | 28.6 | 59.8 | |
| 11. | Describes/imitates action pictures (60m) | | | | 27.6 | 58.7 | |
| 12. | Spots single difference between pairs of pictures (60m) | | | | 26.7 | 57.9 | |
| 13. | Detects absurdities in pictures (60m) | | | | 25.9 | 55.8 | |
| 14. | Arranges pictures sequentially to form a story (72m) | | | | | 25.7 | 62.4 |
| | **Pre-writing** | | | | | | |
| 15. | Holds pencil/crayon/writing instrument safely to scribble (24m) | 64.5 | | | | | |
| 16. | Draws vertical and horizontal strokes on imitation (24m) | 63.3 | | | | | |
| 17. | Draws cross and plus on imitation (24m) | 59.7 | | | | | |
| 18. | Draws circle on imitation (36m) | 24.6 | 56.8 | | | | |
| 19. | Copies a square (48m) | | 32.3 | 63.7 | | | |
| 20. | Draws a man with at least four parts (48m) | | 31.8 | 60.4 | | | |
| 21. | Copies a triangle (60m) | | | | 26.8 | 59.7 | |
| 22. | Draws a man with at least six parts (60m) | | | | 23.7 | 58.7 | |
| 23. | Traces outline of own palm on paper using pencil (72m) | | | | | 23.8 | 61.4 |

*Table 4.14 Contd.*

*Table 4.14 Contd.*

| No. | Preacademic Domain | 24M | 36M | 48M | 50M | 66M | 72M |
|---|---|---|---|---|---|---|---|
| 24. | Copies out an inverted triangle (72m) | | | | | 21.5 | 57.9 |
| | **Pre-arithmetic** | | | | | | |
| 25. | Rote recites numbers up to five (36m) | 22.6 | 58.7 | | | | |
| 26. | Sorts objects according to criteria (colour/shape/use/size) (36m) | 21.5 | 57.7 | | | | |
| 27. | Matches similar numbers of objects/pictures (36m) | 19.5 | 56.6 | | | | |
| 28. | Repeats two digits forward (36m) | 17.8 | 55.6 | | | | |
| 29. | Reads/identifies printed numbers below 12 (48m) | | 27.9 | 63.7 | | | |
| 30. | Understands/uses 'more-less' (48m) | | 25.7 | 58.9 | | | |
| 31. | Rote recites numbers up to nine (48 m) | | 23.5 | 57.8 | | | |
| 32. | Understands/uses 'before-after' (48m) | | 22.7 | 55.8 | | | |
| 33. | Reads/identifies numbers below 10 (48m) | | 21.8 | 54.6 | | | |
| 34. | Repeats three digits forward (48m) | | 19.8 | 53.8 | | | |
| 35. | Repeats two digits backward (48m) | | 18.7 | 52.2 | | | |
| 36. | Reads a cast dice below six (48m) | | 15.7 | 51.8 | | | |
| 37. | Counts and gives objects below nine (54m) | | | 23.4 | 63.7 | | |
| 38. | Differentiates 'big-small' numbers below nine (60m) | | | 22.7 | 59.8 | | |
| 39. | Repeats three digits backward (60m) | | | 21.8 | 57.8 | | |
| 40. | Denotes next number to a specific digit below nine (66m) | | | | 23.7 | 57.9 | |
| 41. | Reads a pair of cast dice below 12 (66m) | | | | 22.8 | 56.7 | |
| 42. | Names values of four coins (66m) | | | | | 24.8 | 56.8 |
| 43. | Enter numbers below nine into calculator (66m) | | | | | 23.5 | 56.4 |
| 44. | Reads cast dice/makes appropriate moves in board games (72m) | | | | | 21.6 | 55.7 |
| 45. | Understands ordinal position of numbers below nine (72m) | | | | | 20.7 | 53.7 |
| 46. | Rote counts by tens up to hundred (72m) | | | | | 19.7 | 52.7 |
| 47. | Repeats four digits forward (72m) | | | | | 13.5 | 51.7 |
| 48. | Adds single digit numbers within 10 (72m) | | | | | | |
| 49. | Subtracts single digit numbers within 10 (72m) | | | | | | |
| 50. | Adds two-digit numbers without carring over (72m) | | | | | | |

**Note:** 'M' and 'm' both indicate months.

**Key for scoring:** NA: Not Applicable (0); TD: Totally Dependent (1); PP: Physical Prompt (2); VP: Verbal Prompt (3); C: Clueing (4); I: Independent (5)—see text page 113.

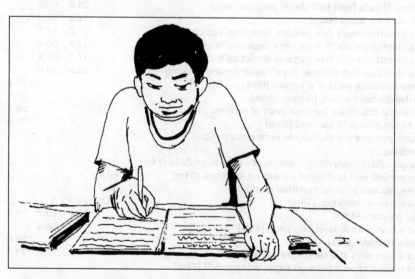

**Illustration 4.11 Reading and Writing Activities under Preacademic Domain**

**Table 4.15**
**Inter-domain Correlation on ACPC-DD**

| No. | Domain | S | GM | FM | C | P | SHS | Cg | PA |
|-----|--------|------|------|------|------|------|------|------|------|
| 1. | S | 1.00 | | | | | | | |
| 2. | GM | 0.94 | 1.00 | | | | | | |
| 3. | FM | 0.91 | 0.84 | 1.00 | | | | | |
| 4. | C | 0.72 | 0.70 | 0.62 | 1.00 | | | | |
| 5. | P | 0.68 | 0.62 | 0.60 | 0.58 | 1.00 | | | |
| 6. | SHS | 0.54 | 0.57 | 0.52 | 0.50 | 0.66 | 1.00 | | |
| 7. | Cg | 0.50 | 0.42 | 0.41 | 0.41 | 0.51 | 0.41 | 1.00 | |
| 8. | Pa | 0.44 | 0.36 | 0.33 | 0.37 | 0.41 | 0.57 | 0.66 | 1.00 |

**Notes:** S: Sensory; GM: Gross motor; FM: Fine motor; C: Communication; P: Play; SHS: Self-help skills; Cg: Cognitive; PA: Preacademics.

**Validity:** Apart from internal validation exercises, concurrent validity of ACPC-DD against Developmental Quotient (DQ) estimates on standardized developmental schedules (Bharatraj, 1983), Social Quotient (SQ) estimates on standardized social-maturity scales (Malin, 1961) and parental/caregiver estimates of developmental age levels of their children with DDs was also carried out. The consideration of parental estimate is justified by a concurrent investigation (Venkatesan and Rao, 1990). The concurrent validity coefficient for ACPC-DD against DQ measures of the same sub-sample of 46 children with DDs on Developmental Screening Test (DST) (Bharatraj, 1983) was found to be 0.847; and those with SQ measures on the Vineland Social Maturity Scale, Indian Adaptation (Malin, 1961) was found to be 0.863. The concurrent validity coefficient for ACPC-DD against parent/caregiver estimates of mental ages was found to be 0.924.

**Sensitivity:** A three month home-based training programme was carried out on a select sub-sample of 52 cases with DDs. This sample included cases with developmental delays (DDs) (N: 18), specific speech delays (SSDs) (N: 9), specific motor-co-ordination disorder (MCDs) (N: 4), pervasive developmental disorder (PDDs) (N: 4) and others (N: 17) (Table 4.16).

**Table 4.16**
**Distribution of Sample Characteristics Used for Sensitivity Analysis**

| No. | Diagnosis | Age Levels in Years (where 'x' indicates age) | | | | | | | Total |
|-----|-----------|------|------|------|------|------|------|-----|-------|
| | | $x \leq 1$ | $1 < x \leq 2$ | $2 < x \leq 3$ | $3 < x \leq 4$ | $4 < x \leq 5$ | $5 < x \leq 6$ | 6+ | |
| 1. | DDs | 6 | 4 | 3 | 2 | 2 | 1 | – | 18 |
| 2. | SSDs | – | 1 | 4 | 3 | 1 | – | – | 9 |
| 3. | MCDs | – | 1 | 2 | 1 | – | – | – | 4 |
| 4. | PDDs | – | – | 1 | 2 | 1 | – | – | 4 |
| 5. | Others | – | – | – | 2 | 4 | 5 | 6 | 17 |
| | Total | 6 | 6 | 10 | 10 | 8 | 6 | 6 | 52 |

There were approximately fortnightly follow-ups of at least half-hour duration each over 12 weeks in order to assess the quarterly gains on ACPC-DD. Thereby, parents/caregivers received counselling/guidance for three hours. The intention was not only to determine the effectiveness of home-based training programmes, but also to find out the sensitivity of ACPC-DD in detecting quantitative gains over the intervening training phase. During home-based training programmes, parents/caregivers were guided in the selection of not more than three to five behavioural objectives from ACPC-DD along with specific instructional tips on activities or procedures to train on chosen target behaviours over the next three months. Appropriate guidance and counselling techniques, bibliographic materials, demonstration therapy, individual discussions, etc. were used to convey the gist of training activities to parents or caregivers of children with DDs. The results indicate statistically significant/substantial changes in scores of sample children for overall, as well as within each domain, scores on ACPC-DD (Table 4.17).

**Table 4.17**
**Sensitivity of ACPC-DD**

| Domain | Mean (N: 289) | SD | Probability |
|---|---|---|---|
| Sensory | | | |
| Pre | 156.78 | 21.41 | t: 8.319 |
| Post | 189.43 | 18.51 | p: <0.001 |
| Gross motor | | | |
| Pre | 142.71 | 18.74 | t: 11.434 |
| Post | 183.41 | 17.54 | p: <0.001 |
| Fine motor | | | |
| Pre | 134.24 | 16.97 | t: 13.471 |
| Post | 177.72 | 15.93 | p: <0.001 |
| Communication | | | |
| Pre | 128.97 | 15.47 | t: 4.725 |
| Post | 144.27 | 17.49 | p: <0.001 |
| Play | | | |
| Pre | 122.67 | 12.79 | t: 5.464 |
| Post | 138.47 | 16.47 | p: <0.001 |
| Self help | | | |
| Pre | 124.83 | 18.97 | t: 7.789 |
| Post | 147.54 | 12.67 | p: <0.001 |
| Cognitive | | | |
| Pre | 124.87 | 12.33 | t: 3.206 |
| Post | 132.54 | 12.07 | p: <0.01 |
| Preacademics | | | |
| Pre | 119.56 | 12.67 | t: 2.517 |
| Post | 126.54 | 15.47 | p: <0.02 |
| Overall | | | |
| Pre | 131.23 | 16.24 | t: 7.727 |
| Post | 154.68 | 14.67 | p: <0.001 |

(p: <0.05 [S]; p: <0.01 [HS]; p: <0.001 [VHS])

**Notes:** 't' is the ratio of a statistic to its standard error, 'p' denotes probability, 'H' means highly significant and 'VHS' means very highly significant.

## (f) Materials Required for Assessment/Training on ACPC-DD

(NOTE: It is advisable for caregivers to develop and maintain a play kit for individual/groups of children with developmental disabilities. The play materials as suggested below need not necessarily be expensive toys and costly game equipment. On many occasions, with a little ingenuity, many of these materials can be prepared by the caregivers at home or within preschool settings.)

ABC books
Balls (large, medium and small sizes)
Binoculars
Bolts
Carom board
Chimes
Coins
Cubes
Dolls
Face mask
Glue
Kaleidoscope
'Ludo' game
Match sticks
Nails
One-inch cubes
Pencil sharpner
Picture books
Pins
Playing cards
Rattles
Safety pin
Shape sorters
Sketch pens
Soap wrappers
Story pictures
Tactile rug
Telescope
Toy carpentry set
Toy telephone
Tracing paper
Visual chimer
Whistle

Action pictures
Bangles
Beads
Blindfold
Calendar
Cellotape
Clay
Coloured dangles
Currency
Earphones
Flash cards
Gum
Kitchen set
Magnifying glass
Mirror
Needle
Painting brushes
Pen torch
Picture cards
Plasticine
Pocket calculator
Rocking horse
Scissors
Shoelace
Slate
Sponge
Straw
Teddy bears
Thread
Toy clock
Toy train
Tricycles
Water colours
Xylophone

Balloons
Bat
Bell
Blunt pair of scissors
Candles
Chalk pieces
Clothes clips
Crayons
Dice
Envelope
Gem clips
Incense sticks
Lock and key
Marbles
Nail clipper
Nuts
Pencils
Perforated sheets
Piggy bank
Plastic nipple
Punching machine
Rubber bands
Sea shells
Size sorters
Snakes and ladders
Stapler
String
Teether
Top
Toy drum
Toy vehicles
Tweezers
Weight box
Zips

# SECTION C

## Assistance Guide for Training on ACPC-DD

# CHAPTER 5

# TRAINING GUIDELINES ON ACPC-DD

*This chapter gives training guidelines and a glossary on ACPC-DD. A 'do-it-yourself' advisor type of presentation is endeavoured for trainers to help them understand the theoretical background for teaching specific behaviours by arranging them into convenient activity clusters. Appropriate references for the activities listed under ACPC-DD are given in brackets throughout the running text.*

## Sensory Domain

The sensory domain of ACPC-DD comprises of activities related to augmentation of vision, audition, olfaction, gustatory, tactile and vestibular senses. The activity clusters under this domain are reflexes, hearing–listening, seeing–looking, use of touch, taste, smell, balance, etc.

### Activity Cluster # 1: Reflexes

The infant begins as a bundle of reflexes which are seemingly spontaneous stimulus-response patterns of reactions. At birth, a normal infant is endowed with over a hundred spontaneous reflexes. Many of them are of great survival value. Within a few weeks of birth, nearly 80 per cent of these reflexes are lost. The remaining need to be optimally activated, particularly in infants 'at risk' or those with DDs. Reflexes constitute a basic foundation on which rests the edifice of sensory-motor development of children. The presence, absence or quality of reflexes reflects the neurological status of an individual. A poor sucking reflex or poor tone of muscles, abnormal posture or asymmetrical movements reflect pathological status. It is ideal, although not practical, to subject every newborn child to a detailed/systematic neurological examination of the reflexes. The various sub-types of reflexes are:

**Foundation Reflexes** form the basis for development of basic movements involving hand skills, bipedal walking and symmetrical body movements. Examples: galant reflex, grasp, automatic standing and walking, protective side-turning reflex, etc.

**Positional Reflexes** help a person assume a body position from which to function with maximum efficiency and minimum effort. Examples: asymmetric tonic neck reflex (ATNR), symmetric tonic neck reflex (STNR), etc.

**Righting Reflexes** are concerned with the maintenance and restoration of balance and equilibrium. They prevent the person from falling and harming him/herself. Examples: placing reactions, Landau reactions, parachute reactions, equilibrium reactions, neck-righting reflex, labyrinthine, body-righting reflex, etc.

**Primitive or Survival Reflexes** are seen in newborns and persist for about a month. They are transient and become dysfunctional by the time the child is about six months old. They are generally lost, or get integrated into more complex patterns of motor functions as the individual matures. However, some of these reflexes (such as Babbinski) reappear again when some neurological pathology sets in in the individual. Examples: birth cry, rooting reflex, sucking, swallowing, biting or gag reflex, etc. A newborn cannot afford to sustain life functions like breathing, nourishing or excreting without these reflexes.

**Autonomic Reflexes** develop over the first two years of life and remain functional almost throughout the life span of an individual unless there is some neurological insult at some time.

## Reflex Training

Place the child on the floor on his back and individually try out the following activities as part of a comprehensive reflex assessment-cum-training programme. Introduce a nipple or the tip of your finger and allow the infant to suck it. This activity enables the child to use the *sucking reflex* (S1). Gently tap the child's cheek. He or she will respond by turning his or her head sideways. Alternate this kind of stimulation from left to right cheek and vice versa. This activity enables the infant to use the *rooting reflex*. Tap on the tip of the child's lips. He will respond with a *pouting reflex* (S3). Reacting with a startle to sudden sounds is *basic reflex activity* (S4), and has implications for most hearing–listening skills in later life. This is analogous to blinking/closing eyes when tapped on the forehead (S5) with implications for later visual-sight skills. Press your index finger on the child's palms. The child will respond by closing his fingers on them. This enables use of rudimentary *palm-grasp reflex* (S6). Press your thumb gently at the anterior (upper) side of the child's toes. He or she responds by bending the toes down. This is *plantar reflex* (S7). Press your thumb gently at the lower end of the child's toes. The child responds by bending his or her toes backwards. This is the *Babbinski reflex* (S8). Hold the infant under the armpits while resting his or her feet firmly on the surface of the floor. The child will respond by making forward stepping movements as though attempting to initiate walking. This facilitates the *stepping reflex*. Repeat each of the above mentioned sequences of exercises at regular intervals.

Some additional reflex-training activities can include tapping sharply with the forefinger on the infant's cheeks. The infant responds by twitching his or her facial muscles on the stimulated side. This involves use of *Chvosteks' reflex* (S2). Place the index finger of your left hand well below the baby's lower lip and deliver a short tap with your right forefinger. The infant will respond with a contraction of the masseter muscles that can be felt rather than seen by the examiner. This is the *Masseter* or *Jaw Jerk reflex*. Hold the infant's head firmly and tap sharply on the glabella (where pituitary is located). The infant responds with tight closure of eyes for short duration. This is the *Glabella reflex*. Scratch a pin in the four quadrants of the abdominal wall around the navel and the infant responds with contraction of abdominal musculature. Scratch a pin on the medial part of the thigh and the baby responds with withdrawal of testis on the stimulated side or bilaterally. This is called *Cremasters' reflex*. Scratch the pin around the peri-anal skin of the supine infant and he responds by contraction of sphincter. This is the *Anal reflex*. Cast a bright ray of light into the eyes of the infant and he responds with quick closure of eyes in demonstration of *Blink reflex* (S5). In related *acoustic blink reflex*, clap your hands about 30 centimetres from the infant's head and he or she responds with quick closure of eyes.

Rotate the infant's head slowly to the right and he or she will respond with an anti-clockwise rotation of the eyeballs. And if the head is rotated to the left, there is a clockwise rotation of the eyeballs. This is the *Dolls Eye Test* which disappears after the infant has achieved visual fixation. Turn the face slowly to the right side and hold it in the extreme position with the jaw over the right shoulder. Repeat by turning face towards the left shoulder. The jaw, arm and legs extend. The occipital arm flexes at the elbow. The responses of the lower limbs are more constant than those of the upper limbs evidencing assymetric tonic neck reflex (ATNR) seen around two to three months of age. Scratch the soles of the infant's feet with a pin and notice simultaneous flexion of hip, knee and foot, often followed by unstimulated leg movement in demonstration of *Withdrawal reflex*. In supine position, start by grasping the infant's hands at the wrist and pulling him or her slowly to the sitting position. If necessary, support the head. The baby responds with resistance to the extension of arms at the elbow when the body is pulled to sitting position and the head is actively lifted. This is *Traction reflex*. Keep the infant in prone position (on the stomach). If he does not crawl spontaneously, try a gentle push on the sole of his feet. He will show spontaneous crawling as evidence for *Beavers' reflex* (S10). Keep the infant prone and slowly scratch with a pin down from the shoulders to buttocks. He or she responds through *Galant's reflex* by arching the trunk with concavity at the stimulated side.

For children 'at risk' and those with DDs, it is advisable for parents to check the existing status of the entire gamut of infant reflexes. A poverty or weakness in elicitation of any specific reflex must immediately point to the need for subjecting them to a comprehensive reflex-training programme. A poor sucking reflex, for example, must suggest various sucking activities for the infant. The reflexes that have their spontaneous demise over time may be ignored. Others need to be targeted for regular or intensive stimulation. It is necessary to understand that an infant's reflexes proceed along four discrete but fairly interconnected stages, viz., reflex, reaction, automation and volition stages. The reflex stage commences around the seventh week intrauterine and proceeds up to two months after birth. In this stage, the infant is incapable of any voluntary action or response. Movements occurring in this stage seldom cover the entire body. Only specific parts of the body are stimulated by specific kinds of stimulus impinged on the infant. During the reaction stage, extending from two to eight months, there are minimum voluntary actions from the infant. In automation stage, beginning around eight months and extending all through a person's life, greater voluntary control on individual or specific parts of the body is achieved. However, the quality, strength, speed, rhythm, duration and budgeting (or economy) of neuromuscular energy in carrying out movements is not as impressive as during the eventual volition stage of reflexes.

## Activity Cluster # 2: Sensory-motor

The healthy/intact status of the senses, viz., vision, hearing, touch, taste and smell, are crucial for diagnosis and commencement of remediation programmes in children with DDs. Hearing refers to the status of the auditory apparatus. The child should be able to hear a normal range of conversational sounds. The child must have normal or corrected vision. The sense of touch should exclude pathological conditions resulting from neurological/CNS disorders like parasthesias, agnosias, apraxias, etc. The sensations of vision, hearing and/or touch progress in children through demarcated developmental phases from sensory fixation, pursuit/tracking, scanning, localization, matching, discrimination, analysis, identification, naming and generalization. An understanding of these background aspects is necessary to appreciate the specific cognitive fixation or developmental stagnation in any given child with DDs. Normal children smoothly progress through these sensory-perceptual developmental processes. In children with DDs, there is marked developmental arrest at one or the other phases leading to some sort of cognitive breakdown.

## Activity Cluster # 2a: Hearing and Listening

A logical offshoot of adequate hearing is listening. Listening is distinguished from hearing. Not all that is heard need be listened. Listening is the active psychological process of attention or selective organization of perceived auditory stimuli. Many external factors influence listening in an individual, such as the size, extensivity, intensity, duration or propensity of the stimuli. Other internal factors include mood or interest of subject, mental set or attitude of the listener, etc. Listening can be improved by practice and training. Listening helps maintain the received impact of auditory stimuli over required periods of time. It includes ability to pay and sustain attention on given instructions for learning target behaviours. It involves attention to, and maintenance of, concentration on perceived auditory stimuli over required periods of time. Listening is a learned ability to pay and sustain attention on given instructions for learning target behaviours. Thus, listening is an important prerequisite and adjuvant for

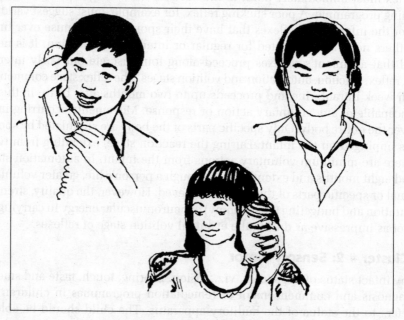

**Illustration 5.1  Hearing and Listening**

both comprehension as well as attention-concentration activities in toddlers. Hearing sensations progress into listening skills in young children through various definite transformational stages, including auditory fixation (S17), pursuit/tracking (S13), scanning, localization (S13; C1; C2), matching, discrimination, analysis, identification, naming and generalization. The beginning infant, for example, begins to train the auditory apparatus towards various sound sources coming from above, below, in front and/or behind him (C2). This is followed by a stage wherein the child pursues or tracks source of sounds in its environment. He or she may do this by turning his or her head (or ears) in the direction of auditory stimuli. The child scans all over or around to localize, and matches similar sounds or differentiates dissimilar ones. During this stage parents should make the same sounds as the child is making to facilitate imitative babbling (C4).

These primitive developments seemingly appear effortlessly and spontaneously in normal children. They are at once ready to extend their attention over time in the form of listening skills. Listening is generally assumed to develop automatically in children. We believe that a word or command to 'listen!' or 'pay attention!', or a silent glare, is enough to bring the child to attention. Such gestures can only force the child physically. His mind will be still at large. Listening is a skill that is to be taught as well as learnt.

Listening is dealt through three phases, viz., pre-listening, while-listening and post-listening. The pre-listening phase consists of introduction to the topic intended to be learnt. The while-listening phase refers to actual delivery of learning materials. The post-listening phase consists of activities to test listening. Most preparatory skills for hearing and listening are to be included at the nursery level itself. The child is exposed to a variety of sounds in his environment, such as the whirr of fans, barking of dogs, mewing of cats, screeching of vehicles and so on. There are many prerecorded cassettes, CDs and audio-aided children's software, not to speak of the humble record player, which can be used to mimic various sounds from the child's milieu. It could be gusts of wind, creaking doors, chirping birds, the cackle of geese, roar of a lion, hiss of snakes and so on.

It is necessary to draw the child's attention to all these and as many sound sources with attending pantomime actions. Additional ear devices (S35) may be used, such as earphones, walkman or toy phones, to convey some of these sounds. The child's own babbling may be recorded and replayed to arouse interest. Whisper games form an absorbing activity for many preschoolers. Whisper small commands or even gibberish talk into the ears of an avid preschooler. It could be a mere pretend play with no meaningful message or instruction. Listening to conversation or directions over the telephone is a specially curious activity for the toddler who hears voices of familiar caregivers in their physical absence. Whisper games involving seemingly 'secret' messages for the child's compliance training is another useful activity in this connection. Some related activities for the interested teacher are given under Table 5.1.

Listening is learned. It is not innate. It is hearing, recognizing and interpreting through previous experiences. The lack of ability to listen, to interpret what is said, is responsible for many speech defects and for much of communication misunderstandings in our times. Some auditory training activities that can be practised for preschool children include creation of awareness about various types of sound in the child's milieu. Aid the child to differentiate various types of sounds. These sounds could even be self-productive in the form of babbling or reproduction of vowel sounds on imitation (C4). Repeat the sounds made by the child

**Table 5.1**

**Prerequisites and Activities for Promoting Hearing and Listening Skills**

**Prerequisites**

Create awareness about various types of sounds.
Help child differentiate between various types of sounds.
Encourage babbling or allied sound production.
Encourage child to respond to name call.

**Activities**

Listens through ear devices like telephone, ear phones and/or walkman.
Participates in simulated whisper games.
Localizes sources of sound.
Matches pairs of similar sounds.
Differentiates dissimilar sounds.
Listens to stories/narration.
Listens to jokes.
Listens to music.
Echo game: whisper a word to a child in a row; the child passes the word to the next and thus the word goes down the line until the last child yells it aloud.
Giving instructions for the child to follow.
Identifying sounds of animals, things, vehicles, etc.
Listening to sea shells.

after or along with him or her. Reinforce repetitions with hugs, kisses or even edibles liked by the child. In case external sounds are provided, the child must simultaneously learn to locate the directional source of these sounds (C2). Clap your hands from left, right, top or bottom directions so that the child responds by looking in the direction of the sound source. Keep calling the child's name frequently to familiarize him or her with specific sounds. It is preferable to use short names or pet names instead at long names. A corollary activity to this is to encourage the child to point to self or various objects in the child's surroundings. Pointing is an important pre-linguistic skill and precedes the activity of pointing to self upon name call. An older child could be allowed to listen to the sounds of various things or events like the roar of waves, rustling of leaves, whirr of machinery, barking of dogs and so on. The scope of this list is endless. It is preferable to take the child on a walk and direct his attention to various sources of sounds. Alternatively, a recorded version is also convenient as an indoor activity for improving listening.

An echo game involves the child passing whispered commands/instructions received from one end in a group of children to another with the suppressed excitement of secrecy and concealment. Echoes are useful for increasing perplexity and bewilderment of young preschoolers even as their listening skills are being trained. Following commands to perform various activities is another way of improving listening. The child's ability to follow commands/instructions progress along a continuum of complexity beginning from an understanding of isolated commands like 'sit', 'stand', 'give', take', 'come', 'go', etc., to more complex levels of verbal instruction like 'give me that box!', 'sit on the chair!', 'open the door!', and so on. Children usually follow single-step instructions before graduating to two, three or multiple instructions (Refer to Activity Cluster 6B).

Listening to narratives, fables, incidents and stories (C41) come as high order listening in preschool children. The beginning narratives should be entirely personalized and centred on the daily activities of the child. It could be fictitious, but necessarily exclusive to the life events of the child. The story of 'Once upon a time, there was a king with three wives ...' may not evoke interest for the beginning story listener. Try to get into the cognitive frame and imaginary world of the child before you commence the narrative. A preschooler interested in toy cars and ice creams may be narrated a fiction on a boy riding an automobile to buy his favourite ice cream. There need not be any strong storyline in the recital. There must be a scatter of familiar persons, acts, images, things or events from the daily life of the preschool child to enable him or her to relate to the narration and sustain listening focus on the presentation.

## Activity Cluster # 2b: Vision and Looking

The difference between vision–looking is analogous to hearing–listening. Not all that is seen may be observed. Much of what has been said for hearing and listening is a relevant extension for vision–looking skills in children. Observation is an active psychological process of attention or selective organization of perceived visual stimuli. Indeed, many factors influence the observation skills of an individual. Looking can also be improved by practice and training. Looking helps maintain the received impact of visual stimuli over required periods of time. It includes ability to pay and sustain attention on given instructions for learning target behaviours. It involves attention to, and maintenance of concentration on, perceived visual stimuli over required periods of time.

Visual sensations progress into looking skills in toddlers much through the same transformational stages like visual fixation (S11), pursuit/tracking (S15; S20), scanning (S14), localization (S12), matching (S38; S40; S41), discrimination, analysis, identification, naming and generalization. The beginning infant starts to train the visual apparatus towards various photic sources in his or her milieu. This is followed by a stage wherein the child pursues visual stimuli in his or her surroundings. It is then that one sees the infant give up an obsession with gazing fixedly at a light source to tracking a light moved across or in front. In this stage, parents are advised to leave a bed lamp on all through the night so that the child learns to fixate by turning his or her eyes in the direction of moving visual stimuli (S16). The child scans visually all over or around to localize moving objects. Rotating toys enamour the child, and he or she matches similar objects or discriminate dissimilar ones.

*Visual fixations* are encouraged by allowing the infant to gaze at the fingers of his or her own hand. You can even tie a colourful band or amulet to attract the infant's attention. In continuation of this activity, present your own smiling or emotionally active face. The faces must vocalize continually and simultaneously. Combine use of brightly coloured toys, sound producing toys, tinkle of bangles, scents and fragrance of flowers to enable multi-sensory stimulation. The emotionally active human faces should include expressions of pretended anger, love, affection, etc. An angry expression is likely to result in responses of weeping by the infant, just as an immediate tickle thereafter will result in giggles, smiles and even loud laughter. All this is preparation for oncoming advanced cognitive processes like discrimination, identification, naming and generalization. An offshoot of adequate visual apparatus necessary for remediation programmes in infants with DDs is visual-gaze (S18). This includes facial gaze and/or eye-to-eye contact (S19) maintenance behaviours. Many of these children show difficulties in paying or sustaining facial/eye gaze when interacting with people around them. This becomes a major impediment in commencing any formal remediation programme. It is necessary to commence with formal eye-to-eye contact training activities before embarking on any other formal programme for skill remediation in children with DDs. The use of mirror (S22) to enhance gazing skills is more than justified. Mirror play (FM10) promotes the visual skills of young infants. Carry the child and place him or her in front of a full-length mirror. Attempt a play by taking him close to the mirror as though pretending to dash him against it. Simultaneously verbalize the approach to the mirror by using the words 'dash … sh … sh …!' The observing child may respond with smile or laughter. Simultaneously, encourage the child to explore, touch or pat his or her own image in the mirror.

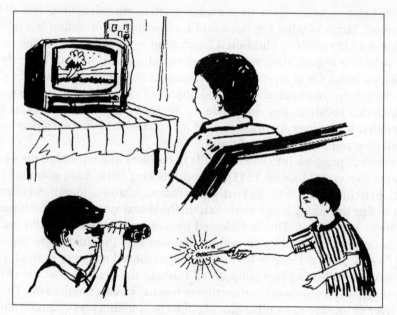

**Illustration 5.2  Vision and Looking**

Very young infants do not have a sense of object permanence. This means that objects or persons in or around their surroundings exist for them only and only so long as they are presented visually in front of them. A face exists when visible in front of the child. A toy exists so long as it is displayed in front of the child. The moment the face is withdrawn or the toys taken away from the line of the child's vision, they cease to exist for the child! This predicament of 'here-and-now' experience of the infant's world may be not easily comprehended by adults since we have reached a stage where we have object permanence. We now assume that objects exist in spite of our perceiving or not perceiving them in our field of vision. Some infants need assistance during this transition phase between their initial sense of not having object permanence to attaining it. This can be done by activities involving 'peek-a-boo' games (S31).

Place the child on the floor (preferably on a soft bed) on his back. Take a colourful cloth and wave it above or in front of the child's line of vision. Bring the cloth playfully towards the child's eyes in an attempt to obscure his vision. Simultaneously verbalize to the child in his native tongue to mean 'not to be seen'. The child may initially show signs of restlessness when his or her face is covered with the piece of cloth. Provide physical prompts by lifting the child's hands to pull away the piece of cloth from his or her face. Gradually fade physical prompts as he learns to pull away the cloth on his own. Repeat this sequence of play several times within every 10 or 15 minute play periods once in three to four hours (S25). Alternatively, infants can be stimulated on an activity wherein the adult abruptly withdraws a toy or doll from the child's line of vision and declares 'all gone!' (C11). As the child begins to achieve object permanence, he or she will eagerly show expressions of seeking the missing toy. A variation of this activity can involve placing a piece of fine thread on the child's face so that he or she grows restless to remove it on his own (FM12). This promotes fine motor/prehension. The role of visual righting reflexes associated with orientation of the head or fixation of objects in visual field is a critical accompaniment in this process.

The development of object permanence in young children is a crucial link and prerequisite between primitive visual skills and later facial gaze proficiencies. Object permanence refers to the child's ability to recognize that objects continue to exist despite their being hidden from view. During their early months, infants are seemingly in a world of here-and-now! Any object (whether it is the image of mother or a doll/toy) exists for infants only as long as it remains within their visual field. The moment an object is moved away from the infants' visual field, it ceases to exist for him or her. Gradually, as rudimentary mental representation of objects set through 'symbolization', the child develops an attitude that objects have an existence independent of his or her involvement with them. The child learns to differentiate himself from the world and is able to maintain a mental image of an object even though it is not present and visible. The acquisition of object permanence and rudimentary symbolization may be purposefully instilled in children with developmental disabilities by means of 'peek-a-boo' games (S31), covering the infants face with a cloth to tempt him to remove them (S25), etc.

Figure-ground discrimination constitutes a special difficulty for many preschool children with DDs. All sensory perceptions are patterned after figure-ground reconciliation during preschool years. In any perceptual experience, there is a 'figure' which stands out, has good contours and gives appearance of solidity and three-dimensionality. The 'ground' is indistinct and its parts are not clearly shaped or patterned. Thus, the reading matter on this page is 'figure' against the background of white of the sheet on which it is printed. The sounds of a teachers' lecture in a classroom is 'figure' against the background of a variety of voices/noises in the teaching milieu. Figure-ground reconciliation occurs spontaneously in most human perception. It seems so easy and natural to most of us that we do not realize the deleterious consequences at not perceiving it until there is a figure-ground discrimination failure in our perceptual systems. Toddlers with figure-ground difficulties have serious problems under teaching conditions that involve simultaneous use of two or more modalities, such as oral and written/visual presentations. They may respond well to singular or modality-specific oral or visual presentations alone. Specific activities to train in figure-ground discrimination skills could make use of identification of objects from embedded/superimposed pictures (S48).

Most elementary skills for vision-looking are to be included at the nursery level itself. The child is exposed to a variety of visual stimuli ranging from colourful lights, sparklers, bright or dim lights, picture books, posters, photographs, television and so on. A beginning visual stimulation may be as simple as placing a dim bedroom lamp adjacent to infants crib or rotator toys just above their line of vision. This aids visual fixation, tracking and pursuit skills, which become foundation skills for later visual development. The maintenance of eye-to-eye contact during conversation is primordial to later development of social skills in infants and toddlers. Many children with DDs show difficulties in initiating or sustaining eye contact skills during conversation. Their direction of eye gaze may be fleeting or even misdirected. They seem to 'looking through' rather than 'looking at' objects and/or persons with whom they are in contact. This problem is not due to any inherent visual defect as many parents are wont to assume. It is poorly trained sensory skills that create problems in later social relationships. Parents and teachers must insist on the child making eye contact or maintaining facial gaze before/during every conversation. The child must be rewarded immediately and only after making such contacts.

Along with eye contact, small and often imperceptible body language communication details are required to be explicitly brought to the attention of children with DDs. As in normal children, it cannot be taken for granted that these children will spontaneously or naturally understand the 'within' meaning of many of these silent messages in any conversation. As a result, gaps occur between what is intended by the adult during conversation and what is actually understood or received by the child with DDs. Body language skills that need to be taught explicitly to these children involve their recognition of particular emotional expressions of others, including anger, fear, sadness, boredom, etc. The child should be able to make out a frown on someone's face from an expression of love or friendliness. He or she should learn to take cues on when to ask, when to speak or when to stop speaking by taking in the expressed or unexpressed signs of boredom in the listener.

Many 'seeing games' are an useful adjuvant to promoting observation in children. The child could be made to look through viewing instruments like binoculars, camera view hole, peep-holes, tubes, kaleidoscope, magnifying glass, masks, bioscope and so on (S34). Aiming and hitting targets kept three to five feet away with a medium-sized ball (GM49) adds to visual skills and concentration in children. A simple game involving the child hurling a ball at a target on the wall or at objects kept at some meaningful distance from the child can improve aiming abilities. Marble games, dart games and the like are also included under this category.

## Activity Cluster # 2c: Touch, Taste, Smell, Balance and Movements

Even though taste and smell are considered as relatively inferior senses for infants, their simultaneous stimulation is an essential ingredient of multi-sensory programmes in children with DDs. The infant must learn to react to different pleasant and unpleasant smells and tastes. Cotton dipped in pleasant odours such as talcum powder, liquid soap and detergent may be waved under the noses of young infants. The sense of smell (olfaction) is encouraged through activities involving exposure to various pleasant/unpleasant odours (S26), breathing exercises (S45), etc. Likewise different tastes, such as sweet lime syrup, tamarind juice, salt or honey can placed on the tip of their tongues (S27). Watch the infant make smacking sounds with his or her lips in relish of these different tastes. The older blindfolded child may

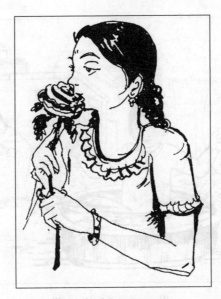

**Illustration 5.3  Sense of Smell**

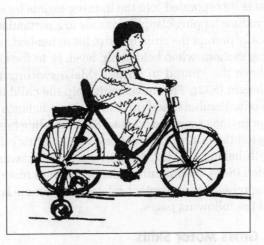

**Illustration 5.4  Cycling**

be taught to identify a given taste even without looking at the item (S39) or seek correction in tastes of food (S49). The child should be able to identify/name salt, sour, bitter, sweet, etc. Activities to promote tactile sensations in infants can include water sports (S23), tickling games (S24), caregiver/parent touches or carrying feet to mouth (S29), flexing of legs to stomach when lying on back (S30), fostering hand preference (S33), discriminating between 'hot–cold' (S37), 'rough–smooth' through tactile rugs (S42), games involving identification of shapes/objects by touch (S43; S47), differentiating 'right–left' (S50), etc.

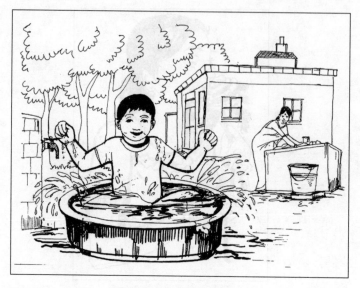

**Illustration 5.5  Water Play**

A sense of movement is incorporated into the training regime by seating the child in front of you or on your lap. Produce tapping/clapping sounds to a particular rhythm or in accompaniment to a song. Physically prompt the child to move his or her body according to the rhythm. The child enjoys swirling motions when held at hip level. Hold the child from underarm and lift him or her high above the ground to do this. Make swirling motions yourself while carrying the child at a height (S32). The movements help the child feel vibratory sensations throughout his or her body. Vestibular activities to promote balance in toddlers include sitting with pillow props or inside protective cradles (S21), nodding head in accompaniment to a rhythm (S28), making toddlers sit on rocking horses (S36) or tricycles and pedal cars (P35), standing on one leg with balance (GM27; GM28), walking backwards (GM37), walking in balance when blindfolded (S46), maintaining balance when in motion (S44) or when blindfolded (S46), etc. A comprehensive movement-related programme is elaborated under gross and fine motor skills in the following pages.

## Activity Cluster # 3: Gross Motor Skills

Motor strength, co-ordination and control skills involve small muscles (fine motor skills) as well as large muscles (gross motor skills). Fine motor skills (Table 4.5) are demonstrated in activities like colouring, cutting (FM47), buttoning (SH28), pasting (FM32), writing (PA15), threading needles (FM46), etc. Gross motor skills (Table 4.4) are demonstrated in activities like running (GM22), jumping (GM19), climbing (GM17), throwing (GM32), etc. The earliest motor skills are gross motor activities beginning with neck holding (GM1), weight bearing (GM2), creeping (GM3), rolling over (GM5), sitting self with support (GM6), bouncing when held by armpits in a standing position (GM10), crawling (GM11), sitting (GM8), pulling self to standing position (GM7) and standing without support (GM12). Additional pre-walking

(GM13) and walking (GM14) routines of the child should be compulsorily included. Children with DDs require assisted or extra stimulation of the appropriate deficit behaviour.

---

**Case Vignettes**

Regishia, a six-year-old, was brought in with complaints of weakness in the upper limbs, slow mental (intellectual) development, inadequate speech-language skills for her age—all consequent to an attack of encephalitis at the age of three. Her current level of intellectual functioning was estimated at around 18 months. A neuromuscular examination revealed low muscle power (grade 2) in the muscles of upper limbs suggestive of paresis. Her hand functions were seriously affected with minimum grasp competency. Even though she could sit, stand or walk around, her postures were incorrect.

Raghu, a two-year-old, was diagnosed with cerebral palsy and moderate mental retardation. Even though he could not sit, stand or walk, his parents had never sought any consultations for a home-based physical training programme. Elders in the family had suggested that Raghu would eventually learn to walk once he grew older. 'After all, some children are slow in the beginning but catch up with other children later', the grandmother in the house mused. A physical examination revealed that the child's limbs had developed rigidity. He would yell in pain when any effort was made to bend his knees.

---

Preschoolers and toddlers require extensive practice in walking (GM14), running (GM22), jumping (GM24), balancing (GM25), climbing (GM17), tunneling, somersaulting (GM16; GM36), kicking (GM20), kneeling (GM21), squatting (GM23), dodging (GM46), bending, marching (GM29), pushing (GM31), rotating, walking backwards (GM37) and so on. The contemporary

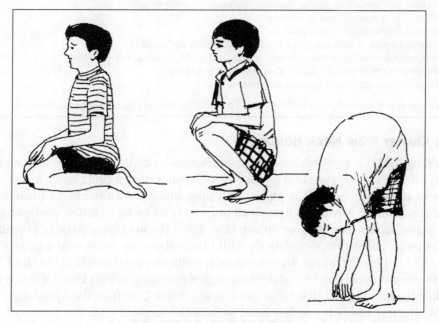

**Illustration 5.6  Gross Motor Skills**

trend of housing nursery, kindergarten and play homes for children in diminutive rooms or enclosed spaces is becoming the calamitous order of urban living. The children seldom get an opportunity to stretch their limbs, leave alone their requirement for exploring nature in its bountiful expanse. Many instances of seeming motor-co-ordination disorders in young children are due to restricted or nil opportunities for motor training. It is equally pathetic to hear of preschoolers being subjected to various fine motor or concentration demanding activities like alphabet/number writing even before they have done enough routine gross motor activities. No wonder such ill-prepared children do terribly on prematurely introduced high-vigilance activities like reading and writing. It is mandatory that preschoolers go through a rigorous training on all nursery level activities listed under gross/fine motor domains of ACPC-DD before commencing on preacademic activities. Infants require extensive practice on pre-walking activities beginning from neck holding, rolling over, creeping, crawling, pulling up self from supine to sitting position, rising from sitting to standing position, etc. While most children with motor problems progress seemingly well on merely being provided with appropriate opportunities for stretching or using their limbs, it may not be so with cases with severe motor disorders. An intensive physical training programme may be required to be prepared under the expert supervision of a psychiatrist, physiotherapist or occupational therapist (Table 5.2).

---

**Table 5.2**

**When is it Time to Seek Help from Physical Therapists?**

Does your child show

1. Poor mobility at the joints (arms, elbow, knees, wrist, ankle, toes, neck, etc.)?
2. Poor strength in muscles in some or all parts of the body?
3. Incorrect postures while sitting, standing, walking, jumping, squatting, etc.?
4. Deformities or contractures of muscles?
5. Wasting or decrease in size of muscles?
6. Decrease in tone of muscles either as spasticity, rigidity or flaccidity?
7. Poor power/strength (paresis) or complete loss of strength (paralysis) of muscles?
8. Poor co-ordination and/or control of muscles and breathing?
9. Pain while making certain types of movements?

If your answer to any of the above questions is, yes, it would be wise to consult a physical therapist.

---

## Activity Cluster # 3a: Neck Holding

Neck holding (GM1) is probably one of the earliest motor control activities that is mastered by young infants. Placing the child on his stomach can induce a proficiency in this activity. A pillow or rolled-up bedsheet is placed as a prop underneath the child's trunk in an inclined plane. Another way of eliciting head prop-up is by using a clothes cradle or the edge of cross-legged lap by the caregiver. In any case, allow the neck/head to be left unsupported by the prop-up. Thereafter, stimulate the child from above by using sound-producing and brightly-coloured toys or rattles. Simultaneously, continue to call or talk to the child. Reward the child's effort at every step by cuddling, kissing or providing similar kinds of tactile rewards that enable the child to feel that he or she is being loved. Continue the stimulation even as the child attempts to lift his or her head to establish contact with the source of stimuli. Repeat the above sequence of exercises at regular intervals.

## Activity Cluster # 3b: Creeping–Crawling

In order to make the infant creep forward (GM3) when he or she is made to lie on the stomach and pressed, her soles are pressed, follow this sequence of training steps. Squat at the feet of the infant and press both soles of the feet gently (S10) but firmly by flexing at the knees. The child will creep forward under pressure. Attractive toys are additionally placed in front of the child to motivate the child to reach for them as he or she moves forward. This activity enables the child to use *Baeuers' response reflex*. Repeat the abovementioned sequence of exercises at regular intervals. Over time, and with repetition of this activity, the child will learn to lift his or her head when lying on the stomach by freeing the nose off the ground. Another related activity involves teaching the infant to bear weight (GM2) on the elbows when lying on the stomach. Placing the child on the floor/mattress on his or her stomach does this. Squat in front of the child. Insert a prop-up (using a pillow or bedspread) underneath the child's trunk in an inclined plane. Flex the child's elbow close to his or her chest and allow the neck or head to be raised. Continue to use physical prompts till the child learns to bear the body's weight on the elbows and raise him or herself.

For teaching the infant to roll over (stomach to back, or vice versa) place the child on his back. Squat behind the child and hold his or her toes together. Gently provide physical assistance to help the child turn onto his or her belly. Alternatively, the child could be playfully tickled and pushed onto his or her back. Repeat each of these sequences of play several times within each 10 to 15 minute play period once in three to four hours daily. Crawling (GM11) is a fairly advanced activity compared to creeping. Lifting the infant under the belly with the support of cloth can enable crawling. Gradually remove the cloth and use your hands to support the crawling child. After the child has learnt to crawl some distance, try placing small obstacles along his or her path, such as a folded piece of cloth, rug, small pillow, etc. Gradually increase the size of the objects being placed along the path of the crawling child. Later, teach the child to crawl upstairs and downstairs.

## Activity Cluster # 3c: Sitting

Though not mandatory, sitting usually follows creeping–crawling motions in infants. The progression to sitting positions (GM8) is facilitated by activities involving the infant carrying his or her fists (GM4), and then feet, to mouth, or flexion of legs to tummy when made to lie on his or her back. Place the child on his back, preferably on a soft bed. Flex the legs at the knees and allow the toes to touch the mouth. Assist the child physically by allowing the palms to grab the toes while they are being pulled towards the mouth. Gradually fade physical prompts after the child learns to hold the toes to the mouth. Many infants enjoy flexion of their legs at the knee which allows their calves to touch their tummy. The pressure on their tummy incites a giggle. Combine this activity with other forms of sensory play like tickling to laughter. The child initially learns to seat self with support (GM6). To train this competency, the child is made to sit against the corner of a wall. Place a large round inverted pot in front of the child and allow the child to rest his or her hands on the pot. Keep the child in the same position for 10 to 15 minutes for every three to four hour cycle until the child learns to sit self-supported. Thereafter, physical support is gradually withdrawn until the child is able to sit in the centre of the floor without support (GM8). Alternatively, instead of the support of the wall, the child can be even seated against the support of rounded pillows or your own body as you sit cross-legged. Placing the child inside a clothes cradle can also enable sitting postures with support. The child may also require practice on seating self on chairs with and without arms (GM15) without losing balance or falling off. Postural sitting, either cross-legged (GM26) or in padmasan position (P32), enhances motor skills in preschool children. Kneeling (GM21), as a special form of sitting, maybe first be attempted on soft mattresses or with assist kneecaps.

## Activity Cluster # 3d: Standing

The transition from sitting to standing is crucial in the development of motor competencies in a child. Squat the child on the floor and hold by the hands. Pull the child up with a physical prompt to 'stand!'. Once the child stands up, allow him or her to collapse by his or her own weight as you say 'sit!'. Initially you may have to provide greater assistance in pulling the child up to the standing position with supports (GM7). The 'sit–stand' instructional game can also foster squatting (GM23) without losing balance. Practice the child to stand against the corner of a wall, cot or chair. Hold the child by the finger. Initially, you have to place yourself close to the standing child. Gradually, place yourself at a distance of two to three feet away from the child with arms extended. Encourage the child to move forward by showing him toys or eatables. Hold the child before he or she collapses into your waiting arms. Continue practice on these sequences until the child learns to stand without support (GM12).

## Activity Cluster # 3e: Walking

A rudimentary form of walking is indicated when infants make stepping movements while being held underarm and upright (S9). Walking with support requires holding the child's hands to practice walking around on a plain surface. The child may initially take a couple of

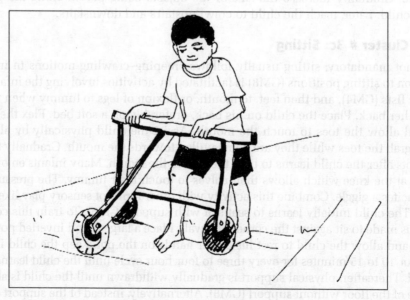

**Illustration 5.7  Using a Push-cart**

steps before collapsing (GM13). Care is taken to adjust toe walking (if present in your child) by placing his feet flat on the surface of the ground. Some children require additional physical exercises to endorse dorsi-flexion (adequate rotation/bending at ankles) and/or plantar flexion (forward bending of toes) before placing their feet on the floor. A few children do not get easily weaned away from walking with supports. In such cases, intermediate steps may be incorporated wherein the child is made to hold an extended scale, wooden rod or ruler as supports. As the child gains confidence for walking, it may be replaced with a rope or cloth which is held at one end by the trainer and at other end by the child. Walking-related activities include running, climbing up and down stairs, walking backwards *(GM37)*, balanced standing/walking, sack walking (GM48), walking while balancing books on the head (GM28), etc. The walking child requires practice on corollary actions like squatting (GM23), kneeling (GM21), sitting cross-legged (GM26), balanced walking (GM25; GM27), jumping (GM19; GM24) and so on. A 'sit–stand' instructional game can foster squatting without loss of balance. The child is held by the arms and instructed to 'sit!' and 'stand!' alternatively by gathering one's own body weight to pull up the child to a standing position.

## Activity Cluster # 3f: Climbing

Climbing (GM17; GM34) is initiated along safe and small heights before difficult heights are taught to be negotiated. The child is encouraged to climb up and down stairs (GM30), ladders (GM34), furniture, playground equipment, grills, gates, trees and so on. Clinging (P31) to an iron rod by supporting the entire weight of one's body is also a crucial associate of climbing activities.

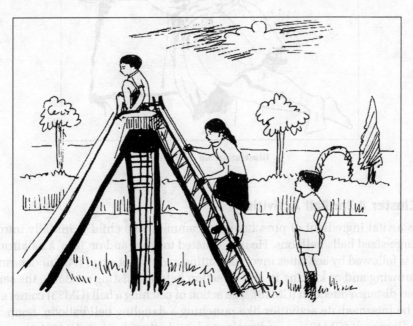

**Illustration 5.8  Climbing**

## Activity Cluster # 3g: Swinging

Swinging (S32) involves use of the vestibular sensations. The initial exposure may involve making swirling or rotating motions by caregivers after holding the child by the underarms. The child may then be seated on rocking cradles, cloth swings or other such protective devices that prevent him or her from falling. Later the child may be seated on garden swings while the adult pushes from behind to enable oscillations. The child has to gradually learn to move from a seated (P13) to a standing (P27) position, or to seat another child beside and swing effectively. Attempting to balance self when in motion on a swing, rocking horse (S36) or moving vehicle is crucial for all preschool children.

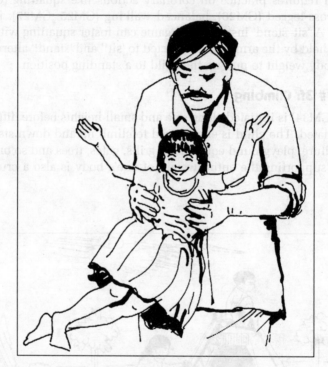

**Illustration 5.9  Swinging**

## Activity Cluster # 3h: Ball Activities

Ball play is a vital ingredient of preschool programmes. The child is initially introduced to handling large-sized balls/balloons. He is instructed to 'give' and/or 'take' a ball from another child. This is followed by activities involving sitting and rolling a ball (P3), underarm pushing, overarm throwing and/or kicking in any direction before insisting on doing the same things in a specified distance/direction (GM18). The action of catching a ball (GM33) comes eventually. There can be intermediate activities like punching a dangling ball/balloon, bouncing a ball against the floor/wall (GM47), co-ordinating to hit a ball with a bat (GM38), throwing a ball

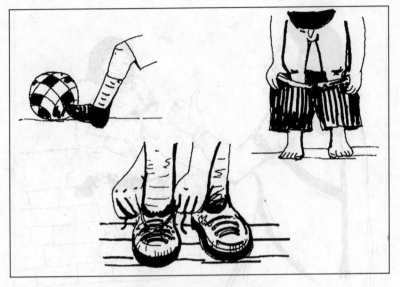

**Illustration 5.10  Kicking a Ball**

beyond a target distance (GM32), aiming and hitting targets using a ball (GM49), dodging (GM46) when another child hurls a ball, etc.

## Activity Cluster # 3i: Balance

Standing and walking (GM27; GM28) exercises stimulate motor co-ordination and concentration in young children. The child is instructed to stand still till an alarm is set off or some numbers are counted. Balancing exercises can be achieved by drawing straight or parallel lines on the floor, placing bricks in zig-zag rows, beam balancing and like activities which favour motor equilibrium. Attempting to stand or balance on one foot is a needed activity for toddlers. Activities involving balancing on a stationary surface (book balancing, lemon-and-spoon walking) (GM28; P50) or walking on the toes (FM27) is followed by similar endeavours on moving planes. It could mean sitting on a moving swing, standing on a rotation disc and/or getting up to a standing position upon moving equipment. A conclusive mastery is achieved when the child is able to swing in sitting as well as standing positions by propelling himself. Additional special types of activities to increase balance are walking along a straight line, on sidewalks or on bricks and on laid-out narrow carpet ways. Walking backwards adds to these balance activities. Blindman's-buff increases directionality and vestibular sensations in the young child. Kneeling (GM21) involves a special type of positioning balance where the child attempts to bear the entire body weight on the kneecaps. Squatting (GM23) is relatively easier since the body weight is placed on the toes/ankles.

## Activity Cluster # 3j: Jumping

Children need to be gradually challenged through increasing heights for jumping (GM24), but depending on their own individual rates of progression rather than in mutual competition

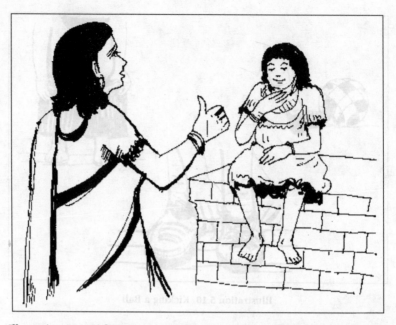

**Illustration 5.11  Girl Sitting on a Wall as Her Mother Calls Out for Her to Jump**

between one another. The beginning child, who has not gone over the founding stage of co-operative play, is simply not yet ready to understand competitive play. Jumping involves taking the whole weight of one's body from the last step of a staircase, or it could simply mean jumping with both feet off the floor (GM19). Two adults can hold the child underarm simultaneously (GM10) on either side before lifting him lightly into the air and dropping him down playfully. The control of the brief sensation of being lifted into the air is titillation for jumping activities in toddlers (GM24). Jumping activities require the child to not only negotiate heights, but also distance. The toddler must first learn to jump up and down in the same place. A dangling balloon can be a useful prop for children to reach for at the beginning stages. If the dangling balloon is dodged, the play could be more interesting for the young child. Thus short and long jumps are to be introduced as well. A hilarious version of jumping is enacted in sack walking (GM48) and leap-frog games (GM40). Skipping (GM42) and hopping (GM41) are an advanced form of a well-co-ordinated sequence of jumping activities in young children.

## Activity Cluster # 3k: Motor Imitation

Motor imitation needs to be goaded purposely. This is especially true for children who are deficient in social skills, such as children with autistic disorders. Simple physical calisthenics, exercises, 'yogasanas' (P32), marching (GM29), individual or group dancing (P6; P21), motor sequences and the like are performed for imitation by children in small groups. A simple illustration is the action of extending the hands up, down, bending them and so on to the tune of 'standing-up line, lying-down line, slanting line, curved line and crooked line', and is sufficient to evoke imitation skills in toddlers. In fact, children can be encouraged to imitate all motor activities among one another.

## Activity Cluster # 3l: Motor Strength

Motor strength activities involve running, lifting, pulling, pushing (GM31), carrying, squeezing, wringing (FM48), wrestling and so on. Through games, the child is enthused to lift objects and pull or push them from one end of a room to another. Squeezing a wet sponge or cloth to dry it is a water sport that toddlers enjoy. Wrestling out objects from the closed fists of adults and grappling in tug-of-war or 'fists-down' games give most young children great joy. It is important to understand that there is an optimum range of motion prescribed for the major joints in the human body. The knee, elbow and hip joints should show a normal flexion of around 140 degrees. The wrist is normally expected to show a maximum flexion of around 80 degrees. Swimming, skating, cycling, skipping, long jump, etc., are semi-formal sports that may be considered for young children depending upon available opportunities (GM44; GM45).

No two children have identical talents for learning. Even in the same child, there are wide differences in the rates/speed of learning for different target activities. However, a general principle while proceeding with any teaching process (especially motor skills) is to gradually offer decreasing levels of assistance during performance of learning activities. Begin initially by providing physical guidance or active physical assistance in a new activity targeted for learning. This is to be associated with simultaneous verbal instructions during the performance of that activity. Eventually, the assistance and instructions should be faded to only hints or clues for performance until the child learns to do the activity on his or her own. While it is one procedure to incorporate motor sequences and activities in isolation, it would be still better to blend them concurrently along with other domestic or social activities of preschoolers. Toddler activities like dusting/wiping furniture on instruction (GM35), sweeping using broom (GM39), polishing shoes/footwear (GM45), clipping nails (GM50), etc., are better incorporated as part of preschool curriculum.

## Activity Cluster # 4: Fine Motor Skills

Fine motor skills involving smaller muscles develop sequentially at a later date after gross motor skills in toddlers. Therefore, caregivers must initially and extensively train them in gross motor skills before beginning to fine-tune a programme for fine motor activities (Table 4.5). Most fine motor activities demand a level of vigilance and concentration that may not be readily available with ill-prepared children and/or those with associated attention problems. Many parents are guilty of attempting high-vigilance activities in young children and failing. Consequently, they blame the child who is unable to match the activities against his or her abilities.

## Activity Cluster # 4a: Grasp

The commencement of activities under fine motor domain begins by converting palm grasp (prehension) (FM7) in infants to finger/pincer grasp (prehension) (FM11). Simple routines involving the child picking up progressively smaller objects (FM14) encourage this transition. Additionally, pincer grasp is fine tuned through activities like holding and inserting a key into a lock

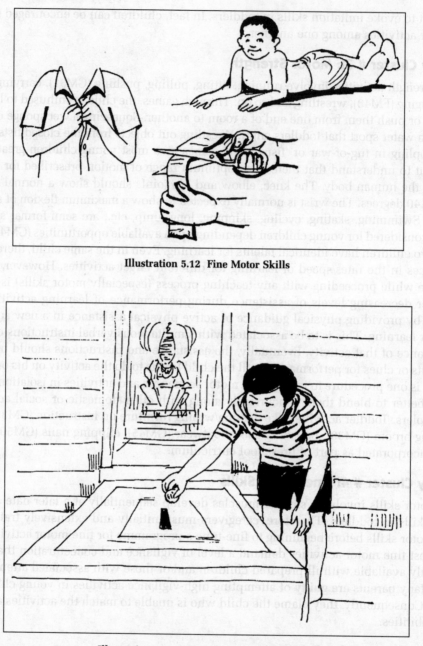

**Illustration 5.12  Fine Motor Skills**

**Illustration 5.13  Inserts Coins into Piggy Box**

(FM23), latching doors (FM17), inserting coins into a piggy bank (FM22), dropping pebbles, pins or pegs into narrow-mouthed bottles (FM15), inverting a small bottle to obtain raisins/peas (GM16), etc. The elimination of fisting (FM6) is crucial to development of grasp skills.

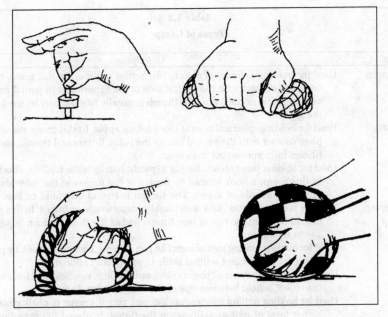

**Illustration 5.14  Types of Grasp**

Other types of grasp are equally important. Cylindrical (FM1) and spherical (FM2) grasp is promoted by holding appropriate objects. Hand functions are an important aspect of the forelimb for object manipulation. The crucial hand functions that need to be rigorously practised in young children are object reaching (FM5; FM8), grasping (FM9), transporting and/or release (FM19) skills. Grasp is the pattern or position in which an object is held. Differentiate 'grasp' from 'grip', which refers to the strength with which an object is held. Different objects require different actions and strength for holding. For example, lifting a pin from a table requires a lighter grip than while pulling out a thorn from the heel. Most hand functions commence with grasping reflex that involves clutching of any small object with the fingers (or toes) that stimulate the palm of the hand (or sole of feet). Children with physical problems, poverty of hand grip and/or spasticity require extensive training in acquisition of all these types of grasp (Table 5.3).

To initiate grasp activities, place small pieces of rolled-up cloth in the fisted palm of the child (FM6). The child must learn to retain small objects in one hand (FM1). Gradually shift to placing smaller objects like an inch cube in the fisted palm of the child. Sometimes, children require physical prompts like the hand being tied with a soft cloth to help them hold on the cube for some time continuously. This is followed by activities involving the infant reaching for objects dangled in front of him (FM5). Take a noisy toy that is brightly coloured and shake it vigorously in front and in the visual line of the child. If the child does not reach for the object, offer it into his or her hands and simultaneously vocalize these actions. Select rattles that easily fit into the infant's grasp before offering rattles wherein the child has to make an effort to hold on to. Later, offer objects in various shapes and sizes,

**Table 5.3**

**Types of Grasp**

| Type of Grasp | Description |
|---|---|
| Cylindrical grasp (FM1) | Used for holding cylindrical objects like bottles or pipes. In this grasp, the object is in complete contact with the ventral side of the fingers and in partial contact with the ventral aspect of the palm. The thumb is usually free but may be used for reinforcing the grasp. |
| Spherical grasp (FM2) | Used for holding spherical objects like a ball or apple. In this grasp, the object is in complete contact with the ventral side of the palm, fingers and thumb, and the palm and fingers fully encompass the object. |
| Hook grasp (FM3) | Used for holding larger objects having a specific handle at the top, like a bucket or suitcase. In this grasp, a hook formed by flexing of the fingers at the inter-pharyngeal joints holds the handle of object. The thumb is free of any hold or load in this grasp. |
| Opponance grasp (FM4) | Used for holding objects like a glass tumbler, paperweight or inkpot. In this grasp the object is held between the tips of four fingers and of the thumb which is positioned opposite to the fingers. |
| Palmar grasp (FM7) | Used for holding writing instruments like pen, pencils, crayons or chalk by palm at a primitive level of emergent writing skills in preschool children. |
| Pincer grasp (FM11) | Used for holding very small objects like peanuts, pins, needles, pebbles, etc. In this grasp, the object is held between tips of the thumb-index finger. |
| Tripod grasp (FM20) | Used for holding writing instruments like pen, pencil, crayon or chalk pieces by palm at a higher level of writing skills when the thumb is placed in opposition to the index finger to imitate adult strokes or grapho-motor skills. |
| Lateral grasp (FM40) | Used for holding objects like a deck of playing cards. In this grasp, the object is held between the adduced thumb and the side of the index finger or palm. |

such as square, triangle, spherical, cube, etc. The infant should learn to eliminate fisting (FM6) in due course of time before he or she begins to use thumb and finger in opposition to pick up large-sized objects. Other related hand/finger activities to facilitate pincer grasp are turning the pages of a book singly (FM13), putting small objects (clips, pins, seeds, coins or pebbles) into a container (FM15). Lateral grasp involves holding six to seven playing cards

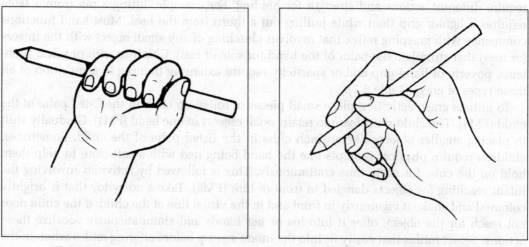

**Illustration 5.15  Palmar Grasp**                    **Illustration 5.16  Tripod Hold**

effectively in the form of a hand fan (FM49). Some advanced activities can include use of punch machine, stapler (FM43), pouring water through a funnel into a bottle (FM41), using a lock and key to bolt a door (FM39), tying knots, assembling nuts and bolts, corking/uncorking lids of bottles, etc.

## Activity Cluster # 4b: Tearing/Shredding

Tearing/shredding of paper by children is generally frowned upon by uninitiated adults as an act of indiscipline. What seems unruly may, in fact, be assiduous finger exercises for toddlers to be purposively trained through activities involving shredding paper into two/four pieces (FM40) and tearing perforated sheets, thick cardboard, felt or drawing paper, ivory sheets, etc. Pasting goes along with tearing activities in preschool children whereby they learn to use gum, paste or glue (FM32), cellotape, etc. Other fine motor activities for preschoolers are beading wire (FM21), threading a needle (FM46), building blocks, rings or bangles into wooden sticks, zipping/unzipping clothing or leather goods (FM24), opening/closing safety pins (FM29), using erasers (FM31), pencil sharpeners (FM36), peeling fruits (SH9), tying tags, laces or knots (FM38), etc.

## Activity Cluster # 4c: Pebble Play

Pebble play (FM44) is a game that requires children to throw up small pebbles in the air at one time and snatch the remaining four pebbles into the palm in one go. There are many varieties to this game. Rangoli (FM50) is a typically south Indian ritual of using colourful rice powder to draw designs in the courtyard. It is both an expression of art as well as of concern for fellow creatures. Supportive squeezing manipulations involving wringing wet cloth/sponge (FM48) can add to fine motor strength. Fine co-ordination is encouraged through screwing (FM26) or unscrewing lids of bottles (FM18), corking/uncorking and closing/opening lids of bottles (FM18).

## Activity Cluster # 4c: Folding

Folding activities ensure achievement of motor control. The first folding actions involve imitation of simple paper/handkerchief folding (FM25) *on observation* of an adult performance. Children are initiated by instructing them to fold old newspapers. The existing creases ease this activity initially. Single folds may then be replaced by double and triple folds, before going onto train the child in origami activities. Children are encouraged to make paper boats, airplanes and the like (P42). Folding is succeeded by insertion of paper or card sheets into punching machines, covers, envelopes or wrappers (FM35). Seat the child in front of you and let him or her watch you spread a handkerchief. Ask the child to imitate your actions with a handkerchief or piece of cloth. Initially, show a single fold to imitate and then proceed to teach double or triple folds. Later, folding of mats, towels, bedspreads, garments, etc., may be shown.

## Activity Cluster # 4d: Cube Assembly

Cube assembly (FM30; FM33; FM37; FM45) forms a series of progressively integrated and accumulative fine motor activity for toddlers. One-inch cubes are to be arranged for stacking towers (level one), bridges (level two), trains (level three) and staircases (level four). To enhance finger agility and co-ordination, activities involving use of rubber bands to strap a box (FM28) can be also considered.

## Activity Cluster # 4e: Cutting and Pasting

Many caregivers are apprehensive about giving scissors (FM47), knives or matchsticks (FM42) to toddlers. Their apprehension deprives the child of the opportunity to learn certain vital motor as well as safety skills that they may otherwise end up learning from other sources. The use of these cutting devices can be shown by using a pair of blunt scissors. The child may be initiated into just inserting his fingers appropriately into the handles of a pair of scissors and making imitative cutting movements. Once he has mastered making these movements, he is initiated into cutting straight lines drawn on old magazines or newspapers. This is done by purposeful straight-line or dotted-line cutting wherein the trainer draws a vertical and/or horizontal stroke on paper for the child to cut along. Cutting out curved lines and facial profiles are fairly advanced activities. The child also needs to be taught to cut butter, fruits, dough and other such soft items using a knife. Pasting (FM32) involves use of cellotape (FM34) to paste gift items, gum or glue pasting to make a collage out of small shreds of paper, pasting of small solids using adhesives, etc.

## Activity Cluster # 4f: Oral Activities

A unique constellation of fine motor competencies involves teaching oral activities to children. Oral or bucco-facial competencies in children should include sucking (SH14), pouting,

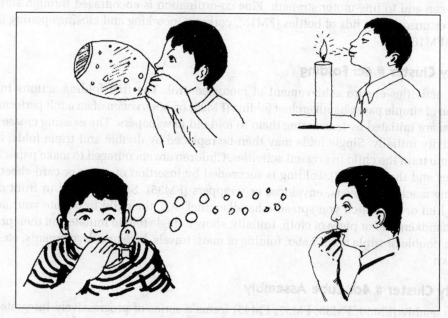

**Illustration 5.17 Oral Activities**

biting, chewing (SH4), swallowing (SH16), spitting (SH15), retaining solids/liquid in mouth (SH8) without gulping or spitting (SH15), sucking through a straw (SH14), blowing (SH12) (balloons, wind instruments, soap bubbles, lighted candles), making a fountain by releasing water from the mouth (SH110), etc. The training of spitting skills is a crucial prerequisite for effective tooth brushing competency in children. When asked to 'spit out!', many children end up gulping or swallowing the water in their mouth. For one thing, the child may not be conversant with the instructions 'in–out' (C24) which the parents may erroneously assume the child knows. A simple way to check this could be to draw a circle on the floor using chalk and attempting a game of 'in!' and 'out!'. When instructed 'in', the child must get into the circle, and when instructed 'out' the child must get out of it. If the child fails to understand this instruction, in all probability he or she does not understand the concept of 'in–out'. Sometimes, children may understand in-out in the above situation, but not in the context of breathing-in and breathing-out. A course on breathing exercises could be practised in preparation for children being taught to spit out. Further, children should be able to retain solids and/or liquids in their mouth before starting a programme that teaches spitting skills. A child who is unable to retain things in the mouth is unlikely to master spitting skills. Once this proficiency is achieved, the child is trained to tilt his head down to bring out the liquid, accompanied with the instruction 'out!' This done repeatedly, along with sufficient rewards following the correct performance of this activity, is likely to result in spitting competencies in children.

## Activity Cluster # 5: Attention-concentration

Many parents complain that their child is 'unable to pay attention' or 'concentrate' on given activities. Implicit in such allegations is an assumption that the locus of the problem is the child and not the teachers/parents themselves. This is not true. Agreed that sometimes the locus of attention problems could be the child. Take for instance children with attention deficit and/or hyperactivity disorders. There is an assumed neuro-behavioural basis for lack of attention or poor concentration in these children. But such cases are few and far in-between. In the majority of cases, problems of attention stem from poor or faulty programming of the skill training schedules.

Attention refers to the selection of stimuli from a wide array of stimuli that impinge on an individual at any point of time. It is one thing to select appropriate stimuli for paying attention and another thing to sustain that attention over a required length of time. Many children have problems in paying or sustaining attention on target stimuli/activities over the required length of time. In fact, this is a problem of concentration. Concentration in children is never an all-or-nothing phenomenon. In other words, children show varying levels/degrees of concentration. The ability to concentrate may be person, situation and activity specific too. Attention-provoking devices like aiming/hitting games (P14; P15; P43), threading a needle, stringing beads (P8), transferring liquids into containers with small mouths (P7), etc., are activities that improve attention-concentration in young children (Table 5.4). Caregivers need to understand the factors that influence attention-concentration of children. The difficulties in sustaining attention upon target behaviours during the teaching process need not always be faulted upon the child. More commonly, it is overexpectation on part of the caregivers. Toddlers are expected to sit with high concentration activities like writing, copying, colouring or reading for hours at a time. It may be that the child is not yet ready for such activities at all. The programme planning must take into account the developmental levels of each child and target low concentration or highly all-inclusive activities like running, jumping, somersaulting, tunneling, sliding, etc.

---

**Table 5.4**

**Activities for Promoting Attention-concentration**

Awaits till a specific verbal command is issued.
Awaits till a specific number count.
Digit/word span activities.
Repeats the last two to three elements of narration.
Cancellation activities (colour or shapes).
Imitative tapping activities.
Remains a 'statue' or 'freeze' game activities.
'Aiming and hitting' target games.

---

## Activity Cluster # 5a: Now–Later

Many parents have the false assumption that children understand or perceive time just as adults do. A mother who tells her nagging toddler, 'mummy will give you toffee *later*', is dismayed to see the child return again (within seconds) to demand for the same thing. 'Did I not tell you *later*?', she continues to insist. The point to be understood in this parent–child interaction is that the subjective frame of reference regarding time is different between the adult and the toddler. For the parent 'later' may mean, subjectively as well as objectively, 'an hour or so'. But, does the child have the same subjective or objective perception of the hour as 60 minutes into 60 seconds? This disparity in the mutual frame of reference leads to a lot of misunderstanding in the parent–child instructional set. Therefore, the child requires to be taught to wait till a specific verbal or non-verbal command is issued. Initially, the time gap is minimal since the child does not and cannot inherently wait for long periods of time. Gradually, the time gap may be increased. When the child has learnt to rote count certain numbers, you may introduce this waiting game up to some specific count, say, 'one, two, three ... now jump!', or 'one, two, three ... now eat!', or 'one, two, three ... now run!', or 'one, two, three ... now take!' and so on.

## Activity Cluster # 5b: Digit/Word Span Activities

For older children, number game activities like forward repetition of digits, presented by the caregiver at the rate of one number per second, can be carried out to improve attention. A set of random numbers is presented at the rate of one digit per second before the child is asked to repeat them (PA28; PA34; PA47). Then, four digit presentations or more can be added. A maximum of five to six digit repetition can be expected from children around six to seven years of age. Alphabets or words like may also be used for forward repetition in place of numerals. Backward repetition of digits (PA35; PA39) is relatively more difficult for pre-school children who have not yet mastered reversal. This involves the presentation of a set of numbers which the child has to repeat backwards. Herein, alphabets, words and sounds are also used for repetition. Children who are unable to understand the beginning concept of forward as well as backward repetitions for numbers, alphabets, words or sound syllables presented orally may be presented with visual or picture cards. Place three picture cards or even real objects, say 'spoon-pencil-key-coin', and cover them behind a screen before asking the child to repeat them in the same order or reversed order of their presentation. Alternatively, some children may even require certain basic practice on sequencing activities for successful performance on digit or word span games. Sequencing games require the caregiver to initially present alternate sequences of objects like 'spoon-plate-spoon-plate-spoon ...' before asking the child to answer or point to which object comes next in the sequence: plate or spoon? A simple alternate sequencing may be replaced at higher levels with double or triple alternate sequencing activities.

## Activity Cluster # 5c: Repetition of Last Two to Three Elements of Narration

This is essentially a game of concentration. The child is presented, orally or visually, with a series of objects, numbers, shapes, colours, sound syllables or just about anything in a predetermined and scheduled manner. For example, the caregiver may call out random numbers at the speed of one digit per second: '5-8-4-3-4-0-4-7-2-9 ...!' He must then abruptly stop without any prior notice, warning or cue. The listening child is expected to repeat the last two digits in that series. This activity requires that the child continually pay attention to the series of stimuli that is being presented before him. Only then will he be able to repeat the last two elements in the narration or presentation. Children must be presented with these and other types of concentration games, along with attendant prizes or rewards for better performance. A correct answer may be reinforced with a token star. A collection of stars may then be exchanged for more tangible rewards, such as 10 stars for a sweet, 25 stars for a cup of ice cream and so on.

## Activity Cluster # 5d: Cancellation Activities

This is an activity that fosters scanning speed and concentration in young children. A paper-and-pencil form of cancellation involves presenting the child with a mixed series of randomly placed red, green, blue and/or yellow dots. The child is asked to strike out as many dots of one colour as possible within 30 or 60 seconds. If the child is not adept with colours, shapes or numbers may be used. At a concrete level, the same game involves asking the child to put in one place all the items in the room which are similar in shape or colour to the ones on a reference card. Time settings are important in these games in order to foster speech and accuracy of performance.

## Activity Cluster # 6: Communication-receptive

A mother picks up her infant when he or she cries. When your friend calls your name, you attend to him. When the calling bell goes on, we know that someone is at the door. All these are common instances of communication. All living creatures communicate for various reasons. If they do it to satisfy their own needs it is called 'instrumental communication'. If it is meant to control others' behaviour, it is called 'regulatory communication'. If it is meant to greet others, it is 'interactive communication', if it is to seek information, it is 'heuristic communication'. If it is to convey information, it is termed as 'informative communication', and if it is meant to become aware of one's own self, it is called 'personal communication'.

Communication between two or more individuals can occur in different modalities, viz., hearing (speaking, alarm, telephone), visual (reading, writing, facial expression, television, body posture), or other senses (handshakes, kisses, hugs, hitting). Language is the main vehicle for communication. Language is a set of arbitrary symbols (mainly conventional, and used by a group of people for purposes of communication). Among other things, there are two dimensions of language; viz., reception and expression. *Receptive language* refers to understanding of spoken or written words and sentences. The most common modes of reception are listening and reading. *Expressive language* is the process of using either speech, words or signs to indicate various needs or meanings to the listener. The most common mode of expression is speech and writing.

*Receptive language* involves grasping/understanding commands and instructions for performance of various teaching activities. A minimum range or level of comprehension is a prerequisite for commencement of remediation programmes in toddlers with DDs. The child must also have skills for comprehension. To begin with, there must comprehension of pre-linguistic gestures, particularly pointing by self or by others.

## Activity Cluster # 6a: Pointing

An ancillary to comprehension of verbal commands/instructions is the understanding of non-verbal or gesture communications. Pointing, an important pre-linguistic skill, comes consequent to development of some minimum level of comprehension. Unless the child understands singular commands or sequences of one, two or more steps of instructions, he

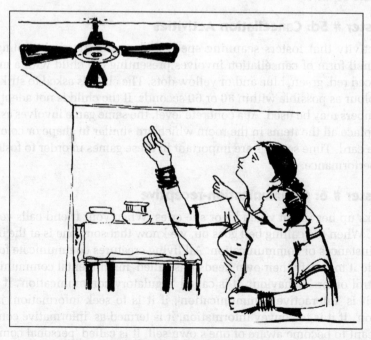

**Illustration 5.18  Pointing**

or she will not be able to point to specific objects around him. Pointing can be taught by selecting commonly captivating objects from the child's surroundings (C5; C22). Often, young children begin by pointing for their primary rewards like edibles, toffees or candies (C9). It is convenient to place such objects within the visual reach of the child and physically guide him to raise his finger/hand before yielding to their demands. A rudimentary pointing activity can be initiated by repeatedly conditioning the child to hear and recognize his own name (C3). On every occasion of the child's name call, he or she can be guided to pat him or herself for the question 'who's ...?', or 'where's ...?' After the child has learnt to point or pat to self on name call, the names of significant others in the child's milieu may be added through queries like 'where's/who's mummy? ... where's/who's papa?' and so on.

## Activity Cluster # 6b: Instructional Sets

As mentioned, listening is a vital accessory to comprehension in young children. There are various levels for comprehension of instructions. Usually, children begin by following simple or direct commands (C7; C12) like 'come', 'go', 'sit', 'stand', 'give', 'take', 'yes', 'no', 'stop' and so on. Later, they comprehend instructions requiring them to perform a series of actions (C32), such as, 'close the door!', 'open your mouth!', etc. Much later, they comprehend two- or three-step instructions (C43) given simultaneously. For example, the child performs two sets of actions (one after the other) after your singular but two-step instruction: 'close the door and then get me that ball!', or three step instruction: 'Give him the ball, close the door and get me that box.' There are specific procedures and techniques for training children to progress over these complex layers of instructional sets. In order to discover the correct level at which a given child is in the continuum of instructional sets, give him the two- or three-step instruction in one go. Do not prompt him at the end of performing only part of the instructions.

## Activity Cluster # 6c: Grammatical Forms-modes

There are a number of paradigms and procedures to look into with regard to language development in young children. Caregivers need to appreciate that grammar components in any language include nouns, verbs, adjectives, prepositions, conjunctions, adverbs, pronouns and so on. Even though one learns to comprehend the formal rules of application in grammar during the later school years, the young child seemingly progresses through gradual stages in the use of grammatical forms. In the earliest stage, the toddler begins to learn various noun forms of a language. This is when teachers must concentrate on building up the noun vocabulary of the child. Point or show the child as many objects, persons, things or events whereby he or she will know their names. This is done by showing pictures of noun forms or, better still, live objects/things themselves. The various categories of noun forms that can be included within this initial phase of the child's vocabulary development are names of animals, vegetables, fruits, vehicles, household articles, garments for daily use, family relationships, occupational headings, etc. The child must attain proficiency in at least over a hundred noun forms before you begin introducing verb forms. Verb forms of language include words or pictures depicting actions, such as running, walking, eating, praying, throwing, picking, catching, falling, spitting, sitting, reading, shouting, etc. A simple procedure to check whether your child is predominantly in the noun mode or verb mode of a given language is to show him or her a picture and ask: 'what is in this picture?' If the child's verbal responses are mere names of various objects in the picture, say, 'dog', 'man', 'umbrella', etc., you can safely conclude that he or she is operating on a nominal level (noun mode) and that she requires extensive training in the verb mode of language operations. The child in verb mode of language use will be more descriptive about actions in the same picture. For the same query, the child will respond as 'dog barks', 'man walks', 'child runs', etc. In the last stage, which is not likely to appear well past the primary school level, the child will be able to make interpretative responses on the same picture cards. This is when the child is able to narrate a story out of the picture card by incorporating emotions. The story-like expressions would contain details on what is happening in the picture, what could have happened that has led to the situation in the picture and what is likely to happen to characters in the future.

In the next stage of language use, the child is trained using adjective forms. This is fairly difficult for many teachers since adjective forms are not tangible, concrete or visible attributes of persons or events as noun forms and/or verb forms. For example, it would be easy to show a particular object or picture and tell its name. It would also be easy to show the activity of an object or person and describe the action. However, it would not be so easy to explain adjective forms like 'beautiful–ugly', 'nice–not nice', 'tall–short', 'fast–slow', 'young–old' (C26), etc. The use of pantomime or actual simulations of objects or events can convey adjective forms to many children. There are various sub-types of adjective forms that qualify noun forms, viz., qualitative adjectives (such as smooth–rough, beautiful–ugly), quantitative adjectives (such as some, more, little, enough, all, sufficient, much), demonstrative adjectives (such as this, that, these, those), interrogative adjectives (such as which, what, where), possessive adjectives (such as our, my, your, his, her, their) and exclamatory adjectives (such as, 'what a movie!').

The use of prepositions/postposition-forms is to be taught to children whereby they would appreciate positional descriptions of objects/events, such as, 'above–below', 'on–under', 'front–back', 'here–there', 'up–down', etc. This follows use of conjunction forms to facilitate correct and longer sentence expositions in the child. The correct use of 'and', 'if', 'then', 'but', 'if', 'unless', 'although', 'since', 'because' or such words in comprehension or conversational language must appear eventually in the agenda for teaching linguistic grammar to young children. The use of pronoun forms appears to be by far more difficult to acquire in speech or language, especially in children with autistic disorders. They need special attention to follow and use expressions like 'I', 'he', 'she', 'they', 'them', etc. These children are likely to show confusions between using 'he' and 'she' to designate a boy or girl appropriately. A girl may be referred to as 'he', or vice versa. A pronoun is a word that is used instead of a noun. There are various sub-types of pronouns, viz., demonstrative pronouns (such as this, that, these, those), indefinite pronouns (such as one, none, some, few, everyone, anyone, anybody, everybody), distinctive pronouns (such as each, either, neither), reciprocal pronouns (such as each other, one another), relative pronouns (such as 'this is the man *who* teaches us', or 'this is the dog *which* bit people'). The uses of interjections come with some difficulty in children with autistic disorders as it involves an expression of sudden or spontaneous feeling. Some examples of interjections are sentences involving use of expressions like 'alas!', 'bravo!', 'hurrah!', 'oh!', 'ah!', 'dear me!', 'well done!', etc.

## Activity Cluster # 6d: Question Forms-modes

Another perspective for viewing the sequence of acquiring language comprehension-expression in children with DDs is question forms. Usually, the child learns to ask question forms involving 'what?', followed by other question forms involving 'where?', 'which?', 'whose?', 'when?' and so on. The question forms involving 'how?' and/or 'why?' may come up fairly slowly (or not at all unless provoked) in children with autistic disorders. It is useful for parents to make a current inventory on the types of question forms their child is predominantly using in day-to-day conversations before commencing a programme for training exclusively in those forms wherein he appears to be deficient.

## Activity Cluster # 6e: Comprehension of Contrasts

From the early toddler phase, children need to be exposed to a variety of opposites. The contrasts may be any of the following categories, viz., positional (up–down, here–there, front–back, inside–outside, near–far, left–right, north–south–east–west, above–below, top–bottom) (C16; C17; C23; C24; C29; S50); aesthetic (nice–not nice, good–bad–ugly) (C28); action (give–take, yes–no, on–off, come–go, sit–stand, open–close) (C14; C27); relational/order (father–mother, uncle–aunt, son–daughter, grandpa–grandma, boy–girl, man–woman); dimensional (big–small, little–greater, heavy–light, thick–thin, more–less, few–many, heavy–light); directional (far–near) and temporal (fast–slow, now–sooner–later), respectively (Table 5.13).

## Activity Cluster # 7: Communication-expression

The activities listed (Table 4.6) serve as a general hierarchical guide for teachers attempting to improve on basic expressive-language competencies of preschool children. Obviously, the list does not take into account all aspects of speech-language development like articulation, intonation, sentence length, vocabulary, grammar, semantics, etc. Admittedly, a well-made speech therapeutic programme takes into account all these and many more correlated aspects of expressive language. For example, a particular strategy for toddlers with specific delays in speech-language development can involve the parents making out a list of words that the child actually uses in day-to-day conversation. If it is observed that there is predominance in the use of noun forms in the linguistic repertoire of a child, specific efforts must be expended to enhance his use of verb forms (action words), adjectives, pronouns and so on.

Expressive language refers to facial, vocal or gesture responses of the child during the communication process. Children with expressive-language disorders show lower than their mental-age level sentence-word-sound production skills in spite of almost adequate receptive/comprehension skills. They may compensate their lack of speech by extensive use of demonstration, gestures, mime or non-speech vocalizations. It is not unusual to encounter expressive-language age levels of some children that are relatively lower than their receptive-language age levels by a measure of few months/years. In any case, these children are unable to perform activities that require them to name or verbalize responses. Many problems between trainers and their children are the result of flawed lines of communication in the dyadic relationship (Table 5.5). The teacher intends one thing in his or her communication; the child understands it in a completely different sense. It is relevant to look into some of these adult foibles before pointing an accusing finger at children for their poor comprehension skills (Table 5.6). Expressive language proceeds through three distinct phases, viz., nominal level through descriptive level to interpretative level, as described earlier.

---

**Table 5.5**

**Characteristics of 'Good' Instructions in Adult–Child Dyad of Communication**

'Good' instructions to ensure candid comprehension in young children and toddlers must follow the following guidelines:

1.  Secure the child's attention before passing any command or instruction.
2.  Be brief, firm (not loud), clear and precise in the instruction.
3.  If possible, use excessive gestures and physical/body language in accompaniment with verbal instructions when conversing with young children. Mime, pantomime, drama and expression have greater impact than dull or drab utterances.
4.  Use positive instructions of 'do this!' more frequently than negative instructions of 'don't do this!' when it comes to dealings with younger children. 'Sit in one place!' is preferable to 'don't keep running around the room!'.
5.  Praise your child or give rewards every time he or she follows an instruction. By the same token, do not reward when he or she is non-compliant.
6.  Never give instructions that you yourself are unable or not prepared to enforce. For example, an empty threat that the child would never be allowed to watch television, hereafter followed by compassionate regret and over-yielding, will assure the child that you do not mean what you say.
7.  Never make prophecy-fulfilling instructions. 'I know, you are like your father who gets angry at the very sight of this dish … now, you don't get angry!' This statement invites the child to get angry and fulfil the expected role model of an angry father.

---

## Activity Cluster # 7a: Levels of Language Expression

Expressive language begins with babbling vowel sounds in young infants (such as a-e-i-o-u) which has to be encouraged by imitating the child's utterance (C4). Later, the child is motivated to imitate sounds of pets, vehicles, machinery (C10; P22) etc., along with their simple beginning word utterances (C8), repetition of songs/rhymes (C21; P24) or allied sequences of actions (C31). Often repeated radio/TV commercials, advertisements or songs (C35) come handy in the interests of the young toddler.

Parents need provide special encouragement towards building narrative abilities of toddlers. Summarizing, paraphrasing, relating and narrating witness accounts of day-to-day events is a crucial practice required for all toddlers. Asking the child to recount what happened during an outing, or on a visit to a store, or the playhouse, or while visiting a friend's house, etc., may be routinely carried out. The actual nature or contents of the personalized events may vary. What is important is that the toddler must have an opportunity for making such verbal expressions in the presence of encouraging adult listeners. During this stage, the child may come up with bits of make-believe or fictitious content (C38) which parents are advised against snubbing or ridiculing. An advanced form of narration could even involve relating a joke in front of a household audience. These narratives can be carried out in person or on the telephone (C39).

Another way of viewing the levels of language expression in young children is the kind of meanings they give to specific terms. For example, when asked 'what is ball?', there are two levels of verbal responses that may be expected. At level one (preschool years), the child may give only 'usefruct' responses (C37), such as 'ball is what we play with', or 'spoon is what we

---

**Table 5.6**

**Common Errors in Adult–Child Dyad of Communication**

**Recognition of individual differences**

No two children are identical. Therefore, direct comparison between two or more children is best avoided. Even though two children may be chronologically/mentally at the same level or class, this does not justify any comparison between them. Each child has his or her own pace of learning and doing things. It is best to recognize these differences and tune oneself to every given child's pace of learning.

**Avoid comparisons**

Implicit in the above proposition is the truth that no child would like to be compared with another for better or worse. A teacher may intend well in comparing a poorly performing child with another better performing child as a model for the first child to emulate. However, in actuality, this may imply a comparison that is resented by the child against the other child. The result could then be a greater tragedy.

**Avoid verbose instructions**

Instructions given to children during any teaching assignment must be necessarily brief. It is always advisable to provide only one instruction at a time. A chain of instructions like: 'get dressed, brush you teeth, have your breakfast, phone grandma before going to school!' can be quite a complex 'information overload' for young children. It is suggested that tasks requiring a chain of activities are best sliced or broken down into smaller parts and instructions are given separately thereof.

**Avoid vague instructions**

Instructions given to children also needs to precise and specific. Often we assume we are being very exact in our instructions with children. Indeed, we are not. Consider the example of a mother telling her child: 'very good!' on observing the daughter's colouring book. However, her timing and precision was lost in the fact that the child was biting her nails when the comment was made! A definitive comment from the mother would have been: 'very good! You have coloured so well!'.

**Avoid question form instructions**

Some of us are accustomed to giving instructions in question form. 'Would you get some milk from the fridge for me?', or 'Would you now do your homework?' and so on. The problem with this kind of instruction is that the child can always say 'no!'. The opportunity for behavioural refusal is invited unwittingly by the adult.

**Avoid explanatory instructions**

Another form of communication anomaly between adults and children is the explanatory type of instructions from the former. 'Clean up your room and start doing your homework soon because you know very well that your class teacher will punish you if you do not do your homework ...!'. The problem in these instructions is that the main message gets garbled in the volley of instructions

**Make it a private affair**

Conveying displeasure, reprimands or negative instructions is a serious business. It is best done privately, but not secretly. In their zeal to discipline children, many parents end up conveying negative instructions in public. Any child would not only resent this, but also would generally end up doing just the opposite of what he or she is being told—only to negate their perceived parental oppression! Further, parents should also avoid arguing, fighting, quarrelling or disagreeing between themselves—especially in front of their own children. There may be differences between parents that need to be resolved. Resolve them by all means. But it should be done privately, outside the purview of the child.

---

eat with' or 'pencil is what we write with' and so on. Beyond the preschool years, responses to the same question transgress beyond giving mere 'uses' of objects or things (Cg45). For example, the answer to the same question may be: 'ball is round in shape ... made of rubber', or that 'pencil is made of wood', or 'spoon is made of stainless steel or plastic ... with scoop and handle'. Preschoolers need to be stimulated to cross over from 'usefruct' modes of verbal operations to beyond by repeated quizzing activities.

## Activity Cluster # 7b: General/Personal Information

Call it a social skill or a language skill, but the child's knowledge and expression of at least some grains of general/personal information is a required inclusion in the preschool curriculum. The child must be able to give details about himself or herself wherein the situation demands. Giving details about name (including surname), age (C34), names of home town, city or village (C40), state or country (C45), giving occupational details of parents (C47), important places of interest in the native town/village (Cg 49) and complete residential address (C50) are pragmatic social-communication skills that need to be taught to all preschool children. In contrast, the child should also be trained to seek information from others, such as asking for a route, the time, permission, etc. (C48).

## Activity Cluster # 8: Social and Play

The development of social skills (interwoven with play skills) constitutes a major area of child development. Deficits, delays or disturbance in social behaviours may either be the cause or consequence of DDs in toddlers and young children. Their felt linguistic, preacademic and/or academic failures distance them from their age peers in many social-play situations. It may be that their social-play skills are deficient, thereby leading to non-acceptance by their peers, or it may be that other children are not accommodating to their vagaries in social situations. In any case, there is need for supervised social activities and superintended preparatory play for these children during their interaction with their peers. More often, such difficulties are multiplied by attitude malformations in caregivers rather than due to inherent impairments of these children.

Man has long been recognized as a social animal. The human infant shows a natural propensity towards pro-social behaviours beginning with spontaneous smiles, eye gaze (S18) and anticipatory motor responses to being picked up by caregivers or crying responses when left unattended. Later, acquired social skills include responses to own name (C3) by turning head, gesticulating 'bye-bye' (GM9), identifying members of the immediate family (C20), indulging in co-operative activities and so on. The typical social responses that can be expected of a child vary with the age/stage of social development.

Play is an important medium for social development in young children. It is a 'voluntary activity engaged for the enjoyment it gives without consideration of the end result' (Piaget, 1962). Play is also a medium through which the child is 'instinctively prepared to take up the role of adulthood' (Jeffree et al., 1977). For younger infants and toddlers, play may simply be a means of 'expending surplus energy ... a method used by children to relieve certain powerful experiences and thus come to terms with them' (Lansdown, 1985). Some investigators have viewed that play 'recapitulates the history of their race', or that it serves an 'adaptive function'. While one may write endlessly on various definitions of play, its importance in the overall development of children can be hardly discounted. Play activities can serve as a recreational as well as a propaedeutic task (Peshawaria et al., 1991). There are many types of play observed in children depending on their age/developmental levels (Venkatesan, 2000) (Table 5.7).

Play activities for kids need to be fostered age appropriately. Obviously, infants' level of autistic play by clasping both fists together and banging at own mouth (GM4) will not appreciate

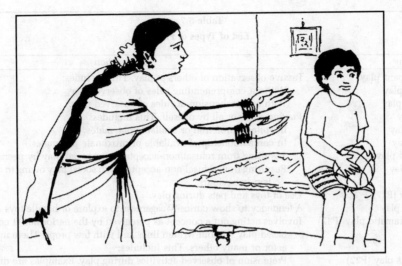

**Illustration 5.19 Mother Calls to Boy Holding a Ball**

the stimulation derived by an older child from doll/pet play. Dragging furniture to make loud noises or banging an object (P1)—a self-stimulatory play activity for beginning toddlers—becomes a source of irritation for an older child. Playing pat-a-cake (P2) or being excited with shadow play (P4) may not evoke the same excitement for an older child who has reached a stage of rule-based kindergarten play (P36). A sample list of play activities is included under Table 4.7. They range from solitary activities like skipping (P5), sliding (P12) and tunnelling (P19) to group activities like leap-frog games (P26), running to catch peers (P34), hide-and-seek games (P35), games of 'freeze/statue' (P39), blindman's-buff (P40), hop-scotch (P44), etc. Preschoolers can be exposed to indoor games like carom (P29), snakes and ladders or elementary card games (P46).

Many caregivers mistakenly consider play as invariably interwoven with the purchase or use of expensive toys, gadgets and teaching aids. Children with DDs require a specific pre-programme of activities to advance their play skills directly and/or their social skills indirectly. These children show marked discrepancies in what is termed as 'pre-social skills' which seemingly appear spontaneously in normal kids and toddlers. Caregivers need to undertake specific pre-training programmes for targeting these skills before embarking on formal training programmes on APCC-DD. Most play and social skills in normal or non-disabled children seemingly develop so spontaneously or effortlessly that no one generally gives a thought about how they are acquired. One realizes the difficulties and challenges involved in the acquisition of these skills only when one interacts with special children. The acquisition of play/social skills in children with special needs pose unique challenges. The limitations imposed by their sensory, physical, intellectual, emotional, social and environmental factors cause considerable deviations or dysfunctions in these children. Additionally, the negative attitudes of others (including parents, caregivers and teachers), faulty expectations (or overexpectations), lack of appreciation of their special needs and difficulties, etc., hinder the smooth development of these skills in children with disabilities.

**Table 5.7**
**List of Types of Play**

| Type of Play | Description |
|---|---|
| Non-participant play | Passive observation of others at play. This includes: |
| Onlooker play | Without comprehending rules of observed play. |
| Spectator play | With comprehension of rules of observed play. |
| Solitary play | Playing alone or all by oneself. This includes: |
| Autistic play | In spite of preferred or available playmates. |
| Parallel play | In companionship of available or proximate playmates. |
| Segregated play | Resulting from refusal/non-acceptance in social play by peers. |
| Isolated play | Resulting from refusal/non-acceptance in social play owing to child's problem behaviours. |
| Toy/pet play (P17) | Use of toys and pets during play. |
| Exploratory play | A tendency to show curiosity/eagerness to explore or handle toys and/or pets. |
| Symbolic/Dramatic play (P37) | Involves acting out a concept as perceived by the performer. It contains rule-based play without written lines and with few props. There may be a lone actor or many others. This includes: |
| Pretentious play (P22) | Pretension of observed activities during play. Examples are drinking milk from cup, eating with spoon, going to sleep, eating chocolates, etc. |
| Representational play | Use of surrogates to represent objects or situations in play. Examples, leaves as money, wooden block as car, spoon as oar, etc. |
| Enactive play | Role-play entire sequences of behaviour of various persons or situations observed around. Example, playing a teacher, father, mother, bus driver, etc. |
| Relational play | Shows ability to relate two or more objects as going together during play situations. Examples are bat and ball, pen and paper, spoon and cup, etc. |
| Social/Associative play | Participatory play with same-aged, younger or older peers occurring at co-operative or competitive levels. This includes: |
| Co-operative pre-rule/ Imitation play | With mutual imitation of play activities and not necessarily governed by complete understanding of their rules by the players. Examples are running, jumping, climbing, sliding, etc. |
| Co-operative rule-based/ Exercise play | With full understanding of rules governing them. Examples are chasing, catching hopscotch, etc. |
| Competitive play | Involving formal rules and active competition between players, either indoor or outdoor. Examples are, chess, carom, cricket, volleyball, tennis, etc. |

**Case Vignettes**

Rahim, a six-year-old diagnosed with mild developmental delay, has difficulty speaking in sentences. He can occasionally utter only some monosyllables which are hardly understood by most people around him except probably his mother! He loves to play with other children of his age and goes near them even though he only half understands what they are playing. The other children do not allow him to play with them and he is left alone to fend for himself.

Rajni, a five-year-old diagnosed with autistic disorder, performs most activities according to her age. Clinical psychologists have measured her intelligence as 'average'. Rajni refuses to look into the eyes of other people when they talk to her. She seems to be in a world of her own despite being put in the company of other children. While children of her age played together, she preferred solitary play. She did not protest if other children took away her belongings.

Rachna, a four-year-old, was on a holiday from the Middle East to her native place in Kerala along with her parents. During her stay, relatives noticed that Rachna was unduly reticent. She did not mix with children of her age. In a group, it was seen that she played by herself rather than with others. She showed poor eye-to-eye contact in conversation with others. She could sometimes speak long sentences, but they were parrot-like repetitions of adult speech or TV commercials, rattled off mechanically and out of context. She appeared cold, aloof, reserved and did not mix in group situations. An inquiry into Rachna's life in Dubai revealed that since her birth, she was brought up almost in isolation. Her parents were both working and she was reared mostly by a baby-sitter at home. She would be fed punctually and tucked away in front of a television or in bed. There was no opportunity for her to interact with her peers. The parents had only weekends to spare for their child—which was also spent on an outing.

The special problems of children with DDs in relation to their social-play activities distance them from their age peers. Either they do not go to their peers or their peers do not find them interesting enough to reciprocate their pro-social attempts. They require supervised play or group activities. Adults need to prompt these children to participate in social/play activities just as non-disabled peers are encouraged to accommodate to the special needs of these children. In this context, integrated education of the disabled seems to be the most relevant strategy for the mutual benefit of disabled and normal children. The prerequisite and/or associated skills to be fostered during or through play in children with DDs are listed under Table 5.8. There are specific activities, training schedules, play procedures, supervised group activities and guided play therapy that needs to be used in the teaching of each of these skills. These strategies are discussed below.

**Table 5.8**
**Associated Areas Related to Social Skills Training**

| | |
|---|---|
| Hearing and listening skills* | Turn-taking skills |
| Looking and seeing skills* | Recognition of body language/expressions |
| Pointing skills* | Sharing skills |
| Eye Gaze-ETE contact skills* | Greeting skills |
| Observation skills* | Elementary safety and first aid skills |
| Imitation skills | Manners/etiquette |
| Procrastination skills | Waiting skills |
| Empathy-sympathy | Participation in group play |
| Recognition of self-others belongings | Social smile |
| Keeping secrets | Pretend cheating in games |
| Guiding younger peers in games | Detecting breach of rules in games |
| Use of leisure | Humour |

Note: *Indicate activity clusters that have been discussed earlier.

## Activity Cluster # 8a: Social Smile

Smiling is the most basic and initial social response of infants. Although smiles appear spontaneously in many disabled children, they are actually learnt through social interactions with the mother. Try to get the eye contact of the infant. Look directly into the child's eyes. Talk to the child pleasantly and keep smiling spontaneously. When the child smiles back, respond with a hug or kiss. More and more people (or faces) need to smile and establish emotional connectivity with the child (S18). Young children, siblings, adults, grandparents, cousins and other people need to show their smiling faces in front of the infant. Gradually, children learn to smile at familiar faces or even reach out for their faces to touch or feel them.

Do not hide or shy away the child with disability from contact with others. This decreases opportunity for social stimulation. Many times parents attempt these exercises for some trials and when the smiling response is not forthcoming within the expected number of attempts, they discontinue their efforts. This is another type of under-stimulation suffered by infants with disabilities as compared to their non-disabled peers. The non-disabled infant soon responds with a smile that reinforces others to play with him more. Since the same type or amount of social response is not forthcoming in children with disabilities, others are also not motivated to stimulate the child. This vicious cycle needs to be broken. Avail all opportunities to expose the child to new places, persons, faces, events, relatives, friends, festivals, etc. All this encourages the infant to develop better social responses and lays a firm foundation for their later robust social development. Social smiles of young infants are distinguished from later development of loud laughter. Tickling games foster loud laughter in children. These activities are eventually the basis for later development of a sense of humour in children, or even as adults.

The roots of social apathy or non-responsiveness in later years may be traced to the early formative years when the child has been left alone by a 'busy' or 'un-attending' mother, or mothers who have been emotionally 'cold' or 'aloof' in their early interactions with their infants. It is not sufficient that mothers merely play the role of a 'nourisher' by providing food periodically to a hungry infant. There is more to building on motherhood—an emotional contact in the mother–child dyad that lays the foundation stone for later development of a strong emotional edifice in the child with disabilities. Most women can *become* mothers, but only a few can *be* mothers!

## Activity Cluster # 8b: Greeting Skills

A starting greeting skill in young children is waving of the arms to say 'bye-bye' or 'ta-ta' (GM9). The infant is still incapable of uttering these words. He can at least perform these actions in accompaniment to adult utterances of these words. Take every opportunity of people leaving the house to wave 'bye-bye' or 'ta-ta' repeatedly. Initially, the adult may have to take the child's hands and literally wave the action. Gradually, the child learns to do it on his or her own, or even with an associated verbalization. Much later, more complex greeting skills to be taught to toddlers may require showing or saying 'good morning!', 'good evening!', 'good night!', 'Adaab!', 'Sat Sri Akaal!', or any other native expressions of courtesies like 'please/thank you' (C36).

## Activity Cluster # 8c: Self and Other Recognition

At birth, no child knows his own name. The repeated use of a name in front of the child conditions him or her to an understanding that it is his or her name. The processes of knowing and/or responding to one's own name (C3) is also an elaborate and sequential process that is developed through arduous learning in young infants. Initially, you may have to repeatedly keep using the child's name during each and every activity that is being carried on or along with the child, like 'Raju! Take this!', 'Raju! Look here!', 'Raju! Come!', 'Raju! Eat this!', and so on. It is almost a sort of a running commentary on the child's activities along with an utterance of his name (or pet name). This can be simultaneously attempted with activities involving the child pointing to self upon utterance of his or her name. 'Where's Raju?' The mother takes the child's hand in hers and points to the child himself with 'This is Raju!'. Each exchange should be followed by a reward such as a hug, smile and/or kiss for the child. On the whole, it should be an enjoyable or pleasurable experience for the child. The awareness or skill to *point to self on name call* (C6) is an important prerequisite for teaching *names or relationships of others in the family* (C20). The child must be taught to point to other members in the family for questions like 'Who's mummy?', 'Who's daddy?', 'Who's uncle?', etc. The child must be then taught to become proficient in recognizing/pointing to self and others in individual photographs as well as group photographs. All these exercises on self and other recognition is an important requirement for later teaching body parts, including left–right orientation.

## Activity Cluster # 8d: Recogniton of Self-Others' Belongings

An extension of knowledge or awareness about oneself is the recognition of one's own and others' belongings (P28). At an early stage, children learn to become possessive about their own belongings. They respond with an emphatic 'mine!' for every question like 'whose frock is this?' or 'whose mummy is this?' or 'whose nose is this?' and so on (C13). There may be a wave of protest behaviour to arguing or confronting 'No! It's my frock!' or 'No! It's my mummy!' and so on. Some children even end up by throwing mild 'tantrums' unless what they perceive as the 'intruder' takes back his or her words. This is a positive and age-appropriate behaviour during the pre-toddler/toddler stages. However, in case of children with autistic disorders, this possessive awareness of one's own belongings is conspicuous by their absence, sometimes even beyond the toddler phase. Even as he or she sees others take away his or her belongings, the child does not register any protest. He bears a countenance of 'indifference' or 'startling unconcern'! A training programme on fostering these skills should repeatedly bring it to the notice of the child that various things or items belong to him or her, or they are better named along with the name of a family member. An opportunity to carry out this exercise is available while folding clothes. The mother can fold each garment and relate it to the name of its user. 'This is mummy's dress!', or 'This is papa's shirt!' or 'This is Dolly's frock!' and so on. At the preschool or play home, teachers could insist the children deposit their belongings at a particular place immediately after reporting at school only to identify them as and when required to do so. At a much later stage, the child may also need to be trained into respecting others' belongings. The child should be taught that the permission of others is required before their belongings can be used, as also that they must be returned safely after their use. He or she should know to thank them appropriately. This skill can be prepared by incorporating several instances wherein the child is guided to request others for their belongings like pencils, erasers, books, etc.

## Activity Cluster # 8e: Procrastination Skills

Procrastination skills are an important ingredient of early social skills. Infants have a strong urge for instantaneous gratification of their needs. A pang of hunger is to be met instantaneously by feeding activity. A parched thirst has to be quenched at once. Any delay in need gratification is intolerable and catastrophic within the phenomenological perception of the child. However, with increasing age, children learn to delay gratification owing to an expansion in their subjective perception of time. Nevertheless, children differ in the extent of time to which they can delay gratification of their needs. In any case, an optimum time lag or waiting sense is an important prerequisite to listening and/or comprehension of instructions by the child. The child should be able to wait at least until a set of instructions are passed on by the tutor. He must comprehend the difference between 'now!' and 'later!' 'Have your breakfast *now*!', or 'We shall be going out *later*!' A lack of clear understanding of these verbal expressions by the child has often become the root cause of many parental frustrations over not being able to convince their child to bear with fortitude. Children with DDs appear to be ever in a hurry. They hardly seem to wait till the entire set of commands or instructions are passed on for any given activity. This may result in errors or incomplete performance of target activities. Therefore, the procrastination training schedule is optimally required to slow down the hurrying child before commencing on a programme of skill remediation. This can be accomplished by adopting simple techniques whereby the child's wants are delayed for varying periods of time between a few seconds to a few minutes. A counting up to some specific number (say, three or five) or the ring of a bell may be used to postpone wish gratification over time. The training programme on waiting skills can be incorporated during meal times, play, conversation, shopping, etc.

## Activity Cluster # 8f: Imitation

Imitation or modelling is a powerful tool in teaching or acquisition of pro-social skills in children. Play becomes the most powerful medium for expression of their imitation skills. Beginning from rudimentary pro-social behaviours like social smiles, giggles and loud laughter; the young infant progresses through activities like pointing to self and/or other significant others upon name calls. The infant learns to recognize facial emotions and expressions of others. A frown is differentiated from a smile. Disgust is not the same as amazement, anger, grief and sadness. Body language, postures and gesticulations of others is also appreciated an understood. While many normal or non-disabled children seem to imitate spontaneously, children with mental retardation, autistic disorders and learning disorders may lose opportunities for normal peer interaction and hence imitation. The imitations of these children become objects of burlesque, parody and rejection owing to their primary impairments. They reflect deficient social play skills, not so much due to any inherent blemish, rather as a consequence of negative attitudes of peers and fellow mates. Imitation games are encouraged in group situations, wherein the deficient child is guided (albeit subtly) to do as other children are doing around him or her (P25). 'Try jumping like Mona!', 'Try reading the newspaper like papa!' or 'Try saying your prayers like grandma!' is a common refrain of many households who enthrall themselves in the childish mimicry of the young toddler (P9). Group work, singing or dancing (P6; P21) induce imitation in toddlers.

## Activity Cluster # 8g: Sharing Skills

Sharing (P23) is a vital ingredient of most social activities in children and adults. The ability to share things develops in toddlers only after the skill to recognize their own belongings has manifested at least to some extent. The child who does not discriminate between his or her own and others' belongings is unlikely to share in the true sense. He may be just giving away things without the same sense of magnanimity or unselfishness that is the hallmark of sharing behaviours. With increasing competitiveness in the contemporary generation, and parental obsessions on their child not loosing out in the race with fellow peers, the value of teaching sharing behaviours is being minimized. The joy of shared group work is being nipped at the bud itself in many play schools. The results can be catastrophic, since each child will become self-centred and selfish. From a very young age, children can be encouraged to share their toys other things with fellow peers and family members. Every occasion for eating an evening snack can be converted into a teaching session/activity for the toddler to go around the house and distribute the edibles to every member in the family. 'Give this piece to papa!', 'Give this piece of cake to granny!', 'Give this piece to sister!' and so on. A sensitive balance needs to be struck between the child's willingness to share things with others and his appreciative sense of belonging or possession about some articles as his own. Older children can be even taught to nurture younger peers during play or feeding time (P41).

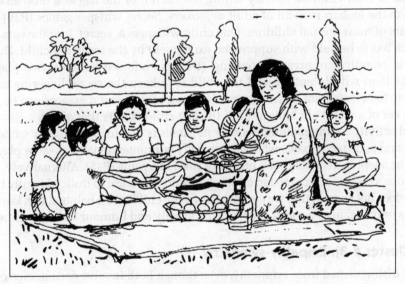

**Illustration 5.20  Sharing Skills**

## Activity Cluster # 8h: Turn-taking Skills

Many occasions for social action require temporary postponement of self-gratification (procrastination skills) as also waiting patiently for one's turn in the group. Whether the occasion is one of getting into a bus in a queue, or to purchase tickets at a counter, throwing dice in a board game, or just about anywhere, the child needs to be oriented that there are turns to be awaited (P10). Indeed, some children may infringe rules and break out of turn in a group play situation. The child should be made aware that this is inappropriate. He or she must not only take notice of such transgressions, but also be taught to protest against it. The child must learn to chide the erring companion (P20). Children deficient in social skills seem either not to take notice of it or are not moved enough to register their protest. Adults guiding social-skill training programmes should contrive such social situations and see that the reticent child comes out of his shell to assert himself adequately in such group situations.

## Activity Cluster # 8i: Keeping Secrets

It is just as important a social skill for young children to approach others (even strangers) and strike up a conversation effectively as it is to keep to oneself to an appropriate degree. The child should be aware of the limits of self-disclosure permitted in each and every relationship. Therefore, the child must have adequate personal information about him or herself, his or her family and the immediate neighbourhood (C34; C40; C45; C47; C50). Over disclosure of details about oneself or others can prove hazardous in competitive social existence. The child needs to be continually made aware of what to talk to others as also how much to talk to others outside the family. Certain adult secrets need to be confined to parents only. They should not be discussed in front of the child. Otherwise, some parents may have to face the consequence of their children naively letting the cat out of the bag at a most inappropriate time much to the embarrassment of adult onlookers. Secret whisper games (P39) are within the repertoire of most normal children. One child whispers a 'secret' into the ears of another child, which has to be held with suppressed excitement by the receiving child. During game situations, a 'secretive connivance cheating' (P48) is endorsed between two players, more out of a joke than with intention, and the child is to keep the secret lingering on for some time much to the excitement of the players. In group play, secret messages can be whispered from ear to ear of a chain of children until the last child shouts that aloud.

A related activity for maintaining secrecy in games is playing foul. In any game situation, there are bound to be participants who, intentionally or unintentionally, cheat or play foul. Your child must be adept in detecting such breach of rules in a game (P45). Alternatively, if one does not stretch one's code of ethics too far, children should also learn to frolic playfully by cheating (P48). This does not suggest that we convert the young child into a habitual liar, law-breaker or cheater. It is only meant as a social skill to bring vitality and humour within a game situation.

## Activity Cluster # 8j: Empathy-sympathy

Empathy is distinguished from sympathy, even though both involve consonance of emotions between two individuals. Sympathy implies that you are subjectively carried away by the condition of the other suffering person. Whereas empathy implies that you are capable of retaining some amount of objectivity regarding the problems and sufferings of the affected person. In allegorical terms, empathy involves getting into the shoes of another person knowing well that the footwear still belongs to the other person. On the other hand, sympathy implies getting into the shoes of the other affected person and assuming them to be your own! Young toddlers are unable to see the world in the perspective of others. They can only see their world, as it appears to them. Without understanding this simple but apparent truth, many adults foist their own perspectives on their children without much success. The mother who pulls her daughters hair in retaliation by saying, 'Now! You will know that this is how it pains!' is trying a futile exercise to communicate her pain. The child is not going to comprehend the pain. Rather, she is going to repeat the misbehaviour once again by imitation of the mother.

## Activity Cluster # 8k: Manner and Etiquette

Manners and etiquette are a matter of relative local customs and norms in different societies. Nevertheless, all human groups have some common denominators of behaviour that are designated as acceptable or unacceptable. From the early formative years, toddlers have to be modelled on those patterns of behaviours that are considered to be socially acceptable. These behaviours could relate to sitting, standing, eating (SH18), greeting, talking, dressing or addressing people, etc. The child is to be taught feeling a sense of shame for appearing dressed shabbily and/or undressed in public, in cultures where it is considered so. He or she is encouraged to make bold but courteous inquiries about a route, bus timings, permission from strangers, etc. (C48).

## Activity Cluster # 8l: Elementary Safety and First-aid Skills

Self care (P47) is an important dimension of social skills in toddlers. The young child should be trained to recognize or realize familiar or common dangers. The child should be aware of the consequences of touching a hot plate, live electric wires, toxic substances, hanging on dangerous places and perilous heights, and playing with fire, crackers, blades, knives or sharp objects. It is one thing for toddlers to have a bitter experience and then learn lessons from them; it is another thing for elders to demonstrate the perils of such endeavours before the child falls prey to them. There is no wisdom in parents attempting to restrict opportunities of children by not exposing them to these so-called 'danger objects'. Some parents of children with DDs do not ever give their children activities involving lighting matchsticks, cutting using a pair of scissors, use of blade or sharpener to sharpen pencils. The denial of these opportunities becomes an impediment for their learning to use these items safely. It has been found that even children with severe handicaps can and do learn to light a candle or use matchsticks provided they are trained safely under supervision. In this context, an extent of training on reading symbols is also relevant for preschoolers. The child should be oriented to identify symbols depicting 'danger' (human skull), 'poison', traffic signals involving 'zebra crossing', holographs depicting 'silence zone', etc. The next aspect of training in safety skills is basic first aid. What must be done if you have a cut? What must be done when you have a fall while running? What ought to be done when you accidently touch a hot plate? The child must know the practical skills of such first-aid management. If possible, the child should also be in a position to guide younger peers on these lessons (P41). A lot of accidents that toddlers suffer can be prevented before they occur—if only adults take certain precautions and also follow some of the guidelines given under Table 5.9.

## Activity Cluster # 8m: Leisure

Correct and constructive self-deployment of leisure (P49) is a vital social skill to be fostered early in the daily regime of toddlers. That an unoccupied mind is a devil's workshop has been long recognized. The peril of an 'unemployed mind' is greater in children with DDs. Either owing to paucity of social skills and/or non-acceptance by age peers, they are at odds in the profitable engagement of leisure time. Further, the development of this social skill requires the child to transgress from external reinforcement to internal or self-reinforcing

Table 5.9
Ten-point Safety Charter for Toddlers

Every year, hundreds of toddlers are injured—sometimes fatally. Often, accidents happen in the presence of adult caregivers. An elementary course of safety skills is an important ingredient in the preschool curriculum of children with DDs. Some common areas for inclusion as part of the curriculum on safety skills for young children are:

1. Electricity: The toddler is made aware of the perils in handling electrical gadgets, touching live electric wires, inserting fingers or sticks into plug sockets, etc.
2. Kitchen: The kitchen is an usual accident spot for toddlers. The child is taught not to play or jump around in the kitchen/cooking area. He or she is made aware of the dangers of touching hot pans/plates, peeping into boiling oil, use of knives/forks and mixer blades, drinking kerosene, etc.
3. Bathroom: The child is to understand dangers of ingesting soaps or detergents; precautions should be taken for checking geysers, hot water baths, etc.
4. Food: There are dangers in toddlers aspirating several foods. They are taught not to talk or laugh while eating, not to put too much food into the mouth, gulp water in large mouthfuls, etc. Children below five should not be given edibles which might choke them.
5. Toys: Toddlers are to be given only age-appropriate toys. Toys with small detachable parts can be ingested by young children. Avoid toys with paints that peel off or may be ingested by toddlers.
6. Baby walkers are best avoided for beginning toddlers. Research has shown that babies who have been given walkers do not walk any more quickly than those not given such aids. There is a danger of toddlers running into furniture or tumbling down the stairs while using baby walkers. Seating them as pillion on bicycles carries the risk of letting their legs get into the spokes of the running wheels.
7. Medicines: Tablets, medicines or drugs must be kept out of reach of young children. They may consume them thinking that they are some kind of sweets. They must be taught that they should not swallow such objects when found in their vicinity.
8. Play: Preschoolers are strongly advised against playing on roads, rooftops or such other non-playing areas in the neighbourhood. They are to be taught the dangers of playing with plastic bags lest they suffocate themselves by wearing them over their heads.
9. Water: Even a small bucket of water can be more dangerous, if a child tumbles headlong into it, than the large expanse of a swimming pool or sea beach. Water sports are always best carried out only under adult supervision.
10. Travel: Adults should avoid carrying toddlers on two wheelers. Headgear or helmets are seldom made for children even if adults choose to protect themselves while riding vehicles. There is greater risk for head injury in toddlers than adults in case of road accidents.

activities. Initially, children work for extrinsic, external and/or tangible rewards, followed thereafter by a stage when they will work for internal/intrinsic rewards. Leisure-time activities for preschoolers can include lessons on environmental science, cleanliness of surroundings, tending plants or pets (Cg48), watering plants, feeding or nursing pets, avoiding pollution, picking up hobbies, sewing, philately, numismatics, etc.

## Activity Cluster # 8n: Humour

Humour is a successful lubricant in many social relationships. Humour eases strain on relationships that tend to rust over time. There are developmental stages in appreciation of humour. What seems humorous to one child at a lower stage may not appear so later. Similarly, adult humour is incomprehensible to children. It is indeed a rare and flexible talent available to some persons that they can cut across all ages and enjoy jokes of all sorts meant for all ages. However, in our interactions with toddlers, it is important to appreciate the stage of humour in a given child and create situations accordingly. At the earliest stage of infancy,

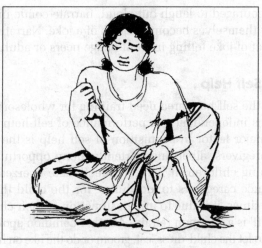

**Illustration 5.21  Sewing**

physical tickling elicits laughter in children (S24). Later, physical actions (acrobatics) invite giggles. Much later, physical incongruities (such as spoon used for writing, or pen for eating) seem humorous to toddlers. This turns into humour for verbal incongruities. Exaggerations induce humour in young children. In one phase, toddlers giggle as adults are annoyed by their actions. The child indulges in those actions that apparently annoy elders. These behaviours appear as acts of infringement in discipline as the child indulges in them for perceived 'fun'. The highest form of humour is when an individual sees himself objectively and is amused by his own infirmities, jealousies or unsocial desires (Table 5.10).

| Table 5.10 | |
| :---: | :---: |
| **List of Various Types of Humour** | |
| *Type of Humour* | *Descriptive Examples* |
| Physical incongruity | Asymmetries like wearing shoe with slippers, etc. |
| Physical stimulation | Tickles, itches, prickles, etc. |
| Exaggerated actions | Belching aloud, etc. |
| Annoying attention seekers | Gurgling, splashing. |
| Teasers | Making faces, gesticulations of persons or animals. |
| Mimicry | Imitation of others. |
| Cartoons | Hand sketches, animated or still pictorials. |
| Overriding authority | Imitating an authority figure, teacher, etc. |
| Vanquishing enemies | Getting even with expression of surrogate humour for unapproved aggression. |
| Comic humour | Laughing at infirmities of others. |
| Transgression of taboos | Sex jokes—outlet for repressed or unfulfilled impulses. |
| Contagious humour | Laughing because others are laughing. |
| Unexpected occurrences | A sudden 'boo'. |
| Peculiar, novel or unusual | Stimuli which are unusual, peculiar or novel arouse humour. |
| Age/sex inappropriate | Inappropriate or Incongruous events. |
| Personal/idiosyncratic | Depends on individual or personal experiences. |
| Laughing at self | Requires ability to see oneself objectively and be amused by one's infirmities, jealousies, un-social desires, etc. |

Toddlers must be encouraged to laugh out aloud, narrate comic incidents, mimic people or take sport when they themselves become objects of a joke. Narrative ability, as discussed earlier, is a crucial aspect of joke telling in front of age peers or adults.

## Activity Cluster # 9: Self Help

Activities pertaining to the self help area need training for wholesome development of toddlers. The child acquires independence in performance of self-help skills through discrete but definite stages. A major factor in acquisition of self help is the provision for learning opportunities. Many caregivers, albeit inadvertently, deny opportunities for learning self-help behaviours by young children. It may be affectionate overzealousness and/or brash overprotection that induce caregivers to 'do things' for the child than enable them to 'do things on their own'. At times, it is due to underestimation of their child's abilities. 'Ah! He's too small to help himself!' is a common refrain. Another common apology given by parents is that there is 'hardly time' to let the child 'dress, eat, groom or do the like on his or her own' during the daily morning bustle to see him or her off to the crèche or playschool. Although justified to some extent, self-help training can be made part of other teaching activities. Table 4.12 lists self-help activities in home training programmes for toddlers.

Self-help skills are often complained to be the most difficult activity to be achieved in toddlers. For example, their refusal to eat cooked food despite surprising preferences for snacks like chocolates, ice creams or biscuits baffles many mothers! Mothers need to introspect upon their feeding habits/practices to overcome these problems. There are many reasons for toddlers' food preferences. It could be an inexperienced mother's overexpectation on the child's food regime, quantity of food intake or timings. It could be one of the several factors that go into acquisition of problem behaviours by young children. Nonetheless, feeding is an important activity in the everyday life of toddlers. It is an occasion for establishing incisive bonding between the mother and child. The verbal exchange that goes on privately between the feeder and fed during the eating process is more crucial than even the food. For example, in children with autistic disorder having feeble eye-to-eye contact, the feeding event can be gainfully used as an occasion for training the deficient skill. The mother could insist before every mouthful that her child looks at her face/eyes. Shaping procedures lead to better eye gaze or contact during conversation, even in non-feeding situations. The distinction between a toddler *not knowing* to carry out a self-help activity and *not wanting* to do it is a very important observation for planning a skill behaviour remediation, or, alternatively, problem-behaviour management, programme. A deficit skill needs to be trained, and a refused behaviour needs to be disciplined.

## Activity Cluster # 9a: Eating

Eating or feeding skills begin by sucking, swallowing, munching, chewing, mastication, spitting, gargling or such other activities. Blowing (SH12) and sucking (SH14) are an important ingredient of most preliminary eating skills. The child should be exposed early to suck through feeding bottles around about the time when he or she is weaned from the mother's nipple. The skill to retain solids or liquids in the mouth (SH8) is an in-between skill between spitting (SH15) and gargling in young children. The toddler must be able to retain liquids without either gulping or spitting. He is then guided to either take the liquid 'in' or spit it 'out'. The child is led to independence in eating through small trifles like unwrapping candies by himself (SH6), holding cup or glass to drink by self, drinking through straw tumblers, eating biscuits from own hands, eating with spoon or fork or with own fingers, etc. There might be initial occasions when the child spills food. This should make the mother think of denying opportunity for the child to learn to eat by self. A large newspaper may be spread beneath the eating plate so that spilled food may be conveniently collected or cleaned.

**Case Vignette**

Anu, a four-year-old diagnosed with an autistic disorder, has a mother who is very fastidious about her child's eating habits. The mother has scheduled timings for feeding that have been scrupulously followed since Anu's birth. Even now, Anu is given only mashed food for fear of indigestion. There is regimented quantity on the menu, which is maintained lest the child becomes undernourished! No spicy foods are entertained, although the family is culturally prone to consume such foods. Snacks are strictly prohibited. No biscuits, chocolates, etc. Only, and only, home-made cooked items are allowed in the specified quantity or during scheduled timings. There were also unwritten rules on who was to feed the child (the mother alone!) or where it was to be done (in front of the television!). Otherwise, the elders at home feared, Anu would cry, throw tantrums and vomit.

Drooling (SH1) is a common problem in toddlers with disabilities, especially in children with cerebral palsy and/or mental retardation. The general weakness of oral musculature or oral malformations (as in Downs syndrome) may be aggravating this problem. Sometimes, a simple and repetitive instruction to continuously keep the mouth closed is sufficient to minimize drooling. But, a majority of these children require supportive oral exercises involving massaging of the lips (Activity Cluster 4f). The application of jam, honey or sweet syrup at the corner of lips so that the child attempts to smack them is a useful exercise to improve bucco-facial control. The child may be instructed periodically to wipe his or her mouth with a piece of cloth. Every small attempt on the part of your child should be consistently and clearly rewarded. Associated oral exercises should include activities involving swallowing (SH6), chewing (SH4), sucking (SH14), blowing (SH12; P11; P18), biting, spitting (SH15), etc. Rotating or sticking out the tongue, and rolling or bending it on imitation from a model can be a further example of oral exercises.

Discrimination of edibles and non-edibles (SH2) is to be exclusively practiced through simulated game activities. Place two or more edible and non-edible items in front of the child. Prompt the child to pick up these items. For the edible items mouthed by the child, being allowed to eat them amounts to a reward. For non-edibles attempted to be mouthed by the child, convey displeasure with a firm and loud 'No!' Conveying displeasure (also called 'reprimand') is not merely telling your child how not to behave. It also means telling your child how to behave. It must be implemented immediately following the target behaviour. The reprimand should be conveyed in a firm voice and with a serious countenance.

To facilitate the child to drink from a cup or glass unassisted (SH3), begin by using a tall glass (Table 5.11). Initially, the parent holds the glass to facilitate the necessary angle of tilt required to sip. Later, the child is taught to drink by holding the glass on own. Eating solid foods with own fingers (or hands) (SH11) precedes competencies for negotiating semi-solids and semi-liquids from a plate. Biscuits or broken pieces of bread may first be laid on a large plate so that the child learns to pick them up and put them into his or her mouth. Simultaneous training on pincer grasp (FM11) is required for learning this activity. Wherever possible, food is placed on the child's palm rather than into the mouth of the child. Still later, the child is trained on mixing food by using the hands (SH13). The skill for using spoon and fork (SH17; SH19) is both a motor and eating skill. It is advisable for parents to encourage their child with a handicap to eat in front of, or alongwith, other members of the family, friends or relatives. Many parents discourage their child from public eating for fear of raillery, ridicule or reprimand. They are apprehensive that the child may project a wrong image in front of others. This apprehension actually deprives the child of an opportunity to watch others eating and imitate them.

---

**Table 5.11**

**Illustrative Samples on Teaching Self-help Activities**

Sample Target Behaviour # 1: Rahim takes off his vest
Steps:

1. Pulls off vest covering his head.
2. Pulls off vest covering his face.
3. Pulls off vest covering about his shoulder.
4. Removes one hand from vest up to shoulders.
5. Removes second hand from vest up to shoulders.
6. Rolls up and pulls off vest around the armpits.

Sample Target Behaviour # 2: Ranjan pulls up elastic shorts on his own
Steps:

1. Pulls elastic shorts up from his thighs to cover front.
2. Pulls elastic shorts up from his thighs to cover back.
3. Pulls elastic shorts up from his knees.
4. Pulls elastic shorts up from below his knees.
5. Pulls elastic shorts up from his ankle.
6. Sits and inserts one leg into elastic shorts.
7. Sits and inserts both legs into elastic shorts.

Sample Target Behaviour # 3: Rajesh drinks from a glass unassisted
Steps:

1. Approaches a tall steel glass and grips it with both palms.
2. Raises steel glass up to his lips.
3. Tilts steel cup containing milk (or water) into mouth.
4. Takes one gulp and returns glass to table.
5. Repeats the same sequence for every gulp thereafter.

---

Blowing, spitting and swallowing (SH12;P11;P18;SH15;SH16) liquids are inter-related oral skills. They are all preceded by the child's skill to retain solids/liquids in the mouth (SH8). The child must be able to retain solid food in the mouth for some time without either swallowing or spitting it out. The child may not be able to retain liquids in the mouth with the same ease or competency. They are taught by tilting the head backward and pouring water into the mouth that is to be retained without gulping or spitting it. With a forward tilt the liquid is likely to spill out. These actions are accompanied with verbal instructions of 'in–out'

The child's inability to follow 'in–out' may also stem from a lack of language comprehension. In such a case, the child needs to be taught receptive language skills. A game requiring the toddler to jump 'in' a circle drawn on the floor and 'out' of it for specific or alternating instructions helps clarify the meanings of these opposites. Blowing can be taught through a variety of activities, such as blowing candles, musical instruments, light feather, thermacol, blowing soap bubbles, whistles, etc. Sucking (SH14) can be practised with the help of straw mugs or water bottles by instructing the child to inhale with one nostril closed. Other eating related activities could include drinking from a cup/glass unassisted (SH3), feeding oneself with solids (SH5) or routine food (SH11), mixing food with own hands (SH13), eating with spoon (SH17), knife and fork (SH19), eating seeded fruits (SH7), etc.

## Activity Cluster # 9b: Dressing

Dressing competencies need to progress simultaneously and gradually from the initial stages of passive co-operation by infants to wearing clothes by extending arms to caregivers. An active endeavour of babies begins with their taking of discomforting headwear (SH20) or other garments obstructing their line of vision. Most dressing skills in toddlers progress in reverse (backward chaining), beginning with mastery in removing dresses (SH21; SH22; SH23) before wearing them (SH27; SH30), unbuttoning before buttoning (SH24), unbuckling before buckling (SH26) and so on. Therefore, the training programme must proceed appropriately and according to this scheme.

Undressing when shirts have been already unbuttoned comes initially and easily (SH21). Pulling off a T-shirt or pullover vest come with more difficulty (Table 5.12). Likewise, taking off elastic shorts and pants are to be taught in progressively backward steps (SH23). The target behaviour is to be sliced into small and simple steps, and each step taught separately to the child. Unbuttoning and buttoning (SH25) skills are fairly complex fine motor activities. Trainers may begin by first introducing press buttons, hooks, velcro fasteners or knots, and then proceed to teach finger manipulation on large coat buttons and small shirt buttons (SH28). Unbuttoning (SH24) generally comes before buttoning skills. Tying knots (SH32) is required for many day-to-day activities, including tying shoelaces. Parents can begin with teaching children to tie a simple knot by placing a thread over the other. They are then practised on tying small objects, books, sheaves of papers, etc. The double knot, tie knot, reef knot or other types of knots may be introduced later. Buckling of sandals (SH26), belts, wristwatches, opening or closing umbrellas and other leather goods are also a skill in regular use for children. Grooming skills (SH33), applying hair oil/creams, combing, plaiting (in case of girls), using toiletries (SH29), talcum powder, etc., may also be included in the dressing training schedules of preschoolers. Using safety pins on own clothing is a special form of buttoning (SH31).

Although teaching all these fine motor activities overlapping on self-care skills is on the usual agenda for preschool children, there is one line of thought which opposes the training of these activities in children with physical disabilities. It is argued that children with cerebral palsy are loaded beyond their physical abilities to negotiate a button or unbutton their garments daily. Rather, it is an adaptive measure to don the child with a robe that does not require buttoning or unbuttoning at all. A haircut would resolve the tedium of plaiting hair for young girls with handicaps. They could be made to use footwear that does not require lacing. The intention is to make life simpler for the child with disability than to make his adjustment with non-disabled world mandatory. A list of dressing activities is given under Table 4.12.

**Table 5.12**

**Guidelines for Teaching Self-help Activities**

1. All children learn easily through small steps. Instead of teaching a self-help skill as a whole, it is apt to teach them in small or simple steps separately to achieve the end objective.
2. Different children require different levels of assistance on their way to learning an objective. Tune your teaching to that level appropriately.
3. The number of steps to lead to your objective in self-help areas cannot be fixed. It is to be tailor-made according to individual cases. Some children may require just three steps to learn a target self-help objective, while another child may require more steps to do the same.
4. There are different ways for proceeding to guide children along the identified route of small steps towards a particular behavioural objective. You could proceed from the last step to the first step in that sequence, or vice versa. In any case, do not forget to reward your child at the end of each step in the identified ladder of teaching tasks towards the behavioural objective.
5. Provide greater or active physical assistance, guidance or instruction initially while teaching a self-help objective. For example, you may have to maximally assist your child to hold the cup or glass while drinking water. Always associate physical guidance procedures along with a running commentary of verbal instructions on whatever activity is being taught to the child.
6. Gradually use more verbal prompts even as you simultaneously decrease physical prompts for the child. Much later, you may have to use only certain verbal or non-verbal cues, before fading them also eventually.
7. Be brief in your instructions while teaching self-care activities. Otherwise, the child will loose sight of the activity being taught in the volley of verbal instructions that you are giving.
8. Children learn a lot of behaviours by imitation. They imitate behaviours of persons whom they consider important. It may be their favourite teacher, parent, film star, friend, etc. Imitation becomes a powerful tool for teaching children self-help skills by demonstration.
9. Do not confuse imitation or modelling with comparison. No one likes to be compared with others, more so if the comparison is based on one's weakness. Avoid comparisons for good or bad. Use modelling as a means to demonstrate how or what your child is required to do while performing a skill behaviour.
10. If a complex series of activity is being taught, slice it into smaller steps or components and demonstrate each part separately. The model itself should be free from flaws or imperfections. Otherwise, the learner will imbibe the same errors in his learning too.
11. Privacy is a basic corollary to teaching dressing and toilet skills in toddlers. A playful utterance of 'Shame! Shame!' for every attempt by the child to undress in public will send signals that dressing or toilet activities need to be carried out in private or appropriate places.

## Activity Cluster # 9c: Toilet and Cleansing

The area of toilet training needs careful consideration by parents. There must be neither extreme fastidious stricture on toilet accidents, nor too permissive overindulgence during toilet-control practices. There is also a need for parents to set apart considerable time for teaching the act of defecation itself so that the child goes through the ritual in a relaxed manner without undue haste. Many bowel/bladder control disorders in toddlers have been ravages of psychological warfare between toddlers and caregivers developing from such negative experiences as apprehension, anxiety, guilt or antagonism to nature's call, rather than actual physiological reasons.

Toddlers need to be led through toilet training protocols whereby they learn to indicate toilet consistently with gestures/words (SH35), followed by activities involving sitting on the toilet seat (SH36), washing self when water is poured (SH39) or on one's own from a running tap (SH41), etc. Toilet training is a time-consuming process. Some amount of readiness is required before toilet control can be introduced for toddlers. The child should be able to communicate some wants either through gestures or words. Many parents mistake the facial grimaces or changes that accompany toilet sensations as the child's ability to indicate such needs. There is no communicative intent in these actions. Further, not all in the child's milieu understand these signals. Usually it is only the mother who is able to decipher these signals.

It is customary to associate a sound or utterance, such as 'Su ... su!' or 'Ka ... ka!' to indicate toilet in most children. Many children with expressive language problems may not be able to utter these sound syllables. It is advisable that parents select only those sounds that the child can utter. For example, if the child can utter a sound like 'Oo ...' this sound could be associated to the toilet activity. Keep uttering the same word in front of the child as many times as possible during the toilet activity. Keep talking with the child: 'What are you doing? You are doing "Oo ... oo".' Use every similar opportunity to connect this word with toilet activities, the toilet place and so on. Use the same word to designate toilet activities of others. 'Where is papa going? He is going for "Oo ... oo!"' Wherever possible, insist the child utter the same sound syllable in the context of toilet activities and not in other situations. Reward correct and successful utterances. Soon the child will learn to associate that particular sound syllable with toilet activity. Some parents are particular about teaching two separate indications for urine and faeces. While such discriminations may be introduced at later stages, begin by using the same sound indication for both activities. Later, two different indications may be introduced.

Observe or note the timings during the day when your child usually goes to toilet. Prepare a toilet training chart. Seat the child on the toilet seat at least 15 minutes before the scheduled time. An elder must remain near the child all through the time till the child passes toilet. In case the child does pass toilet, he or she must be immediately rewarded with a thing or event that he or she likes. The successful activity must be reported to everyone in the house. The child must be made to feel as though he or she has achieved something very impressive by successfully using the toilet. A star may be marked on a chart for each successful occasion. A collection of five or 10 stars may then be exchanged for a thing or event that your child loves. A failure to use the toilet on any occasion is to be ignored. No rewards are given, and no punishments or humiliating comments are to be passed. The child will learn over time that successful toilet experiences bring forth rewards, and failures deprive him of these rewards. This discrimination learning will set the right tempo for successful toilet training in your child.

Bathing is an extension of washing/toilet skills. This activity can commence with simple actions like wiping one's nose with a handkerchief (SH37; SH40), rinsing fingers in running water from a tap, pouring water on self during a bath (SH45), washing face with soap and water (SH38; SH47; SH48), bathing self on instruction, applying soap on body (SH49), etc. This self-help skill has to be taught through small steps like washing hands under running tap water, applying soap on hands, rinsing hands, applying soap on face, washing face, etc. Each sub-skill may be further sliced as per the individual requirements of a child with disability. Towelling (SH46), grooming and brushing (SH42; SH43; SH44) are also part of the cleansing skills to be taught to children during the preschool years. Brushing involves sub-components like tongue cleaning (SH43), gargling, rinsing, application of paste on toothbrush (SH44), gargling, etc. These activities are to be taught separately. Table 5.12 gives guidelines on training in self-help activities.

## Activity Cluster # 10: Cognitive

Cognitive activities for preschoolers emerge after, or in consonance with, basic integration of sensory-motor activities. The activities under cognitive domain of ACPC-DD are broadly divided into four sub-domains, viz., clock-time, calendar, money and general respectively.

## Activity Cluster # 10a: Clock and Time

Toddlers achieve a rudimentary representation of time when they understand the instruction involving 'now' and 'later' (Cg3; Activity Cluster 5a). It is often erroneously assumed that toddlers have almost the same sense of subjective time as adults. Infants and initial toddlers must be assumed to have no sense of time at all. They live in a world of 'now or never'. In this stage, the child shows impatience in any situation requiring procrastination or delay. Their demands have to be met instantaneously, or, in their view, it is assumed that their wants will never be met. Therefore, the child will present negative behavioural reactions when told to wait. The beginning training for the child to wait or postpone the fulfilment of their demands can involve gratification delay of only a few seconds. 'You will get your toffee only after I count three!' can be an initial refrain. The commitment must be definitely honoured. Otherwise, the child is likely to loose trust, and also not properly comprehend the meanings of 'now' and 'later'. The lag in delay gratification can gradually be increased from a few seconds to a few minutes, or even hours. Sometimes, it may be necessary to use a tangible cue like a metronome or alarm bell to signal gratification of their demands. 'You will get your doll only after that bell rings!', can be a means of cue conditioning in training the child on waiting skills. Meanwhile, the acquisition of the notion that there is a 'now' and a 'later' reinforces the idea that there is a temporal spread from what is imminent and what could come afterwards.

Through experience and training in waiting and procrastination skills (Activity Cluster 8e), children begin to appreciate the meaning of 'now' and 'later' (Cg3). The appreciation of 'day–night' (Cg4) requires an understanding of the more tangible concept of 'darkness–light' (Cg1). This is taught by helping the toddler differentiate between rooms having lights 'on' as opposed to 'off'. 'It is dark inside the cellar' or 'Put the lights on' eases this comprehension. A dark box with a slit for peeping in can explain darkness, in contrast with a lighted torch placed inside it, when there is 'light'! It becomes relatively easy to shift to an understanding of 'day–night' after grasping the concept of 'darkness' and 'light'. Descriptive verbal explanations like 'There is light during the day', or 'There is darkness at the night', may clarify the distinction readily to most children. Sometimes, they may require more concrete clues. 'The sky is blue when it is day!', 'The sky is black when it is night!', 'There are stars/moon in the sky when it night!'. The child is instructed to verify each time by looking outside before answering the question as to whether it is day or night.

Thereafter, the teaching of more specialized concepts related to parts of the day, such as 'morning-afternoon-evening' (Cg5), 'breakfast-lunch-dinner' (Cg7) and 'yesterday-today-tomorrow' (Cg8) needs to be associated with specific activities of the child throughout the day. 'Morning' can be associated with breakfast, waking up, going to school and so on. 'Afternoon' can be connected to lunch, a nap or siesta. 'Evening' can be linked to outdoor play, return of 'papa' from office or any activity that happens around the child during those timings.

For the child to understand the concept of 'then–now', we can proceed with the use of pictures to reinforce the understanding that the child's babyhood is separate from his or contemporary toddler phase. In this connection, the use of one's own babyhood photographs could be advantageous. By around three years, the child develops the notion that there are several points of time. Birthdays are important events to convey the concept of year and the idea of growing up through time. It is important to realize that early preschoolers do not really understand morning, afternoon and/or evening. Some activities can be left half fin-ished to convey to the child that it would be continued the next day. Children are encouraged to develop a sense of time at their own rate of development. The toddler is taught to associate time with clocks or watches (Cg2). A frequent association of time with these instruments will bring about an understanding that time is related to clocks. The concept of time begins to dawn on children on frequent association of clocks/watches with the word 'time'. Children intrinsically connect the term 'time' to looking at clocks. The first step in teaching clock read-ing requires the child's proficiency with numbers up to at least 12. The child must be able to rote recite numbers to 12, read or identify them and discriminate between the size of 'big–small' needle on a clock. Given these prerequisites, the child can be taught to tell time to the hour by the small hand/needle on a clock (Cg6). A related math skill for this activity is 'count-ing by fives' (Cg9) or recitation of multiplication tables by fives. Though accurate time-telling ability to the nearest minute/second is seldom achieved, or is an over-expectation for pre-school years, preparatory skills can be fairly imparted in these ages. Advanced time/clock skills like telling time to the nearest minute, reporting hours in a given day, discrimination between ante meridiam (am) and post meridiam (pm), etc. can be targets for inclusion beyond preschool years. For severely disabled children, the tradition of teaching clock/time skills on conventional clocks maybe shelved and reading time from digital devices may be considered advantageous.

The first step in teaching clock-reading skills to young children requires their proficiency in negotiating with numbers up to at least 12. The child must be able to rote recite, read and identify numbers to 12 *(PA25)*. He or she must also have a clear discrimination of size between 'big–small' (PA35). Once the child has acquired these skills, he or she could be initiated into clock- reading skills. Begin with a manually adjustable clock face and set the small hand to a specific number (say, four or six). Train the child to identify or name the exact the numerical location of the small hand of the clock. After this has been accomplished, set the small hand of the clock to positions between two numbers (say, six and seven). At this stage, children may show confusion in numerical location of small hand of the clock. The bafflement may be whether to identify it as six or seven. A practice lesson must then make the child realize that the numeri-cal location of the small hand of the clock is six and NOT seven since it has not crossed the latter number. The child has to comprehend that telling time to the hour involves recognition of the small hand of clock, location of its numerical position at or before it crosses over to the next number. This phase of training may require special attention over several sessions.

After the child has understood to denote or tell time to the nearest hour, proceed to help him or her read the minute (long) hand of the clock. There are many ways of doing this. One simple but tedious procedure can involve asking the child to count the number of dots/ dashes the minute hand has crossed over from 12. For reading the time at 11.10, he could locate the hour (small) hand at 11 and count from the dot after 12 as eleven-one, eleven-two, eleven-three ... up to eleven-ten! Another procedure can involve enabling the child to count or calculate by fives for each number on the clock. One is five, two is 10, three is 15, four is 20 and so on. This means that the child should be proficient in counting by fives or multiplication tables of five.

Yet another procedure can involve teaching the child to identify or read specific anchor points on the clock's face, such as three stands for 15 minutes, six stands for 30 minutes, nine stands for 45 minutes and so on. When the child is familiar with these anchor points, he or her would find it easy to tell time to the nearest half-hour and/or quarter-hour. This can become the prerequisite for later telling time to the specific minute. A relatively easier and assistive technique in case of children with severe arithmetic problems can be to directly assist them to learn to read time from digital watches. There are some protagonists of this approach who believe that life can be made easier and simpler by using assistive devices rather than burdening the already different child with traditional time-telling practices, procedures and devices.

Clock-reading proficiency can be followed by teaching facts on time such as number of hours that make a day, number of minutes that make an hour and/or number of seconds that make a minute. Additional explanations on how it takes 365 days for the earth to go once round the sun, or that it takes 24 hours (one day) for the earth to make one full rotation on its own axis can be added with concrete models and experiments. Still more advanced time skills can include facts on the time of midnight and before noon being referred as ante meridiam (am) and the time after noon and before midnight being referred to as post meridiam (pm). A highly pragmatic and higher order time-negotiating skill can involve teaching the reading of railway time, time tables, solving mathematical problems involving temporal relationships, etc. Several artifacts of time like calendars, clocks, egg-timers, sundials and sandglasses can be used to convey the elementary concept of time to children.

## Activity Cluster # 10b: Calendar

The sequence for teaching the concept of weekdays must begin in preschoolers by the activity of rote recitation of days of the week (Cg10). This is a serial and mechanical rendition of the days of the week with little or no understanding of the recitation. Rote recitation can be inculcated in a spaced manner. The child learns by heart the first three days of the week followed by other days, rather than going on in a single stretch to remember all seven days in one go. Rote recitation of days in a week is followed by an activity involving random check of the day 'after' a specified day. 'What day comes after Friday? Thursday? Monday?' (Cg11). The same procedure is followed for rote recitation of the months in a year (Cg12) and with random checks on a month 'after' a specific month (Cg13). A correct grasp on 'before' checks for days in a week (Cg14) and months in a year (Cg15) requires mastery of reversal operations by the child (Activity Cluster 10d–h). Other related calendar skills which can be considered for inclusion during the preschool years is reporting the seasons in a year (Cg16), identifying or naming the day (Cg17) or specific days for dates on a calendar (Cg18). Common difficulties encountered by children within each level of performance on this operation may be a complete inability to recite days of the week, recitation up to some specific day only, circuitous repetitions or substitutions of some days, etc. Training on months in a year should commence only after the child has achieved sufficient competency in days of the week. A curious problem presents itself in some children who assume that there are no more days after 'Saturday' since they have commenced rote recitation from 'Sunday'. It may be necessary to highlight the circuitous nature in the repeat occurrence of days of the week. In other words, the child is to realize that every 'Saturday' is followed again by another 'Sunday'. This notion can be reinforced by having the days of the week printed/written on a circle to demonstrate their cyclical nature of occurrence. The same problem can be encountered in some children when teaching months of year, when they may assume that there are no more months after 'December'.

### Tables of Time

| | |
|---|---|
| 60 Seconds | : 1 Minute |
| 60 Minutes | : 1 Hour |
| 24 Hours | : 1 Day |
| 7 Days | : 1 Week |
| 30 Days | : 1 month |
| 365 Days | : 1 Year or 12 Months |
| 366 Days | : 1 Leap Year or 12 Months |
| 10 Years | : 1 Decade |
| 100 Years | : 1 Century |
| 1,000 Years | : 10 Centuries or 1 Millennium |

### Jubilee Table

| | |
|---|---|
| 1 Year | : Anniversary |
| 10 Years | : Decade |
| 25 Years | : Silver Jubilee |
| 50 Years | : Golden Jubilee |
| 75 Years | : Diamond Jubilee |
| 100 Years | : Centenary |

It is one thing to merely rote recite days of the week/months, answer by rote to questions like 'How many days are there in a week?' or 'How many months are there in a year?'. It is quite another thing to grasp the practical meaning or relevance of these concepts to everyday calendar-reading skills. To begin with, several children may show confusion between the two areas. They may confuse and add names of months in the list of days of the week, and/ or vice versa. These aspects need careful observation by caregivers before they are remedied. The pragmatics of applying rote knowledge of days of week/months to calendar-reading skills or day-to-day life is achieved by associating significant events for specific days to that particular day. For example, going to church on Sundays, father remains at home on Sundays, the favourite mythological serial on television appears on Thursdays, sister's music lessons are on Wednesdays. A routine of insisting the child tear a single sheet from a daily tear-off calendar or write the dates in a daily activity book associated with verbalizations from caregivers on the day, date and year can provide practical understanding on changing dates. A critical activity around this time is calendar-reading skills. The child requires to be explained the technique of identifying given date/s for specified days or reading particular dates for specified date/s in a month's calendar. Eventually, older children require teaching on concepts of seasons in a year, leap year, meaning of a decade, centenary, and millennium from a jubilee table, calculation of exact age when told the date of birth, etc.

## Activity Cluster # 10c: Money

The concept of money begins with toddlers' recognition/identification of objects in their milieu, including coins/notes. Among other noun forms commonly introduced in naming/identification training sessions (example, 'fan', 'light', 'television', etc.), the child is acquainted with 'money'. At this stage, the child may still not be in a position to appreciate the various elementary dimensions of 'money' like its use, value and denominations. It is probably only an initial appraisal of an object from the other things in his surroundings. The initial acquaintance with money is to be accompanied or followed by repeat instruction and exhortation enabling the child to comprehend that it is an object to be kept carefully (Cg19). This introductory lesson on 'money' can be reinforced by repeat instructions or exhortations on preserving objects like coins and notes and sorting them from other things (Cg20). Another valuable lesson should involve associating activities of shopping, giving or receiving change, buying things for tender of money to shopkeepers in front of the child (Cg21). This frequent experience/observation of elders during business transactions can enlighten the child on the value of money in receiving things during shopping. The child can even be given small change to tender to shopkeepers for exchange of goods like toffees, sweets, snacks, etc. (Cg43).

The discrimination between 'small–big' (Cg22) money may have to be done initially on the basis of apparent size of the coins rather than their inherent denominational value. The child learns that a rupee is 'bigger' money than 50 paise or 25 paise coins. The child is also to learn that notes are different from coins as another form of currency (Cg24). After these initial try-outs, the child may be even commissioned on small errands to buy a thing or two with chits from known neighbourhood shops (Cg23). This is at once an activity related to teaching money skills and community orientation or social skills in toddlers.

As the child learns to read or recognize numbers up to at least 10 or 100, he or she can be taught to read values of coins (Cg25). During this stage, the child may be only able to read the number/s on coins or notes to identify their specific values. Later, a series of exercises are given on inverting and placing the numbers on coins/notes to enable the child to identify values of coins (Cg26). A relatively high-order money skill can involve teaching that a rupee holds 100 paise, two rupees hold 200 paise (and so on) or vice versa. Once the child has been introduced to simple additions (Cg27), either on paper or calculator, he can be given small bills to calculate. For example, 'a toffee costs 20 paise and another titbit costs 30 paise, so how much do you pay the shopkeeper?' Additional practice and elaboration on money-handling skills can be incorporated by games like 'business' and 'trade' or by playing 'shop-shop' (Cg28), discrimination of rupee against paise, knowing values of coins, etc.

## Activity Cluster # 10d: General Skills

Under this sub-domain of ACPC-DD is included an assortment of cognitive activities including classification and categorization through sorting, matching, identification and naming of objects or events. Classification involves grouping objects according to some distinguishing or common characteristic. For example, consider the list 'dog-cat-horse-cow-pig'. They may be classified as a group of 'animals'. To make any classification, the child must be first able to identify similar attributes between objects, such as, their size, shape, colour, etc. The ability to classify objects by their distinguishing characteristics is a key element in understanding many conceptual relationships. This skill develops eventually by about the second or third grade, although the rudiments of such competency facilitate objects and/or pictures. The specific varieties of activities possible under this operation are:

| Examiner | Subject |
| --- | --- |
| Presents one of a pair of objects. | Points or picks up another of the pair of objects. |
| Presents a picture of a pair of objects. | Points or picks up another of the pair of objects. |
| Presents model number of objects. | Places identical number of objects. |

**Matching:** Matching is a discovery of an equivalence between two or more stimulus elements. Matching operations may be carried out between concrete objects (object to object) (Cg29) and/or pictures (object to picture, or picture to picture) (Cg30). Additional activities can include attribute matching involving colour, shapes, size, quantity or other dimensions of objects or pictures (PA1). A wide assortment of picture cards having representations of pet animals, fruits, vegetables, household furniture, dresses, printed numbers, vehicles or things can be kept ready at hand for teaching these matching activities. Attribute matching is a basic preliminary to higher-order matching activities. If the target is to teach the concept of size, begin by giving pairs of objects similar in all other dimensions (such as, shape, colour, material and/or weight) except size. If the target is to teach the concept of shape, begin by giving pairs of objects similar in all other dimensions (such as size, colour, material and/or weight) except shape and so on. The child is instructed to match and sort the objects in two-choice situations (example, red-green) before proceeding along the gradient of three choice situations (example, red-green-yellow), four choice situations (example, red-green-yellow-blue) and so on.

**Sorting:** Sorting follows matching activities during teaching of size, shape and/or colours. Sorting is separating target stimuli according to some definite criteria and arranging them systematically (PA26). Optimum training in sorting is an important condition in young children for development of their concept formation. If the target is to teach the concept of size, begin by giving pairs of objects similar in all dimensions (shape, colour, material and/or weight) except size. If the target is to teach the concept of shape (S38), start with pairs of objects similar in all dimensions (size, colour, material and/or weight) except shape and so on. It is recommended not to use the same objects/teaching materials for teaching two or more concepts simultaneously.

The child is instructed to match and sort objects on the chosen criteria (colour) (S41) in two-choice situations (example, red-green) before proceeding along the gradient of three-choice situations (example, red-green-yellow), four-choice situations (example, red-green-yellow-blue) and so on. Once again the opportunities for teaching sorting through live objects, pictures or articles is limitless, and is left to the ingenuity of the teacher. The same variety of pictures having representations of pet animals, fruits, vegetables, household furniture, dresses, printed number and vehicles can be used for category sorting. Sorting and matching can have photos of family members or the child for sifting 'my family' from 'others' or 'relatives'.

**Identification:** After the child has mastered basic sorting of pairs of objects at a given dimension (size, shape, colour, weights or materials), begin with activities requiring identification of the said dimension (Cg33; Cg34; Cg44). In other words, the child should point to the said dimension (example, 'Show me red!'), again with the gradient progression of two-choice situations, three-choice situations, four-choice situations and so on.

**Naming:** Naming objects on the said dimension (example, 'What color is this?') follows identification (Cg39; Cg50). Once again, the gradient progression of two-choice, three-choice, four-choice situations and so on should be maintained. Children with expressive language problems may be exempted from naming activities. Their pointing/identification may be taken as equivalent for naming activities on ACPC-DD.

**Discrimination:** Discrimination involves choice and distinction between two or more alternatives. The choice is according to some distinguishing or common characteristic within one of the discriminants (Cg31; Cg37; Cg43; Cg47). For example, consider the words 'hot–cold' (S37). They are differentiated based on certain properties that account for what is termed as either 'hot' and/or 'cold'. Toddlers are able to make contradistinctions only after they have achieved some semblance of mastery over classification-categorization through sorting, matching, identification and naming activities. Discrimination training implies a subtle understanding of the law of contrast. Since most of the discriminants are not visible or tangible entities (unlike colour or shape) many children with DDs show a profound puzzlement when dealing with these opposites. This is often reflected in their inadequacy at task execution involving several conceptual operations. A child who does not show you the difference between 'big–small' objects cannot be expected to appreciate 'big–small' numbers or concepts of 'greater–smaller than'. Likewise, the child who fails to understand positional discriminants like 'over–under' or 'above–below–next to' can find great difficulty when carrying out arithmetic operations involving subtraction, division or multiplication. There is a fairly long list of discriminants that young children need to master in their preschool training programme (Table 5.13). Some of these concepts are fairly simple to educate the toddler about, either owing to their 'visibility' and/or ability to 'experience' them. For example, the child can discriminate between 'hot–cold', 'rough–smooth' (S42) or 'heavy–light' before making appropriate decisions. The discrimination of 'big–small' (S39), or 'long–short' is clarified or taught by visual experience. However, discrimination of 'left–right' (S50), 'north–south–east–west' and other positional attributes are neither visible nor can be experienced. Many children show greater bafflement when dealing with such discrimination.

**Sequencing-ordering:** Sequencing refers to the act of negotiating a temporal series of stimuli presented aurally or visually. Sequencing operation, carried out on imitation or modelling, requires a student to repeat a specific order of stimuli presented aurally or visually by the examiner (Table 5.14). The specific activities under these operations (Cg38; Cg42; Cg46) may include repeating digits, sound syllables, alphabets or words presented at a prescribed speed of one stimulus per second (PA28; PA34; PA47). The various levels of actual performance under this category depend upon the number of elements within a stimulus that can be repeated by the student. When a child shows difficulty in negotiating or repeating stimulus

**Table 5.13**

**Discrimination Categories for Inclusion in Preschool Programmes**

| No. | Type of Operant | Item Samples |
|-----|-----------------|--------------|
| 1. | Positional | Up–Down; Here–There; Front–Back; Inside–Outside; Near–Far; Left–Right; North–South–East–West; Above–Below; Top–Bottom; High–Low; Next to–In between; Over–Under; On–Under; Before–After. |
| 2. | Aesthetic | Nice–Not Nice; Good–Bad–Ugly. |
| 3. | Action | Give–Take; Yes–No; On–Off; Come–Go; Sit–Stand; Open–Close. |
| 4. | Emotional | Sad–Happy; Angry–Calm. |
| 5. | Relational/Gender | Father–Mother; Uncle–Aunt; Son–Daughter; Grandpa–Grandma; Boy–Girl; Man–Woman. |
| 6. | Dimensional | Big–Small; Little–Greater; Heavy–Light; Thick–Thin; More–Less; Few–Many; Heavy–Light; Long–Short; Wide–Narrow. |
| 7. | Directional | Far–Near; In–Out. |
| 8. | Temporal | Fast–Slow; Now–Sooner–Later. |
| 9. | Sensory | Hot–Cold; Rough–Smooth; Hard–Soft; Fragrance–Malodour; Tasty–Insipid. |
| 10. | Numeral | Odd–Even; Greater than–Smaller than. |

**Table 5.14**

**Sample List of Stimulus for Sequencing-ordering Tasks**

| Sample Digit Series | Sample Sound Syllable Series |
|---------------------|------------------------------|
| 6-2 | Pa-Ga |
| 7-4-1 | Sa-Ri-Mo |
| 3-7-5-8 | Ri-Po-La-Me |
| 1-7-8-5-2 | Na-Si-Do-Bu-Li |
| 7-4-1-9-5-3 | Ta-So-La-Ja-Gu-Fi |

| Sample Word Series | Sample Alphabet |
|--------------------|-----------------|
| Red-Pink | M-P |
| Cat-Cow-Sheep | V-L-T |
| Rose-Lily-Pansy-Jasmine | S-Q-M-Y |
| Table-Pen-Paper-Spoon-TV | W-Z-O-Y-X |
| Car-Auto-Bus-Plane-Ship-Car | A-D-F-N-R-E |

for oral presentations, the examiner could consider presenting the same visually through a tachistoscope or flash cards. These activities involve immediate sequential memory.

Sequencing operations can be exercised using action pictures like these of waking, brushing, bathing, eating, reading, sleeping, etc. The child would be required to arrange these pictures in a sequence corresponding to his or her daily routines. Sequencing operations at higher levels can incorporate arrangement of story pictures (Cg38). Popular fables (such as, 'fox and crow', 'thirsty crow', 'grapes are sour', etc.) familiar to children and depicted on picture cards are to be arranged to complete the story. Further, printed numbers in units, tens or hundreds may be jumbled up and presented on flash cards for the child to rearrange in a sequence of ascending–descending order. The students may be exercised to identify missing components in a series of numbers below or above tens presented visually in print format. Wherein a child is underway to achieve concepts of size, he may be instructed to make sequential arrangement of various objects (like spoons, coins or pencils) on the basis of increasing or decreasing orders of size. Sequencing patterns in enumerating or identifying alternating odd–even numbers need exclusive emphasis for many students. They could be instructed to highlight, cancel or mark odd (or even) numbers from a sequence of serially-arranged units or tens of numerals. Pragmatic skills are practised during stringing of colour beads in particular sequences (say red-red-blue-red-red-blue, and so on) or by insisting children draw sequences of geometric patterns (say circle-circle-circle-square-circle-circle-circle-square). As ordering pattern, sequencing operations invariably involve some degree of prediction. In a given order in presentation of stimuli, the child must predict what element is to come next at the end of a given sequence. For example, the child should know that a series of 'red-red-green-red-red-green-' will be followed by 'red', or that a '2-4-6-' series is followed by '8'. Exercises involving predictions on what comes next in a sequential series of units, tens and hundreds require extensive practice.

A special category of higher-order sequencing activity is recognition or arrangement of ordinal adjectives (such as first, second, third, and so on). The child should be able to identify or designate descriptive numerical adjectives below five, then below 10 and later above 10, respectively. Another sequencing activity can involve giving numbers in units ($<=9$) at random or in a jumbled fashion to be arranged in an order of increasing (ascending) and/or decreasing (descending) value. The number can be later tried in hundreds ($<=99$), thousands ($<=999$) and so on. Although intimately linked with sequencing operations, ordering is distinguished insofar as the elements in its sequence will be either arranged in an ascending and/or descending pattern. Ordering by increasing size or decreasing size is already hinted at earlier. When the child is presented individual numbers in print form on flash cards, he or she can be trained to order them sequentially in increasing (ascending) pattern of numbers in units, tens and/or hundreds. Simultaneously, the child should also be tutored in ordering them sequentially in decreasing (descending) patterns of numbers in units, tens and/or hundreds.

**Substitution:** Substitutions involve mutual switching/shuffling of acquired concepts where one represents a symbol replacement for another. The act of substitution requires replacement of one set of symbols with another. Symbol substitution involves designation of certain notations (such as $< > - + = \# *$) for specific numerals and asking the child to decode them. Older children need to be taught math symbols for addition, subtraction, division and multiplication. They can be taught roman numbers, entry of digits or symbols into calculators. A concrete activity for inclusion under this operation is dice play (PA44). The child has to count the number cast on a single dice (PA36) or a pair of them (PA41) before making appropriate moves on a checker board, snakes and ladders, ludo, etc. The understanding and use of dice is a basic substitution activity. Dices come in several shapes and forms. Seashells and cowries are commonly used in various board games to count dice. A six/eight cowrie can be used to enable the child to count open dice and make the appropriate number of moves in a board game. Alternatively, numbered dice are easier to use if the child can read printed numbers. Dotted roller dices require the child to count the number of dots tossed.

As the child acquires an understanding of 'big' and 'small' numbers, he or she is introduced to substitutions of symbols like greater than ($>$), less than ($<$) and/or equal to ($=$). Distinguish that mere replacement of the appropriate symbols for these terms is one thing; understanding whether a given number between a pair is 'big'/'small' before denoting these symbols is another step ahead of basic substitution operations. A written exercise involving symbol substitution is an understanding of the < > and = symbols for numbers and/or numbers for symbols respectively. This activity is to usually follow children grasping seriation and ordering of numbers, or that specific numbers come after/before certain other specific numbers. Five is less than seven. Seven is greater than two. The child is to understand that the term less than (<) or greater than (>) is substituted by an appropriate symbol.

The introduction of math symbols does not necessarily mean complete comprehension of all math operations like addition, subtraction, multiplication and/or division. Herein, it simply means that the child is able to denote instructions to 'Add!', 'Sum!' or 'Total!' with the appropriate notation (+). Likewise, the child should denote 'Subtract!', 'Minus!', 'Deduct!', 'Take Away!' or 'Remove!' with a minus sign. The child is to understand all the synonyms that go in with additions, subtraction, multiplication and/or division. Some related substitution activities can be contrived by assigning certain symbols to specific numerals (such as 5 as #, 7 as %, 8 as &, 2 as *, and so on) before asking the student to replace symbols for these numbers or numbers for these symbols. The introduction of meaningful math symbols (+ – x) for identification/naming can begin as the child starts performing these basic math operations. A related practice activity can be carried out by introduction of calculators for making appropriate data entry of numbers and/or basic math symbols. Roman-number substitution (or other native-language-number substitution) for English numerals should be introduced only after the student has acquired sufficient mastery in writing numbers up to 100.

**Reversals:** Reversals refer to tasks involving inversion of forward-moving sequences. Before undertaking these activities, students must be adept at front-sequencing operations. Reversals, a more difficult property, involves travelling backwards or in the opposite direction. It is a vital concept in regrouping, carrying numbers and commutative and associative properties of mathematical operations. A beginning activity can involve inverse rote counting of numbers from nine to one, followed by counting backwards in tens from 99 to 1 or parts thereof like 20 to 1, 50 to 1, and so on. At higher levels, the child is taught to reverse rote count in hundreds from 900 and 99 to 1 or parts thereof. A significant practice activity to foster reversal operations in children is verbal games involving repetition of digits backward akin to repeating digits forward as discussed earlier. Although non-functional, some of these activities may be used for fostering reversal abilities in young children. An understanding of the concept of 'before–after' (PA32; PA40) is critical for enabling successful reversal operations in young children. 'What number comes after five?', 'Who entered the room before you came in?', 'What number comes before six?', 'Which alphabet comes before S?', 'Which day of week comes before Friday?'. Positional discrimination may have to be taught by actually placing concrete objects in front of the child or mapping them on a piece of paper. Reverse-sequencing operations are carried out by imitation. The student is required to reverse and repeat a specific sequence of stimuli presented either aurally or visually by the caregiver. The specific activities under these operations include reverse repetition of digits, sound syllables, alphabets or words presented at a prescribed speed of one stimulus per second. The various levels of actual performance under this category depend upon the number of elements within stimuli that can be repeated by the student. The same list of sample stimulus activities used for forward sequencing can be used in this activity too.

Wherein a child shows difficulty in negotiating or reverse repeating stimuli for oral presentations, caregivers could consider presenting the same stimuli visually through a tachistoscope or through flash cards. Such concrete presentations are easier for the uninitiated child than oral presentations. These activities involve immediately reversed sequential memory. Rote recitation of the alphabets A to Z may be achieved early. An optional, though not again functionally useful reversal game, can incorporate reverse recitation of Z to A. A special form of reverse counting activity for children who have attained basic mastery of arithmetic operations of addition and subtraction is serial subtraction in twos from 20 to 0 and in fours from 40 to 0. A fairly difficult game for children beyond preschool ages involves reversing the hands on a clock. The child is given a specific time set. For example, at quarter-past-nine, the short hand on a clock is at nine and the long hand is at three. The child is asked to reverse the position of the needles and report the time (3:45 in this example).

**Generalization:** The teaching of cognitive concept is incomplete unless the child learns to generalize the acquired concepts in real-life situations. Generalization refers to the process of forming an idea or judgement applicable to an entire class of objects, people or events. It is a process of application of a general idea to new ideas or situations. For example, the child who has learnt to name the colour 'red' using pegs or buttons during a teaching situation must apply or generalize the same concept to name the said colour to any or all objects in the immediate milieu.

## Activity Cluster # 10e: Size Concept

The concept of size is basic in children in learning later notions like magnitude, mass, measurements, volume and proportions. A beginning discrimination between 'big–small' objects is introduced by size-matching activities. The child is instructed to match and sort pairs of objects (such as 20 small- and big-sized buttons each, or 30 small- and big-sized pencils each). He or she could stack similar-sized objects one upon another, contrasting it with another pile of a different size of the same object. The other properties of the matched objects like shape, colour, material or weights should be retained constant to avoid confusion with other dimensions of the objects.

After sufficient practice on sorting and matching sizes, the child is led to identify/point when questioned: 'Which is big?' or 'Which is small?' (Cg39). Be wary of misinterpreting random guesses as correct answers. Eventually, proceed to teach naming 'big–small'. Of course, generalization of size discrimination learnt on specific puzzles, boards, objects, game situations and/or paper-pencil tasks to the real world are targeted as a distinct and necessary culmination for acquisition of this concept. It is no use if a child can point/name 'big' and/or 'small' only on the used teaching materials. The child must know application of similar rules while discriminating size in the real world around. A corollary activity related to acquisition of discrimination between 'big–small' objects is an understanding of 'more–less' (PA30) quantities. This is taught by enabling the child to differentiate liquids as 'more' water is one jug and 'less' in another. The 'visibility' of size could serve as an excellent clue in grabbing the rudiments of the concept of size. Later, this could be extended to discriminating between 'more' and/or 'less' (Cg31) using solids. After learning to name 'big–small' sizes of objects, the child may be guided to arrange similar objects in increasing or decreasing order of size.

## Activity Cluster # 10f: Shape Concept

Shapes (also called 'forms' or 'gestalts') are arbitrarily classified into primary, secondary and tertiary categories. Primary forms are circle, square and triangle. Secondary forms are diamond, rectangle, semi-circle and cross. Tertiary forms are combined derivatives of primary and secondary forms like polygons, hexagons or star patterns. The development of form perception in children approximates progression along these categories beginning with mastery of primary shapes, followed by secondary and tertiary shapes respectively. Perceptual training on form perception should take into account not only the complexity of shapes, but also sequential algorithm or teaching gradient procedures highlighted as matching, sorting, identification, naming and generalization. Form training may begin with matching or sorting primary shapes, to be continued with secondary shapes and tertiary shapes. Cardboard cut-outs of different shapes in the same size or material dimensions are easily made using old greeting cards or wooden chips. The child is instructed to pile one on the other to make a tower of the similar shapes. Three-form boards or paper-form boards can be used. Drawing an outline of these shapes on the floor upon which the child is instructed to pile identical shapes may provide additional cues.

After sufficient trials on sorting and matching shapes, the child is led to identify/point when told 'Show me a circle' (or square or triangle). Be wary of misinterpreting random guesses by a child as correct answers. Proceed from pointing/identification primary shapes through secondary to tertiary shapes. Later, proceed to teach naming primary (Cg34), secondary and tertiary shapes. Some adjuvant activities for training of form perception can involve cutting out various shapes using paper cutters, knives, blades or scissors, enabling recognition of shapes through touch, construction of shapes using match sticks, etc. Towards the end, focus on achieving generalization of shapes from teaching situations and/or paper-pencil tasks to the real world. Asking the child to fetch/identify those objects around his or her surroundings that match a particular shape does this. For example, a ball is round, a bangle is round, the moon is round, a lid is round and so on. Making geometrical shapes using matchsticks can be an absorbing activity for many toddlers (P30).

## Activity Cluster # 10g: Colour

Colour, an important attribute of objects in the outer world, can be theoretically distinguished into two categories, viz., primary and secondary colours. Primary colours are those when mixed in proper proportions yield all other colours including white. Within this definition, red, blue and green are primary colours. Secondary colours are derivatives like yellow, orange, pink, black and white. Perceptual training in colour concepts must necessarily proceed through the same algorithmic sequence of matching, sorting, identification, naming and generalization. Begin on activities involving matching and/or sorting similar objects with primary colours. The child is instructed to match/sort similar sized or shaped, but differently coloured, objects (say, beads or buttons) into appropriate heaps or cups of identical colours. Start with two colour-choice situations (preferably red and green) for matching or sorting. Then proceed matching or sorting fewer than three choice situations (red, green and blue beads or buttons). After the child has achieved sufficient mastery with primary colours, add on similar objects and activities with secondary colours through the progression of two choice situations, three choice situations and so on.

Matching or sorting is followed by identification of colours. Herein, the child is expected to point to specific colours on request ('Show me red!' or 'Show me green!'). Colour identification (Cg33) schemes are usually introduced towards the terminal stages of colour matching activities by repeated verbal pairing; a given sorting action by the child with name of the said primary colour. If possible, make the child repeat aloud the name of colour during each sorting or matching action. Proceed to identification of secondary colours only after mastery of primary colours sufficiently by the child. Naming colours (Cg50) follow wherein children can verbalize or express linguistically. The child is expected to name a given colour on being asked ('What colour is this?'). Primary colours (Cg33) are named before secondary colours (Cg44). Naming colours of specific target objects used in training (such as beads or buttons) is one thing; application of this concept to name primary and secondary colours of other objects in the child's surroundings (generalization) is quite another end activity that needs to be undertaken separately. Contrive situations wherein similar coloured small objects are placed around the child and ask him or her to match, identify and name their colours.

## Activity Cluster # 10h: Body Concept

Activities related to teaching concept of self and others, followed by parts of the body, is an essential ingredient of any preschool programme. The child must begin by knowing to respond to his or her name as a unique property in communication between persons (C3). This is to be followed by names and relationships of immediate family members and other relatives or friends (C20; C30). It is always advisable to commence a generic teaching programme on parts of the body by beginning with pointing (C15) or identification of 'head-hands-legs' before proceeding to specifics like 'mouth-ears-eyes-nose', or still later to 'eyebrows-eyelashes-eyelids', and so on. After the toddler has achieved minimum competence in pointing to parts of his or her own body, later activities can advance to identifying same parts in others, on a favourite doll (or teddy bear) and on pictures, charts or human posters. It will be seen presently that clear understanding of one's body parts is an important prerequisite to later teaching 'left–right' discrimination.

## Activity Cluster # 10i: Left–Right Discrimination

Nature has made us bilaterally symmetrical. We have two eyes, two ears, two legs, two arms, two lungs, etc. Within our complex nervous system is a signal mechanism that relates which side of the body is alerted to action; there is then a corresponding counter-action on the opposite side. There is a counterbalance for every body movement that is made. This is an internal system that is denoted by laterality. The center axis of this laterality is the vertical midline of the body. If the right and left neurological patterns have not been adequately organized, children find it difficult to cross this midline. Children who are unable to perform bilateral tasks smoothly and easily are those who need specific training to bring this equal side about. The ability to cross the midline enables the child to achieve a balanced kinesthetic visual matching. If this is not organized effectively, it may show up in reading problems or reversal difficulties.

Laterality is a matter of balanced internal functioning. It must be achieved before the child can achieve directionality, that is, the 'outside-of-the-body' manifestation of laterality.

Directionality is derived from kinesthetic awareness in our own body. As kinesthetic awareness is taking place, spatial concepts are being built and visual information relating to direction is received. The notion of 'left–right' commonly causes confusion in most children with DDs. Discrimination training for 'left–right' confusions must begin at concrete levels. The establishment of laterality or preferential/consistent use of a particular hand in performance of certain daily activities is a necessary prerequisite to commence this training. For instance, the child must have to consistently use the right hand while eating or when waving 'ta-ta'/'bye-bye'. This eases the imminent task of associating that given activity with the word 'right'. After achieving considerable association between the word 'right' and the preferred hand, the same may be extended to other parts on the right side of the child's body (right eye, right ear, right leg, and so on). Later, the child is made aware of things on the right side of his or her surroundings. Even contrived practice sessions may be invoked by deliberately placing certain objects on the right side of the child for his or her to identify/name regularly. Additional practice activities can involve asking the child to hold a doll in the same direction as he or she faces the caregiver, before asking to point to its specific body parts on the left or right.

After achieving a meaningful measure of success consistently in the child's recognition of 'right', the concept of 'left' is initiated as contra-lateral or opposite side of one's own body parts or objects on that side in the immediate milieu. In this stage, progress from simple direct commands like 'Show me your left hand!' or 'Show me your right eye!', and 'Put your left hand on your left eye!' or 'Put your right hand on your right eye!' to cross-over commands like 'Put your left hand on your right eye!' or 'Put your right hand on left eye!'. Ostensibly, these instructions are intended to eliminate confusions between 'left–right' on or in relation to one's own body. Eventually, the child has to negotiate 'left–right' on own mirror images or others facing him or her. This is a fairly difficult proposition unless the child can conceptually put herself in the shoes of others and view the world from others' perspective rather than on his or her own. Usually, the untutored child may naively point to his or her same side as 'right' or 'left' in the person facing him or her. It is useful to communicate how 'right–left' cross-over occurs by practicing pointing, discrimination or identification exercises in front of a mirror. The activities in this stage progress from instructions like 'Touch my right hand!' or 'Touch my left knee!' through 'Put your left hand on my right hand!' or 'Put your right hand on my left knee!' to 'Put your left hand on my left knee!' or 'Put your right hand on my right knee!'. Table 5.15 summarizes the sequence of left–right discrimination training progressing from self reference to reference on others through various mental-age approximations. A confirmed acquisition of 'left–right' discrimination is essential for attempting teaching of advanced concepts like discrimination of 'north–south–east–west' directions with appropriate reference to oneself.

## Activity Cluster #10j: Positional Concepts

Objects lie at various locations or positions in space. Position refers to the spatial location of an object in reference to an observer or to other objects. Children with difficulties in responding to vocabulary which is specially relevant to temporal, spatial and orientation relationships require extensive exercises on use of pre-positional phrases such as 'high–low', 'front–in between–behind', 'next to', 'up–down', 'over–under/above–below/on–under' and 'far–near'.

**Table 5.15**
**Left–Right Discrimination Training**

Show me your left hand (54m).
Show me your right eye (54m).
Put your left hand on your left eye (54m).
Put your right hand on your right eye (54m).
Put your left hand on your right eye (66m).
Put your right hand on your left eye (66m).
Touch my right hand (90m).
Touch my left knee (90m).
Put your left hand on my right hand (90m).
Put your left hand on my left knee (90m).
Put your left hand on my left knee (90m).
Put your right hand on my right knee (90m).

Note: 'm' signifies months.

The teaching activities for these target behaviours must consider three attitudinal levels, viz., concrete, semi-concrete/pictorial and abstract respectively. The first two levels are particularly crucial for younger children. The concrete attitude for negotiating pre-positional vocabulary refers to manipulation of actual objects or tangible entities on specific commands during activities like 'Put this pencil in front of the box!', 'Keep this umbrella next to that cupboard!', 'Bring the box under that cot!', and so on. The *semi-concrete attitude* for negotiating pre-positional vocabulary refers to manipulation of pictures depicting various positional-directional relationships. For example, between various figures of familiar objects depicted pictorially, the child may be asked to indicate those objects which are 'below' a line, 'inside' a box, 'outside' a circle, and so on. The abstract attitude for negotiating pre-positional vocabulary may come up in situations depicting a hierarchy of positions, such as principal is 'higher' in position than a school attendant or that pupils in a class are 'lower' in status than their monitor/leader and so on. However, this cognitive attitude may not be achieved until after primary school in children. The child is led to gain an understanding of these positional concepts through situation-specific experiences. For example, the concept of 'up' is repeatedly associated with pointing the child's hands upwards, or holding it downward in association with use of the word 'down'. The inceptive accompaniment of gestures must be gradually tapered over trials until the child fully understands just the verbal instruction of either 'up' or 'down'. Several instructional activities like asking the child to keep an object 'over' and/or 'under' the table, stand 'in front of' a mirror, 'in between' two chairs, etc., sharpen knowledge and use of these positional words in children.

## Activity Cluster # 10k: Directional Concepts

Direction refers to the course of movement. Position-direction related concepts are important pre-requirements for teaching advanced math operations like addition and subtraction. They constitute an essential ingredient of visual, spatial and perceptual skills in geometry, graph representations, route finding, map reading, etc. Although intimately associated with positional vocabulary, directional vocabulary is distinct as it refers to a certain course of movement by the subject in relation to an object. This is evidenced in activities involving a child imitating motor actions of a caregiver. The directional rhyme linked with the child's actions of 'standing up line-lying down line-slanting line-curved line-crooked line' is a familiar example.

The two dimensions of 'before–after' concepts are closely related to establishment of directionality in toddlers. Between these, it is easier to convey the idea of 'after' objects, events or numbers in sequence. In a series of numbers from 1 to 10, for example, questions may be asked on what comes 'after' four? In a series of rote recitation of days of the week, what comes 'after' a given day (Monday)? In a series of objects placed visually (pen-eraser-clip-bead), the child is asked to identify what comes 'after' a specific object (eraser)? In a series of words presented aurally (dog-cat-pig-hen), the child is asked to indicate what was said 'after' a specific word (pig)?

The concept of 'before', albeit more difficult, is proceeded preferably at concrete levels in the beginning. A series of objects (pen-eraser-clip-bead) is placed in front of the child, who is instructed to point to, identify or name an item preceding ('before') a target question: 'What comes before the clip?'. After the child has achieved enough practice in negotiating tangible object series, pictorial presentations may be attempted. Later, this is replaced by flash cards depicting printed numerals below 10 from which the child is asked to point, identify or name specific numbers 'before' another given number: 'What comes before seven?'.

## Activity Cluster # 10I: Weight Concepts

There are three major activity components to be conveyed to the child in relation to the concept of mass or weight as a property of things in his or her surroundings. The discrimination or identification of 'heavy–light' is a confusing predicament for the beginning child. The child is likely to view weight as a visible property of objects (like size, shape or colour). When two or more identical objects are placed in front of the child and he or she is asked to identify the 'heavy' (or 'light') one, the child is likely to err by pointing to any one of them arbitrarily without even lifting or 'feeling' their weights. This is a sufficient clue to infer that the child is completely unaware of the concept of weights.

Immediate cueing to 'lift' or 'feel' the objects to infer on their 'heaviness' or 'lightness' may facilitate some beginning notion on this concept. This can be associated with activities involving 'pushing' or 'lifting' of two or more visibly similar, but differently weighted sacks/bags filled with masses of things. Each time, caution must be exercised to maintain constant size, shape, colour and other visible properties of the objects. Otherwise, the child is likely to confuse those properties with weights of the said objects. A more 'visible' procedure could involve the child measuring out weights of identical objects on a weighing scale or weighing balance. Apparently, the tilt of a balance towards one side can provide sufficient visual indication for the child to discriminate between an object which is 'heavy' and an object which is 'light'.

## Activity Cluster # 11: Preacademics

The preacademic activities are usually targeted towards the terminal end of preschool years. They are broadly divided into sub-domains, viz., pre-reading, pre-writing and pre-arithmetic.

**Pre-reading:** While formal reading of alphabets, words and sentences in a given language rightfully commences during primary school levels, preparatory pre-reading activities may begin at preschool ages. Pre-reading activities include negotiating with figures/pictures by means of matching (PA1), picture memory (PA2), pointing or identification of various categories of pictures (PA3; PA6; PA7; PA8; PA9), discovering objects from half-closed pictures or missing parts of a picture (PA10), etc. Other activities related to enhancing pre-reading skills in preschool children could involve negotiating pictures by way of describing/imitating action pictures (PA11), spotting differences between pairs of pictures (PA12), detecting absurdities in pictures (PA13), arranging pictures sequentially to form a story (PA14), etc. Reading one's own name may be introduced as sight-reading activity.

## Activity Cluster # 11a: Dealing with Pictures

From a very young age, toddlers are drawn towards bright and colourful pictures. There is a great ease and economy in getting them interested in pictures since it obviates the tedium of showing actual or live objects for each and every concept that is taught to them. Though preferable, it may not always be possible to get the actual object or thing in person every time a new concept is introduced to the child. Where can the teacher go to show an airplane or helicopter unless one goes to the neighbourhood aerodrome. How would one give an impression of a zebra, giraffe or hippopotamus to the child unless one visits the local zoo! Under such circumstances, pictures come handy for classroom teachers even though it is not to be taken as a substitute for live teaching. Luckily, most young children are fascinated by colourful picture books. The choice of books is to be done with care. It is preferable to opt for near-to-natural pictures to begin with before cartoons or line drawings are shown to toddlers.

There are three sequential levels that all children go through in their dealing with pictures, viz., nominal, descriptive and interpretative, respectively. Initially, toddlers can be taught to name, point or identify specific objects only in pictures shown to them. For example, the child may only name 'Catty!', 'Doggy!' or 'Aunty!' in a picture frame having two women chatting and pets dozing by the sofa. This is a nominal response. During this stage, the child should be introduced to various categories of pictures depicting vegetables, vehicles, fruits, animals, household articles, etc. This is also a stage when the child is grammatically in the 'noun form' mode (Activity Cluster 6c). When the child has attained sufficient proficiency in identifying/naming pictures, he or she could be given activities involving assembly of two or three or more piece jigsaw puzzles and identifying objects from parts of pictures (PA4). At the next level, the same child may give descriptive responses for the same card. 'Doggie sleeps!' or 'Aunts are chatting!' and so on. This is a descriptive response (C42). At a higher level, the child adds interpretation for the same picture by investing emotional embellishments in the descriptions: 'Aunty's face appears to be angry!' or 'She seems to be disturbed'. This is an interpretative response. Children need to be guided meticulously over these increasing stages of dealing effectively with picture cards from nominal through descriptive to interpretative levels of responses. The primary activities involving the child dealing with various categories of pictures can later be replaced by action pictures wherein the child has to describe: 'The boy is bathing ... He's sleeping ... She's writing ...!'. The emphasis needs to be on verbs and actions rather than on nouns or names in the pictures. This achievement is a necessary precondition to later introduction of story pictures or training in sequential narration.

An auxiliary to picture activities can include identification of objects from half-closed pictures, detecting missing features or absurdities in pictures, reporting similarities or differences between pictures, arranging pictures in a sequential order and so on.

## Activity Cluster # 11b: Alphabet/Word Reading

The introduction of alphabets (either upper or lower case) in a language must be commenced only during the later part of preschool years. The child must first become adept at all precognitive concepts including size, shape, colour, weight, position, direction, etc., before starting formal letter reading activities. The phonics (or phonetics) technique for teaching reading skills at preschool levels involves step-by-step progression in mastery of oral skills (Figure 5.1). In this procedure, the toddler is first introduced to identification/reading of all basic alphabets in a given language. This is followed by the procedure of pairing each alphabet to their respective phonic sound/s. For example, 'a' is for 'aa', 'b' is for 'ba', 'c' is for 'ka', 'p' is for 'pa', and so on. All vowel as well as consonant sounds are introduced. Thereafter, combinations of vowels with consonants (such as, at-it-un-ed-ob-or-in, etc.) or consonants with vowels (such as, ca-ba-de-me-pi-di-ro-so, etc.) are practiced with the given child. This is followed by reading practice on meaningful two-letter words like of-on-if-so-in-at-or-it, etc.

**Figure 5.1**
**Steps in Elementary Word-reading Skills**

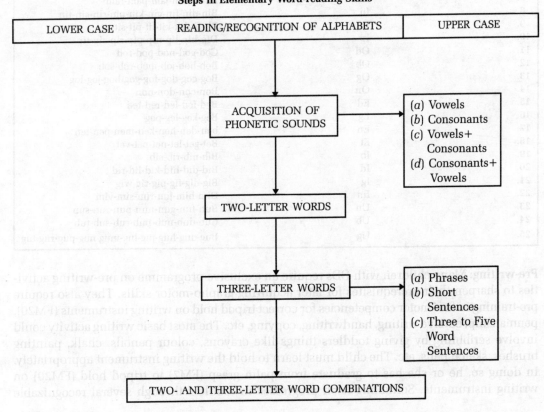

A minimum mastery of these words is sufficient to begin on three-letter word combinations along with the two-letter word sounds. Examples of this level are given in Table 5.16. After the child has acquired three-letter word reading skills, the teacher can try short phrases made from combinations of two-letter and three-letter words. These combinations may be even worked out individually to meet the needs of given child with reading difficulties. Short sentences, phrases and narratives with associated figure-presentations can be more enlivening for preschool readers. Irrespective of any advanced reading skills, the child must be able to read his or her own name (PA5) or allied functional sight words like 'Danger', 'Fire', 'Exit', 'Ladies', 'Gents', 'Poison', etc. These are essential living skills for community adjustment of persons with disability.

**Table 5.16**
**Three-letter Word Reading Lists for Beginners**

| No. | Sound | Word Samples |
| --- | --- | --- |
| 1. | At | Bat-mat-rat-sat-pat-cat-fat-hat-tat |
| 2. | Ap | Cap-gap-lap-map-nap-rap-sap-tap |
| 3. | An | Ban-can-fan-man-pan-ran-tan-van |
| 4. | Ab | Cab-dab-fab-jab-lab-nab-sab-tab |
| 5. | Ad | Bad-dad-fad-had-lad-mad-pad-sad |
| 6. | Ag | Bag-fag-gag-lag-mag-nag-rag-sag-tag-wag |
| 7. | Am | Dam-ham-jam-pam-ram |
| 8. | In | Bin-din-fin-gin-kin-pin-rin-sin-tin |
| 9. | It | Bit-fit-hit-kit-lit-pit-sit-tit |
| 10. | Ip | Dip-hip-lip-nip-pip-rip-sip-tip |
| 11. | Od | Cod-god-nod-pod-rod |
| 12. | Ob | Bob-hob-job-mob-rob-sob |
| 13. | Og | Bog-cog-dog-fog-gog-hog-jog-log |
| 14. | On | Bon-con-don-non |
| 15. | Ed | Bed-fed-led-red-ted |
| 16. | Eg | Beg-keg-leg-peg |
| 17. | En | ben-den-hen-ken-men-pen-ten |
| 18. | Et | Bet-get-let-net-pet-vet |
| 19. | Ib | Bib-nib-rib-sib |
| 20. | Id | Bid-did-hid-kid-lid-rid |
| 21. | Ig | Big-dig-fig-pig-rig-wig |
| 22. | Im | Dim-him-jim-rim-sim-vim |
| 23. | Un | Bun-fun-gun-nun-pun-run-sun |
| 24. | Ub | Cub-dub-nub-pub-rub-sub-tub |
| 25. | Ug | Bug-dug-hug-jug-lug-mug-nug-pug-rug-tug |

**Pre-writing:** Many children with DDs require an exclusive programme on pre-writing activities to sharpen their prerequisites for later acquiring grapho-motor skills. They also require pre-training in fine motor competencies for correct tripod hold on writing instruments (FM20), penmanship, cursive writing, handwriting, copying, etc. The most basic writing activity could involve scribbling by giving toddlers things like crayons, colour pencils, chalk, painting brushes, sketch pens, etc. The child must learn to hold the writing instrument appropriately. In doing so, he or she has to graduate from palm grasp (FM7) to tripod hold (FM20) on writing instruments. Scribbling itself progresses in toddlers through several recognizable phases. It is important for teachers to be aware of these subtle stages in emergent writing skills of toddlers and preschoolers so that intervention activities are targeted age/level appropriately. Other associated pre-writing activities for toddlers can include various forms of finger painting, block printing, leaf painting, thread printing, vegetable painting, etc. These activities will bring the child closer to the world of pen, ink, print and paper.

The achievement of tripod hold on writing instruments can mark the beginning of making dots and dashes, joining pairs of dots, copying vertical/horizontal strokes (PA16), copying a plus or cross on imitation (PA17), and then circles (PA18), squares (PA19), triangles (PA21) and inverted triangles (PA24) in the same order. There are more complex geometric forms that a child may have to master with increasing age/maturation, and which become a pre-requirement for better writing skills during the primary school years. Copying of these shapes like diamond, hospital cross, hexagons, pentagons, honeycomb designs, complex stars, etc., justifiably come under the purview of curriculum for primary school children. Creative skills could be imparted by asking toddlers to draw human figures with various body parts (PA20; PA22), tracing objects or figures using transparent oil papers (PA23), etc.

## Activity Cluster # 11c: Scribbling

The most basic writing activity can involve giving the toddler sketch pens, pencils, painting brushes or crayons to scribble with. The child must begin to hold the writing device appropriately. He has to graduate from palm hold on writing instrument to tripod hold. Beginners around one-and-half to two years scribble with anything in hand or nearby. Their first marks are aimless groups of lines, but are related to later drawing, like babbling is related to later speech. The crayon may be held upside down or sideways with the fist or clenched fingers. Toddlers get enjoyment from doing scribbling. During this stage, the activity itself, and not the final end result, is important for the child. It is a mere sensory motor activity. The process of scribbling, and not the end result, is important for the toddler during this phase. Early scribbling is a disordered or random activity. The child does not have control on hand movements or on the page upon which he or she writing. The child cannot make the crayon move with a specific purpose, nor shows any desire to control or direct the movements of the crayon. He or she does not even recognize the scribbles made on the paper. The child receives comfort just by handling the writing materials, putting crayons in a box, bringing them out, putting them back, rolling them across the table, and so on.

It is useful to keep a portfolio of the visual record of the child's scribbling and progress. A portfolio is a sample or representative collection of their work. It reduces the subjectivity of discussions and helps look at the child's productions objectively. A later stage is controlled scribbling. This occurs when the toddler finds a connection between the writing motions and what gets imprinted on the page. This stage, usually after six months of beginning to scribble, is characterized by relatively better motor control over the scribbling activity. Many adults generally cannot differentiate between controlled and uncontrolled scribbling. But this is a vital difference from the perspective of the child since he or she has gained a semblance of control over the scribbling activity. The scribbling stage is the right occasion to provide the child with a wide variety of writing materials and different shapes or textures of paper. It is always advisable to give as few colours of crayons as possible since a large variety of colours may be too distracting for the child.

**Table 5.17**

**Pre-writing Activities for Toddlers**

Makes impression prints.
Scribbles using tripod hold.
Uses sketch pen to make dots.
Uses sketch pen to extends tail to dots.
Uses sketch pen to joins two dots.
Imitates/copies vertical and horizontal lines.
Traces/copies own palm or small objects on paper.
Colours within circles or squares.
Paints water colours within figures.
Imitates cross and circle.
Copies cross and circle.
Copies square, triangle and inverted triangle.

**Additional forms for primary school years:**

Copies 'Union Jack' and simple star.
Traces/copies diamond, maltese cross and pentagon.
Copies spiked hexagon and complex star.
Copies 3D figures (cylinder, cube, cone and prism).
Copies star in square.
Duplicates patterns by linking dots on a grid.
Works through paper mazes.
Visually scans/cancels specific numbers on array.
Makes own signature.
Fills railway reservation forms and bank forms.
Reads and draws maps.
Reads and draws graphs.
Reads and draws flow diagrams/charts.

The primary aim of these activities is to enrich the child's motor control, switch from palm to tripod hold and reduce exaggerated arm movements from wide or jabbing actions. Some associated pre-writing activities for preschool children (Figure 5.2) could include finger, thread or leaf embossing, sand or block painting, vegetable or string printing, etc. (P16). Some children may not like the feel of finger or palm paint. If so, never force the child. Instead, find some other art activity that interests the child. The technique of rubbing peel-off crayon on paper is loved by children below three years of age.

## Activity Cluster # 11d: Copying Shapes

Purposeful and co-ordinated scribbling in toddlers can gradually be turned towards imitative scribbling. The child may be instructed to imitate dot or jabs made on paper using thick felt pens. He or she could be shaped into modelling dots with a tail in different directions. Associated rhymes like the 'standing up line, lying down line, slanting line, curved line and crooked line' can exhilarate toddlers performing these activities. Making geometrical shapes using matchsticks encourages form perception (P30). Tracing is another absorbing activity for toddlers. The impressions of a dark felt pen through tracing sheet for the child to run his writing instrument over is a curious play to be indulged in over several minutes. The child should begin tracing and copying simple or primary forms like circle, square and triangles.

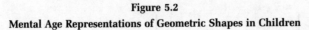

**Figure 5.2**
**Mental Age Representations of Geometric Shapes in Children**

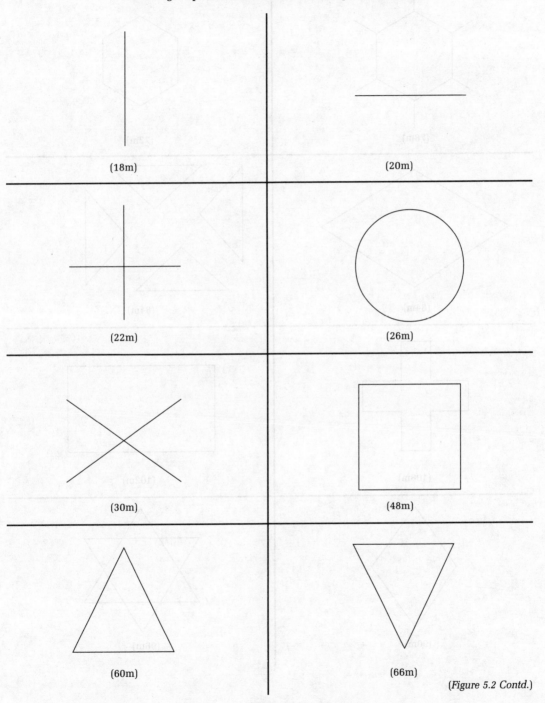

(18m)

(20m)

(22m)

(26m)

(30m)

(48m)

(60m)

(66m)

(*Figure 5.2 Contd.*)

(*Figure 5.2 Contd.*)

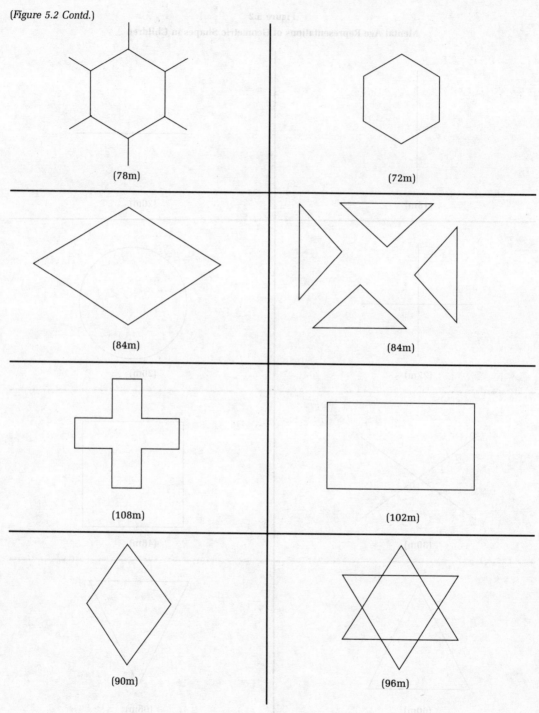

(78m)          (72m)

(84m)          (84m)

(108m)          (102m)

(90m)          (96m)

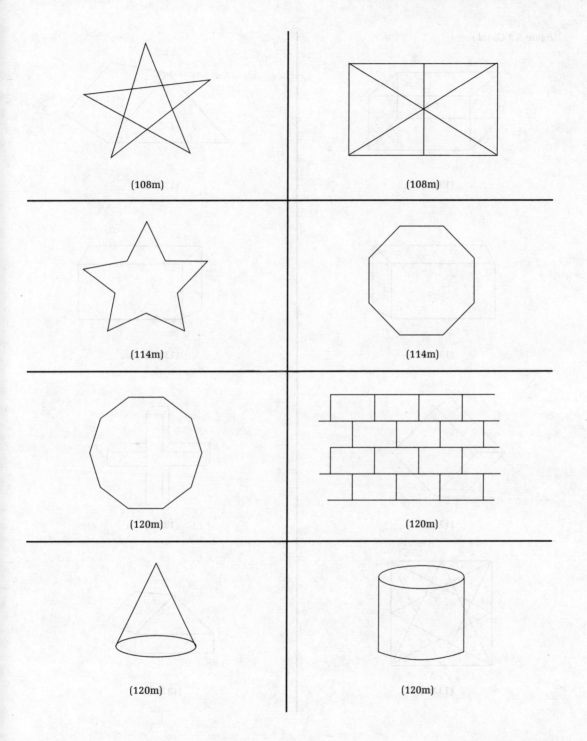

(108m)

(108m)

(114m)

(114m)

(120m)

(120m)

(120m)

(120m)

(*Figure 5.2 Contd.*)

*(Figure 5.2 Contd.)*

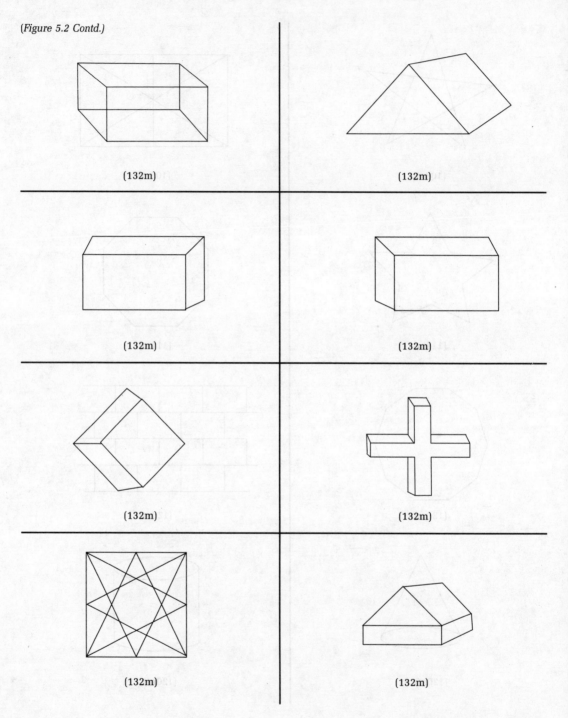

(132m)

(132m)

(132m)

(132m)

(132m)

(132m)

(132m)

(132m)

Then go ahead with inverted or rotated triangles before superimposing two equilateral triangles to form a simple star pattern. Ovals, curved lines or arcs can be added at the primary school or elementary stage. Proceed to secondary shapes like vertical and horizontal diamond, trapezium, parallelogram, honeycomb designs, simple and spiked polygons, hexagon, octagon and the like. Eventually, proceed to enable the child to learn copying complex tertiary shapes like star, three-dimensional cube, cylinder, cone, prism, and so on. A sample representation of various forms is given in Figure 5.2 (Venkatesan, 2002a). Additional and advanced writing skills may be given in the form of duplicating and joining dots on a graphical grid, working through paper mazes, reading and drawing maps, graphs, flow diagrams/charts, etc. Drawing competencies can be encouraged through draw-a-person activities involving the child drawing human figures with as many body parts. The number and quality of details in human figure drawings are usually proportional to the developmental level of any given child.

**Pre-arithmetic:** Upon cursory glance, it may appear that toddlers learn rote recitation of numbers either up to five or 10 (PA25) 'spontaneously' and hence do not require any formal training in this activity. Indeed, most preschoolers learn the basics of numeration on their own from their environment through imitation. In children with DDs, an exclusive programme on number skills has to be imparted. Linking number counts with activities of the toddler can make a beginning exposure to the world of numbers. For example, instruct a toddler to 'jump only after I say start!' or 'run after I count 1–2–3!' These games will not only help the child learn postponement/waiting skills, but also, simultaneously, expose him to numbers. Rote recitation of numbers is a distinct activity from meaningful counting of numbers. A child may be proficient in rote recitation of numbers even till 100 and yet be incapable of counting and giving away five carrots from an array of 10 or more (PA37). Meaningful counting

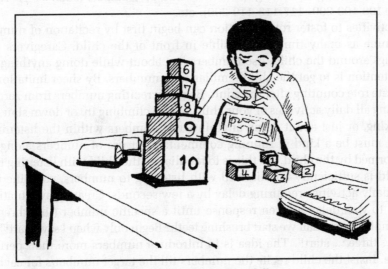

**Illustration 5.22  Number Skills**

carries with it an ability to make one-to-one correspondence between numbers and each object in front of the child. Concurrently, the toddler must also learn to differentiate between 'more–less' from two heaps of objects (PA30). The child could also learn to identify ordinal position on a series of objects beginning from 'first-second-third-fourth' (PA45) and so on. Recognition of printed numbers is quite another activity from rote recitation of numbers and/or meaningful counting of objects by children. Flash cards depicting numbers below 100 or 10 are used to observe whether the child can read a given numeral (PA33) (Venkatesan and Vepuri, 1993b).

## Activity Cluster # 11e: Rote Recitation

Rote recitation is a serial and mechanical rendition of numbers with little or no understanding of the recitation. As a beginning exercise under pre-arithmetic operations, there are various levels of performance. At the lowest level, the child recites numerals in units from one to nine (PA31). This is followed by recitation of numerals in tens from 10 to 99 or higher. Rote recitation must eventually cover the Indian system and the million system. The common difficulties encountered by children within each level of performance in this operation may be complete inability to recite numbers at all, recitation up to some specific number only, circuitous repetitions within some numbers, transgression problems around tens, hundreds or thousands, etc. The baseline assessment of this target behaviour involves instructing the child to recite numbers from one to whatever upper-end limit that he or she can go to. Do not confuse this number recitation activity with meaningful counting, object counting and/or other forms of number work. Observe or hear the child recite till those numbers are reached where he or she commits mistakes. Do not correct the mistakes at once. Just note down the errors without passing any comments/judgements. The common errors in number recitation are inability to recite numbers, recitation only up to 5, 10, 20, 99 or some such specific number, utterance of numbers at random (like 5-8-2-7), jumping/skipping numbers (like 1-2-3-4-5-9-10-11-15), halting or making mistakes at turn off numbers (such as, 18-19-10, 28-29-20, 38-39-50, 108-109-200, 117-118-119-200), etc.

Specific activities to foster rote recitation can begin first by recitation of numbers beginning one to nine as many times as possible in front of the child. Caregivers could keep counting things around the child, use numbers just about while doing anything and everything. The intention is to get the child familiar with numbers. By sheer imitation, the child learns to imitate rote counting after the adult. Begin by reciting numbers from zero to three or five only during all daily activities of your child. While climbing up or down stairs, brushing, bathing, walking, or just about doing anything, use numbers within the listening range of your child. It must be a kind of running commentary on use of numbers along with daily routines performed by the child. All this is to familiarize the child with listening to numbers. After the child is sufficiently familiarized with listening to numbers, combine using them with certain daily activities requiring delay by a few seconds. Create play situations requiring the child to wait/delay a given response until a specific number (like three or five) is counted. Example: 'Now, shall we start brushing teeth? Begin only when I say "start!" ... Ready ... one ... two ... three ... start!'. The idea is to introduce numbers more than performing the activity per se. Insist the child recite the numbers till the target number/s for each and every activity is met. Initially, begin with the maximum number as 'three!', then proceed to expand the upper limit to 5, 10, 20, 50 and so on. Combine number recitation activities of your child with game situations, such as 'One … Two … Three … Run!'.

A higher form of rote recitation is reciting numbers in a specified sequence. This must be distinguished from earlier mechanical recitation under rote counting. Herein, the child has to count in a specific sequence of twos, fives (PA42) and tens (PA46). A precursor to later recitation of multiplication tables and time concepts, this activity is not to be confused with writing specific numbers to dictation, writing in words or other forms of number work. During baseline assessment, instruct the child to 'Rote recite numbers 2 … 4 … 6 … and so on till 20'. Then, proceed to 'Rote recite numbers 5 … 10 … 15 … and so on till 60', still later to 'Rote recite numbers 10 … 20 … 30 … and so on'. The next higher activity related to rote recitation is mechanical (often rhythmic) recitation of mathematical tables. The sing-song fashion of rendition facilitates easy acquisition, retention and recall. Over-learning or acquisition beyond trials of errorless repetition prevents occurrence of errors. Over-learning goes beyond the criterion for learning. Thus, if it takes 20 trials to learn a multiplication table, practice of 20 additional trials is recognized as 100 per cent over-learning. Recitation of tables is an important precursor to later math application skills like multiplication, division and time reading. There are various levels of performance on the task of rote recitation of multiplication tables. An introduction to the concept of recitation of tables one and two is followed by acquisition of tables 3 to 10 respectively. This activity is not to be confused with writing down tables. All that the child is required to achieve under this target behaviour is to orally recite the tables, preferably in rhythm. During baseline assessment, instruct the child to 'Rote recite tables $1 \times 1$: 1, $2 \times 1$: 2, and so on'. Elicit the maximum numbers up to which the child can recite tables.

## Activity Cluster # 11f: Object Counting

Usually following rote counting, object counting refers to the activity of the child meaningfully counting objects placed in front of him or her. There can be various levels of performance on this operation. At the lowest level, the child counts objects in units from 1 to 9. This is followed by object counting in tens from 10 to 99 and hundreds from 100 to 999. During baseline assessment, place some identical objects (say four beads). Instruct the child to count them aloud. An important prerequisite for object counting is rote counting. The child must have the skill to rote recite numbers at least up to 10 before you take up teaching this target behaviour. Another prerequisite for meaningful object counting is one-to-one correspondence. This refers to the ability to assign one numeral to one object at a time, rather than confusing or assigning two or more numbers for the same object. Errors can occur in this activity while assigning numerals singly to each object. To teach this target behaviour, begin by placing less than five objects in front of the child for meaningful counting. Assist the child physically by holding his or her hands and pointing the index finger individually to each object placed in front and saying the number aloud. Use physical guidance and verbal instructions simultaneously as the child is performing the task. Later, increase the number of objects for counting. Generalize the object-counting skills learnt in classroom situations to real life counting in various situations like counting cars in a parking lot, trees along the pavement, spoons on a table, books on a shelf, etc.

## Activity Cluster # 11g: Number Matching

A useful activity following achievement on rote counting and meaningful counting up to around 10 or 20 is matching model number of objects. A prerequisite for this activity is rote counting and visual matching. The child must match objects/pictures of identical animals, vegetables, fruits and/or domestic appliances. Place three objects, say cubes, in front of the child. Instruct him to place an identical number of cubes against each of them. Use physical guidance and verbal instructions simultaneously as the child performs the task. Later, add more and more objects for the child to match against them. Use familiar objects like safety pins, pencils, erasers, pegs, beads, etc. Corollary activities can involve instructing the child to place as many objects as shown on fingers or extending as many fingers as objects in front of him or her (Table 5.18).

**Table 5.18**
**Number Matching Activities for Preschoolers**

| Caregiver | Subject |
|---|---|
| Raises certain number of fingers | Arranges identical model number of objects |
| Shows flash card with a printed number | Raises identical number of fingers |
| Raises certain number of fingers | Raises identical number of fingers |
| Presents model number of objects | Raises identical number of fingers |
| Presents model number of objects | Shows card with identical printed number |
| Raises certain number of fingers | Shows card with identical printed number |
| Shows flash card with a printed number | Shows card with identical printed number |

## Activity Cluster # 11h: Number Naming/Identification

It is one thing to rote recite numbers or even meaningfully count off objects placed before the child. It is quite another thing to read, identify or name printed numerical figures or symbols (such as 1, 2, 3). An important prerequisite to number naming is picture naming or identification. The child should be adept at pointing to pictures of familiar animals, vegetables, vehicles, household articles and so on. During baseline assessment, present single and/or two-digit figures on a paper and ask the child to read them (PA29). Begin with random checks, say by presenting numbers below five; later, proceed to numbers between 5 and 10. The upper limits or maximum level for reading written numbers could be anywhere up to 99 (or 999), proceeding only by increase of tens. The transition from rote recitation of numbers or even meaningful counting of numbers to number reading/identification is critical. There is an initial phase when the child confuses meaningful counting of objects with actual numerical symbols. For example, when asked to point to the number 'three' out of five numbered cards kept before the child, the child may pick up three cards! It is important to clarify that he or she has to point to the number 'three' and not count to pick up three cards. Apart from object counting, the child should also understand ordinal positions of numbers. The child should know that two is a bigger number than one, seven is smaller than nine and so on (PA38).

## Activity Cluster # 11i: Number Writing

Number-writing skills must go hand-in-hand or follow rote recitation of numbers. When the child has mastered rote recitation of numbers up to 100, he or she could be trained in writing numbers serially up to 10. These target behaviours refer to the action of writing numbers serially from one to whatever upper limits that a child can write. Do not confuse this serial number writing activity to writing specific numbers to dictation, writing in words or other forms of number work. During baseline assessment, instruct the child to 'Write numbers serially from one, two, three ... start!'. Observe the child writing numbers till he or she commits mistakes. Note down the child's errors without correcting them or passing any comments/judgements immediately. The common types of errors children make in serial number writing are an inability to write numbers at all; writing to 5, 10, 20, 99 or some such specific number before stopping; writing numbers at random (example: 5-8-2-7-24-16); jumping/skipping numbers (example: 1-2-3-4-5-9-10-11-15); halting/making mistakes at tens, hundreds or turn off numbers (example: 18-19-10, 28-29-20, 38-39-50, 108-109-200, 117-118-119-200). A correction programme for these errors must precede by first ascertaining whether the child can rote recite numbers. The child must also have adequate grapho-motor skills like tripod hold on writing instruments and be able to copy primary shapes.

Start by asking the beginning child to imitate numbers one to three written by you on a slate or paper. Insist on the child saying the number/s aloud as he or she writes each one of them for practice again and again. Combine use of finger-tracing activities on specific number shape cut-outs made of sandpaper or thick cardboard. The child must be made to feel or appreciate the shapes, outlines, contours and curves of each number. Initially, begin with the maximum number as 'Three!', then proceed to expand the upper limits to 10, 20, 50 and so on. Proceed in small steps. Add on according to the individual requirements or speed of learning in each child. Combine number recitation exercises along with serial number-writing activities. After the child has reached numeration facility up to tens of thousand, he or she may have to be taught to rote learn the sequence of 'units (ones)-tens-hundreds-thousand-ten thousand-lakh-ten lakh-crore-ten crore' in the Indian system and/or 'units (ones)-tens-hundreds-thousand-ten thousand-hundred thousand (million)-ten million-hundred million (billion)' in the American system respectively. Appropriate tables may be drawn to provide visual clues for the child to write whole numbers to dictation. The whole number sequences may then be replaced with zeroes at specific place values. The use of a calculator to entry numbers on dictation is a variation to induce interest in young children (PA43).

## Activity Cluster # 11j: Arithmetic Operations

Basic arithmetic operations like addition, subtraction, multiplication and division rightly fall under the domain of primary school curriculum. Yet, if some preschool children are able to master numeration up to 100, single or two digit additions without involving carry-over operations may be introduced at preschool levels too. Single digit addition operations (PA48) are introduced by concrete means by counters, abacus, counting beads, use of fingers or dots/dashes made on paper. Begin with single-digit additions whose answers do not cross over 10. Two-digit additions are one step ahead since the child has to understand to proceed from right to left and not vice versa. Calculators help in making appropriate entries of numbers or math symbols like plus and minus. Single- or-two-digit subtractions (PA49; PA50) are relatively difficult to impress on preschoolers. The numbers or their products should be intentionally kept below 10 so that there is no need to use 'borrow' operations from a neighbouring digit. Again, the use of concrete cues is strongly recommended for teaching subtraction to preschool children.

## Epilogue

With the broad and generic outlines given above, the trainer of children is expected to be proficient in deciding on both questions: 'What to teach?' as well as 'How to teach?' infants, preschoolers and toddlers with DDs. Obviously, the contents in this chapter are to be read in conjunction with the guidelines made available in the other chapters and the steps in skill training programmes delineated in the earlier chapters.

# CHAPTER 6

# RIGHTS FOR THE DISABLED IN INDIA: CONTEMPORARY PROBLEMS AND ISSUES

*This chapter addresses the contemporary trends, problems and issues regarding the rights, immunities and privileges of persons with disabilities in India. A brief sketch on service delivery systems for the disabled, including government initiative, is outlined before discussing possible areas for improvement in the field of disability rehabilitation in the country.*

Organized services for disabled persons are of recent origin in India. Persons with disabilities have always been an integral part of Indian society. The origins and evolution of services in the field of disability rehabilitation in India can be broadly conceptualized as falling under the following distinct but related phases.

## Individualized or Stagnant Personal Services

The prevalent common sense does not distinguish handicaps from illness. Indian folklore is replete with references to a category of individuals in society who are *Mandukas* (inferior in intellect) as against *Paithyams* (transient insanity). Prevailing Indian society in the early days did not find any great need for regular institutional systems to meet the special needs of these persons. The behavioural anomalies of handicapped persons have always been tolerated either as inevitable aberrations of human nature or as justified consequences of one's sins in previous births. The attitude of society, especially towards mild levels of handicaps, has generally been positive, if not overindulgent. Despite overt expressions of pejorative remarks, prank or ridicule against the conventional 'village idiot', 'dud', 'lame', 'crippled', 'blind', etc. (*sic*), the underlying feelings of society towards these persons is one of overwhelming concern. It is only persons with severe forms of disability that society fails to integrate attitudinally (Murthy et al., 1980; Gandhi and Agarwal, 1969). In fact, Indian social systems react with intense vehemence and even enforce confinement, isolation or incarceration of such persons. Often these negative feelings spill over to their close kith and kin. The affected families are understood as the inescapable consequence of past sins in previous births, or punishment meted out by preternatural forces to equalize their balance sheets for all their acts of omission and commission. Popular opinion assuages their unfortunate predicament as benevolent gifts of divine forces attempting to test their resilience in withstanding or overcoming the troubles and travails of their contemporary existence. Most readymade common-sense perceptions on disabilities are based on sop sentimentalism or lofty spiritual excuses. A rationally thought out scientific reflection of this social problem is conspicuous by its absence in lay minds. This ambivalence between over-pity, indulgence and blind patronage for the disabled versus their absolute rejection, ridicule or reprehension dominates the masses even today (Ramdas and Mishra, 1987).

Unorganized, individualized or stagnant personal services for the handicapped exist in the form of traditional healers, magico-religious heads and/or family 'gurus' dispensing non-scientific palliatives such as sermons or preaching. Sometimes, they are couched in semi-scientific advice by family physicians or individual consulting doctors prescribing brain-stimulating tonics or suggesting parents to wait and watch the disabled child develop on his or her own. The major difficulty in these form of services is their prohibitive cost, and the inherent difficulty in shipment of such services beyond certain circumscribed geographical limits. Hence, the reach of these services is restricted to the privileged sections of contemporary society (Narasimhan and Mukherjee, 1995).

## Non-government or Voluntary Services

A background of sentimentalism, lack of scientific temper and inability of stagnant services to cope with the increasing demand has led to development of formal or organized institution-based services for the disabled. Organized institutional services for the disabled are of recent origin in India. For instance, the Home for Mentally Deficient Children, Mumbai, established by the Children's Aid Society in 1941, is said to be the first voluntary agency for mentally retarded persons in India. Even now, many voluntary organizations thrive on the sentimentalism of well-meaning philanthropists. Organized voluntary services for disabled persons in contemporary India is beset with problems. Social activists organize most voluntary organizations with humanitarian concerns. Many of them, especially in earlier periods, were raised on religious zeal and sentimentalism with an eye on doing 'good' for the 'unfortunately disabled'. Their services were seen as acts of service for God. Even today, many institutions project the overt guise of a team of governing-body members/trustees. In actuality, one encounters idolization or even unabashed hero worship of an individual in place of the cause for which these organizations exist.

The individual elements of such systems fail to match perceptions with the broad goals or objectives for which these institutions exist. Decision-making within such systems function in a way to promote success of a particular individual, while there are no mechanisms in place to guarantee the cause for which the entire system is supposed to stand. They invest all individual energies to aggrandize the icons of their dominating masters. The bane of such organizations is aggravated when the individual (around whom the system exists) is myopic, odd or has idiosyncratic quirks that interfere in smooth realization of welfare goals for the handicapped. Also, the longevity of such organizations get circumscribed to the life span of such individuals owing to their incapacity to generate longitudinal leadership that can carry on their activities over generations. Thus, one observes an intense ascendancy of these leaders or their organizations only to culminate in their demise. Most voluntary organizations suffer great strain on their fiscal resources. If they rely on individual donations of philanthropists, they find these resources becoming increasingly scarce in view of the changing outlook favouring materialism, self-centredness and unwillingness to part with economic wealth. Some agencies secure financial aid from the government to run their activities. However, this is not easily achieved owing to bureaucratization of grant-in-aid release procedures.

Organizations have neither the manpower nor the expertise to meander their ways through the corridors of funding agencies.

## Government-aided/Sponsored Services

Before Independence, there was no initiation from the government to partake in services for handicapped persons in the country. There was no demand for such services as public awareness and social consciousness on issues related to disability rehabilitation were dismally low. In 1950, for the first time, the Government of India recognized disabled persons as equal and rightful participants in social and economic activities of the nation. This was guaranteed in the Constitution of India before central and state governments started expressing concern for the welfare of these sections of society. In the early post-Independence years, the government invested on establishment of institutions for care or training of handicapped persons in various parts of the country. Of late, there has been a growing emphasis on disinvestment of such infrastructure building projects (Pandey and Advani, 1996; Chowdhry, 1995). Rather, several support schemes/programmes are being adopted for the welfare of the handicapped by the Government of India in the current scene. The International Year of the Disabled (1981) may be taken as a turning point to draw the attention of the government towards problems of disabled within the country. Owing to international pressure rather than due to domestic activism, last minute deadlines were honoured to promulgate various policies, programmes and laws for the handicapped (Table 6.1).

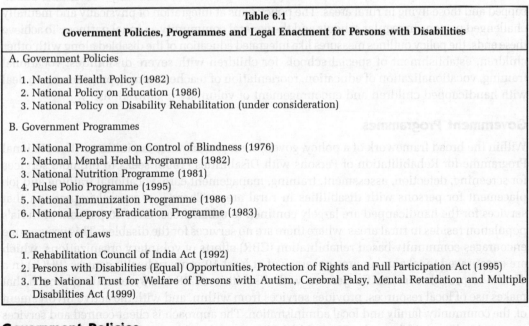

**Table 6.1**

**Government Policies, Programmes and Legal Enactment for Persons with Disabilities**

A. Government Policies

1. National Health Policy (1982)
2. National Policy on Education (1986)
3. National Policy on Disability Rehabilitation (under consideration)

B. Government Programmes

1. National Programme on Control of Blindness (1976)
2. National Mental Health Programme (1982)
3. National Nutrition Programme (1981)
4. Pulse Polio Programme (1995)
5. National Immunization Programme (1986 )
6. National Leprosy Eradication Programme (1983)

C. Enactment of Laws

1. Rehabilitation Council of India Act (1992)
2. Persons with Disabilities (Equal) Opportunities, Protection of Rights and Full Participation Act (1995)
3. The National Trust for Welfare of Persons with Autism, Cerebral Palsy, Mental Retardation and Multiple Disabilities Act (1999)

## Government Policies

A National Policy on Disability Rehabilitation is on the anvil. A couple of drafts of this policy have been in circulation since 1979. A policy document indicates commitment of the government towards programmes and schemes to be formulated and implemented for rehabilitation of persons with disabilities. This policy aims at enablement, empowerment and emancipation of persons with disabilities. There is commitment to take necessary administrative, executive and legislative measures for achieving the objectives of equal opportunities, providing full participation, creating non-handicapping environments and sensitizing the community at large on the needs, potential and contributions of people with disabilities. There is also a resolution to work in close collaboration and partnership with voluntary organizations or parents of persons with disabilities. The major areas for intervention enunciated in the policy includes public awareness, prevention, early detection and intervention, free access to education (with appropriate curricular adaptation and examination reforms), vocational training, employment, etc. There is emphasis on providing social security, concessions, access to recreation and sports facilities and providing or promoting assistive devices for handicapped. The slogan of the document is 'Rehabilitation for all by 2025'.

When this policy comes through eventually, it will have to be read in consonance with other existing government policies. The National Health Policy (1982) outlines approaches and components on a comprehensive network of services, transfer of knowledge, simple skills and technologies to health volunteers, building up of individual self-reliance and effective community participation, provision of services in an integrated manner, organization of domiciliary services and active involvement of voluntary organizations in the process of spreading health care in the country. The National Policy on Education (1986) emphasizes removal of disparities and equalizing educational opportunities for all, including women, the handicapped and those living in rural areas. The policy aims at integration of physically and mentally challenged persons in regular schools and the general community as equal partners. To achieve these ends, the policy outlines measures like integrated education of the disabled along with other children, establishment of special schools for children with severe disabilities, vocational training, vocationalization of education, reorientation of teacher training programmes to deal with handicapped children and encouragement of voluntary organizations.

## Government Programmes

Within the broad framework of a policy, government programmes are initiated. The National Programme for Rehabilitation of Persons with Disabilities (1995) seeks to promote services for screening, detection, assessment, training, management care, vocational training and job placement for persons with disabilities in rural areas. There is a general impression that services for the handicapped are largely confined to urban areas. Over 60 per cent of India's population resides in rural areas, where there are no services for the disabled. This programme encourages community-based rehabilitation (CBR) efforts of voluntary organizations, which are encouraged to take up an area coverage of at least 10 primary health centres (PHCs) in a district to provide services for persons with disabilities. CBR is a systematic approach that makes use of local resources, provides services from within, and with the active involvement of, the community, family and local administration. The approach is client-centred and services are provided for the felt needs of individual or groups of persons with disabilities. The thrust of CBR is also to simplify or demystify technology for training or rehabilitation of disabled persons (Hanumantharao et al., 1993). The *Viklang Bandhu* Training Programme, for example, is a typical CBR activity encouraged by the Ministry of Social Justice and Empowerment, Government of India. Under this programme, people with disabilities, or their relatives in a given locality, *taluk* or district, are selected on a voluntary basis and given training for a period of four months with an objective to help people with disabilities in their own region. The course content includes basic information on all disabilities.

As another part of the National Programme for Rehabilitation of Persons with Disabilities, more than a hundred districts have been selected for setting up district disability rehabilitation centres (DDRCs) monitored by composite regional rehabilitation centres (CRRCs) spread over half-a-dozen zones in the country. The programme thrust is similar to an earlier district rehabilitation centre (DRC) scheme started in 1983. The DRC scheme involved establishment of centres, preferably in the premises of district hospitals, as primary rehabilitation units. The DRCs are manned at three levels by workers at district, PHC and village levels. At the district level, there is a director of the DRC supported by physicians/surgeons, prosthetic and orthotic technicians, physical/occupational therapists, psychologists, vocational counselors/social workers and sensory specialists. At the PHC level, there are multipurpose rehabilitation workers/assistants, therapists, workers and technicians. At the village level, there are village rehabilitation workers. Twelve DRCs were started on an experimental basis in 1983. The regional rehabilitation training centers (RRTCs) were set up to provide technical support to DRCs in the area of training professional manpower, paramedical and field workers. The four RRTC were given jurisdiction over three to four DRCs under each of them. While the existing DRCs are still functional, no further expansion on this line of programme appears to be taking place. Now, the DDRC and the CRRC are expected to continue work at village levels in the future. Other government programmes with direct or indirect bearing to the field of disability rehabilitation are the National Mental Health Programme (1982), National Nutrition Programme (1981), Pulse Polio Programme (1995), National Immunization Programme (1986), National Leprosy Eradication Programme (1983), etc.

## Laws and Legal Enactment

In recent times, the Government of India has initiated a few legislative measures with direct or indirect impact on the overall scenario in disability rehabilitation in our country (Dhanda, 2000). Some of the relevant laws are summarized below.

**Rehabilitation Council of India Act (1992):** The Rehabilitation Council of India Act (1992) came into effect from July 1993 as a corporate body with specific aims (Table 6.2). Among other things, the major achievement of this Council is accreditation of various categories of rehabilitation professionals into the central register and conduct of a joint entrance examination for admission into various levels of professional rehabilitation courses offered by national institutes across the country. In short, the Council is an apex body to further professionalism in the field of disability rehabilitation. For long, semi-professional courses were being marketed by various private organizations and giving rise to quackery. This has now changed. Condensed-level diploma/certificate/bridge courses or long-term degree/post graduate/pre-doctoral/doctoral and post-doctoral courses are now available for aspirants. Further, qualified professionals now have to be formally and legally registered with the Council and display their registration numbers and certificates during their practice. But till now, no audit measures have been undertaken to evaluate utilization of these neo-professionals for the direct benefit of disabled persons. There is an imperative need to develop procedures for reviewing professional behaviour, for cost-benefit analysis of manpower development, to develop accountability checks on their activities, etc.

---

**Table 6.2**

**Aims of the Rehabilitation Council of India**

1. To regulate training policies and programmes in the field of disability rehabilitation.
2. To prescribe minimum standards and regulate them in all training institutions throughout the country.
3. To recognize institutions/universities running degree/diploma/certificate courses in the field of disability rehabilitation and to withdraw recognition wherever facilities are not satisfactory.
4. To recognize foreign degree/diploma/certificates awarded by universities/institutions on a reciprocal basis.
5. To maintain a central rehabilitation register of persons possessing recognized rehabilitation qualifications in the country.
6. To encourage continuing rehabilitation education in collaboration with organizations working in the field of disability rehabilitation in the country.

---

**Persons with Disabilities (Equal) Opportunities, Protection of Rights and Full Participation Act (1995):** This Act received assent from the President of India on 1 January 1996. The promulgation of this Act was a sequel to the meeting to launch the Asian and Pacific Decade of Disabled Persons (1993–2002) by the Social and Economic Commission for Asia and the Pacific, held at Beijing between 1–5 December 1992; and the adoption of Full Participation and Equality of People with Disabilities in these regions. India is a signatory to this proclamation. The contents of this Act are elaborated under various clauses in 14 chapters with sections and sub-sections. In its preliminary section, the Act clarifies various terms, definitions and standard nomenclature. The Act provides for constitution of two committees, viz., central co-ordination committee and state co-ordination committee by notification along with their respective executive committees. The Act emphasizes adoption of several measures such as those listed under 'Government Schemes and Individual Benefits/Concessions for Persons with Disabilities'. A significant detail of the Act is that it seeks to identify, check or monitor and control government and voluntary organizations working with disabled persons. Such organizations must be registered. Their time-bound registration is subject to renewal after a periodic audit of their available facilities and/or performance. To cap it all, the government is committed to appoint a chief commissioner and state level commissioner for persons with disabilities along with other categories of officers and employees to assist in achievement of broad goals and policies envisaged in the Act.

While the enactment of this Act is laudable, there are many criticisms about it. For example, a sizeable number of children with specific learning disabilities and autistic disorders stand no consideration in the present definition of disability within this Act. While it seems sensible to demarcate more than 40 per cent of any disability (as certified by a medical authority) as operational definition of disability, precise numerical markers are not easily available for certain types of disability (like mental retardation). For example, in case of mental retardation, wherein below –2.00 standard deviation from the mean on standardized intelligence tests (such as 70 on Wechslers' Scale) is taken as international criteria, what would be the precise national norm? There are several anomalies in this criterion than what meets the untrained eye. While railway travel concessions are being offered for escorts as well as mentally handicapped persons with an IQ below 70, income tax rebates are offered only to parents of children whose IQ is less than 50.

There are additional problems and constraints in the implementation of this Act. According to the provisions of this Act, steps have to be taken to ensure a barrier-free environment in public places, general utility buildings like schools, cinema theatres, etc., by removal of architectural barriers. There is a need to pursue vigorous programmes to ensure equality for, and full participation of, people with disabilities. Although the Act was passed in 1996, the provisions of the Act are yet to be fully implemented. For example, the 3 per cent reservation of jobs in service sectors has not yet been realized. There are arrangements to be made for transport facilities, or alternatively, provide financial incentives for disabled children.

The Persons with Disabilities (Equal) Opportunities, Protection of Rights and Full Participation Act (1995) of India actually follows the American Disabilities Act (ADA). But there are also some crucial differences. The ADA has clear and specific guidelines for implementation of its provisions along with specific dates, deadlines, alternatives, temporary relief, and so on. The Indian Act does not have such features. For example, there are specifications that one coach per train is reserved for persons with disabilities. The Indian Act has granted this right, but not the means for its implementation. There is an escape clause which says that the government is bound to execute the provisions in the Act to the fullest 'economic capacity', something which is being used to shield or excuse non-performance! There is an ADA watch system to monitor implementation of the Act. This watchdog files suit for and represents the rights of the disabled. For example, television programmes started providing sign language interpreters during elections. A step was removed from a Philadelphia restaurant following litigation since it prevented the use of wheelchairs. In the Indian Act, the Chief Commissioner for Disabilities is supposed to be the watchdog and disseminate information on rights of the disabled across the country. ADA requires compliance and affirmative action by all agencies that receive financial assistance from the federal government. Unfortunately, the Indian Act has no such provisions. The ADA has a strong research agenda which continues to provide ongoing data on various aspects of implementation of the provisions under the Act. There is no research agenda at all in the Indian Act.

**The National Trust for Welfare of Persons with Autism, Cerebral Palsy, Mental Retardation and Multiple Disabilities Act (1999):** This Act was passed with the objective of providing guardianship rights to persons with disabilities. The nagging doubt of many parents on the fate of their handicapped children when they would be no more there to take care of them is answered to some extent by the provisions in this Act. Among other things, the Trust aims to take care of and protect persons with disabilities in the event of death of their parent/guardian. It deals with problems of persons with disabilities without family support. The Trust aims to evolve procedures for appointment of guardians/trustees for persons with disabilities requiring such protection. The Trust works through a Board specially constituted by the government for this purpose. A large number of local level committees have already been set up and are soon to be activated across various districts in the country.

## Government Schemes

A host of government schemes are now made available for service/rehabilitation of persons with handicaps in the country (Table 6.3). Many of these schemes are implemented through voluntary organizations. Probably, the idea is to use existing infrastructure available with most voluntary organizations rather than placing huge investments under such heads by the government. Further, it absolves the government from the trouble of raising a huge manpower force in the form of permanent employees with all their salaries and perks. The salient features of these schemes are presented below.

**Table 6.3**

**Government Schemes for Persons with Disabilities**

Government Schemes (Individual)

1. Scholarship for disabled persons, amanuensis allowance, transport allowance, etc.
2. Reservation of posts for physically handicapped persons in Groups C and D under central services.
3. Unemployment allowance/assistance for self employment for adults with disabilities.
4. Scheme for claim of family pension with respect to mentally retarded children.
5. Insurance schemes for the disabled

   (a) Jeevan Adhar LIC Policy
   (b) Jeevan Vishwas LIC Policy
   (c) Special plan for the handicapped formulated under UTI Children's Gift Growth Fund, 1986

Government Schemes (Institutional)

1. Scheme to promote voluntary action for persons with disabilities.
2. Integrated child development scheme (ICDS).
3. Schemes under ministry of rural development.
4. Scheme under ministry of education for integrated education of disabled.
5. Financial assistance under national handicapped finance corporation (1997).

**Scheme to Promote Voluntary Action for Persons with Disabilities:** This scheme, run by the Disability Division of the Ministry of Social Justice and Empowerment (MSJE), Government of India, provides nearly 90 per cent financial assistance to registered voluntary organizations providing vocational training and rehabilitation services to disabled persons. The specific activities eligible for assistance include primary prevention, detection and tertiary care of the disabled, parent counselling, education and rehabilitation. This is a revised scheme following the merger of four similar schemes of assistance to organizations under one umbrella with effect from January 1999. The four earlier schemes that have been merged under this revised scheme are:

(i)   Scheme of Assistance to Organizations for the Disabled.
(ii)  Scheme of Assistance to Voluntary Organizations for Rehabilitation of Leprosy Cured Persons.
(iii) Scheme of Assistance to Voluntary Organizations for Special School for Handicapped Children.
(iv)  Scheme of Assistance to Organizations for Persons with Cerebral and Mental Retardation.

**Scheme of Assistance to Disabled Persons for Purchase/Fitting of Aids and Appliances:** This scheme offered by the Disability Division of the MSJE, Government of India, assists needy physical and sensory challenged persons in procuring durable, sophisticated and scientifically-manufactured modern aids and appliances to promote their physical, economic and psycho-social rehabilitation. On the basis of monthly income levels of disabled persons or their families, their type or severity of handicap, place of residence, etc., various modalities of subsidies are earmarked under these schemes to be implemented by recognized and registered companies, trusts and societies in the country.

**Integrated Child Development Scheme:** The Integrated Child Development Scheme (ICDS), started in 1975 under the Ministry of Women and Child Development, Government of India, caters to children below six years by providing supplementary nutrition, immunization, health check-ups, referral, preschool and non-formal education. There are sporadic attempts to integrate disability components into this scheme to initiate early infant stimulation for children with disabilities. There is an onerous responsibility on the government to initiate in-service training programmes for *anganwadi* workers, who constitute grass-roots contacts under ICDS projects, so that they are sufficiently oriented on the disability components of early childhood management in rural settings.

**Schemes for Handicapped under Ministry of Rural Development:** Three per cent reservation for persons with disabilities is earmarked under various schemes for poverty alleviation and economic rehabilitation of persons living in rural areas:

(*i*)   Integrated Rural Development Programmes (IRDP)
(*ii*)  Training of Rural Youth for Self-employment (TRYSEM)
(*iii*) Development of Women and Children in Rural Areas (DWCRA)
(*iv*)  Indira Awaz Yojana and Jawahar Rozgar Yojana (JRY)
(*v*)   Swarnajayanthi Gramin Swarojgar Yojana

**Scheme for Integrated Education of Disabled Children:** This is a centrally-sponsored Scheme, launched in 1974 by the then Department of Social Welfare. The Scheme has been transferred to the Department of Education since 1982. Under this Scheme, mildly handicapped children are to be integrated within the normal school system. Hundred per cent assistance is provided for education of children with mild disabilities (including physical handicaps, mild or moderate hearing handicaps, partially sighted, educable group of mental handicaps, multiple and learning handicaps) in normal schools with the help of necessary aid, incentives and specially trained teachers. These children are provided allowances for purchase of books and stationery, uniforms, transport, equipment, etc. 'Resource room facilities' is an emerging concept under this scheme. The resource teacher is specially trained to teach disabled children systematically in co-ordination with the regular class teacher in the general school.

**Scheme for Financial Assistance under National Handicapped Finance Corporation:** To promote economic development activities, provide self-employment avenues, pursue general, professional or technical education and assist groups of individuals or co-operatives of persons with disabilities, the Government of India (under the MSJE) set up the National Handicapped Finance Development Corporation (NHFDC) in 1997 with a share capital of Rs 500 crore.

Loans are provided for amounts up to Rs 5 lakh with a repayment period subject to a maximum of seven years.

**Institutional Facilities:** The Government of India has also established apex bodies or national centres for each type of disability. The objectives of these institutions is to develop manpower, conduct research, provide models of clinical services and serve as information and documentation centres in their respective areas of disability. The six major institutions in this category are:

(*i*)   National Institute for the Visually Handicapped, Dehra Dun
(*ii*)  Ali Yavur Jung National Institute for the Hearing Handicapped, Mumbai
(*iii*) National Institute for the Mentally Handicapped, Secunderabad
(*iv*)  National Institute for Rehabilitation Training and Research, Cuttack
(*v*)   National Institute for the Orthopaedically Handicapped, Kolkata
(*vi*)  Institute for Physically Handicapped, Delhi

Each National Institute has its own regional centres (either direct, affiliated or franchisees) spread across the country. They all work in close co-ordination for achievement of the broad objectives proposed for them. There is also the Artificial Limbs Manufacturing Corporation (ALIMCO) set up in 1972 at Kanpur with the sole objective of promoting, developing, manufacturing and marketing artificial limbs and aids and appliances. ALIMCO is the only public sector company of its type in the country. It manufactures wheelchairs, crutches, tricycles and other aids/appliances matching international standards. They have limb fitting centres and implementing agencies spread across various parts of the country which carry out distribution of aids/appliances. A National Information Centre on Disability and Rehabilitation (NICDR), established in 1987, provides a database for comprehensive information on all facilities and welfare activities for the disabled in the country. It is a nodal agency for awareness creation and preparation, and collection and dissemination of materials or information regarding disability relief and rehabilitation.

## Individual Benefits/Concessions for Persons with Disabilities

A host of individual benefits/concessions for persons with disabilities are provided by the central and state governments (Table 6.4). These benefits accrue directly to individual persons with handicaps subject to proper certification by medical/rehabilitation professionals. Some common benefits/concessions for all categories of handicaps are travel concessions by rail/road, income tax rebate for parents of children with disabilities, customs concessions for individuals and institutions procuring equipment for disabled persons, loans at concession rates from nationalized banks, preferential allotment of house sites or PCO/STD booths, family pension, preferential place of posting for parents of children with mental retardation, etc. Some concessions that are available only in a few states are free braille lessons for blind students (Tamil Nadu), relaxation in age of retirement (Punjab), grace marks in examinations (Uttar Pradesh, Rajasthan and Kerala), financial assistance of Rs 100 to bedridden blind persons (Nagaland), priority in allotment of quarters for blind government employees (Haryana), exemption from the study of a second language in the seventh and tenth class board examinations (Karnataka), etc.

---

**Table 6.4**

**Individual Benefits/Concessions for Persons with Disabilities**

**Benefits and Concessions (Central Government)**

1. Travel concessions by rail or road
2. Awards and honours for persons with disabilities and/or their employers
3. Customs concessions for individuals and institutions
4. Income tax concessions
5. Loans at concession rates from nationalized banks for starting self-employment
6. Family/disability pension
7. Preferential allotment of STD/PCO
8. Preferential allotment of sites
9. Preferential place of posting for government employees having children with mental retardation
10. Children's educational allowance for government employees having children with mental retardation
11. One per cent reservation of jobs in central and state service for physical, hearing and visually handicapped persons
12. Exemption from payment of application or examination fee as prescribed by UPSC/SSC for physically handicapped persons
13. Relaxation in typing qualifications for appointment to posts of lower division clerk in services

**Benefits and Concessions (State Government)**

1. Scholarships
2. Disability pension
3. Unemployment allowance
4. Marriage incentives
5. Free braille for blind students (Tamil Nadu)
6. Relaxation in age of retirement (Punjab)
7. Grace marks in examinations (Uttar Pradesh, Rajasthan and Kerala)
8. Financial assistance of Rs 100 to blind persons who are bedridden (Nagaland)
9. Priority in allotment of quarters for blind government employees (Haryana)
10. Exemption from study of second language subjects in seventh or tenth class board examinations (Karnataka)

---

## Consumer-based Self Support Services

Despite oddities and travails in quality, the momentum to raise voluntary services for individuals with handicaps is gradually gaining ground in India. Simultaneously, one discovers a new trend in the handicapped-care industry from movements initiated by philanthropists to directly by consumers (parents or caregivers of handicapped persons). At times, parents' self-help groups have evolved as a consequence of their dissatisfaction or disgust with philanthropist activities. The present emphasis is on building awareness among consumers and enabling them to form their own self-help groups. Consumers are encouraged to register their associations and even enlist professional support to run services for themselves or their children with disabilities. Initial experiments along these lines are proving popular and successful. There are over a hundred registered parents' self-help groups for mentally handicapped persons. Some of them have even availed of group insurance to ensure adequate economic and social security benefits.

Self-help consumer movements hold great promise for the future of rehabilitation. They have the potential to become strong pressure groups or advocacy nodes to fight for the cause of disabled persons. In due course, they could even become watchdogs to challenge professional behaviour; they could also signal a death knell for pseudo-philanthropist activities by increasing their consumer controls and consciousness. A system of third-party payers to sponsor their expenses must also be invoked. Overt competition between self-help services and voluntary organizations is beginning to appear. Another deviation is that the care industry is shifting from in-patient to ambulatory or itinerant services. The eventual shape that this movement is likely to take in the future is difficult to forecast. The present scenario demonstrates considerable uncertainty. No specific prognostic indicators are now available. More research is now required to increase understanding of these changes so as to frame a perspective that can improve the rehabilitation care system in the country.

## Recommendations

Against the backdrop of available service facilities for persons with disabilities in the country, it would be apt to seriously introspect on the state of affairs and provide reflective recommendations for bettering the qualities of lives of these individuals.

### Converting Attitudinal Fixedness

A beginning anomaly exists in the attitude of the public at large towards persons with disabilities, as well as in professional caregivers/organizations working for the disabled in our country. While professional knowledge condemns the contemporary attitudes of ridicule, pity, charity or sympathy for the disabled as primitive, it is an equally unfortunate predicament that most voluntary organizations work for the handicapped only with charitable or philanthropic contributions from a privileged few. Further, most of them are registered as 'not-for-profit, non-commercial voluntary agencies'. This conveys that they are only consumptive units awaiting benevolent dispensations from the more productive sections of society. Such contributions come in cash or kind, grants-in-aid from the government, funds from national/international agencies, donations from the public, loans from financial institutions, etc. In any case, they have to beg or borrow for their sustenance—leave alone earmarking additional monies for developmental activities and programmes. There is a need to break this traditional bondage of services for the disabled from the clutches of their financial slavery under those sections of society with the means, money or resources that may or may not be parted at their will and mercy. It is time to review and revolutionize the very framework of service delivery for the disabled by shedding the guise of 'not-for-profit, non-commercial voluntary agencies' to profit-making commercial ventures. There is a need for these organizations to give up their 'not-for-profit' attitude in creating or formulating registered societies and/or trusts. There could be a trend towards association of persons under the Companies Act (1956). The enterprise of services for disabled persons needs to be looked upon as an industry or joint business venture having its own distinct name and limited liability.

### Lessons from the Health Sector

In this regard, it is pertinent to take cue from recent developments in the health sector of our country. About a decade ago, extension of health services was mostly in the hands of government agencies and mushrooming private medical practitioners, dispensaries, hospitals and nursing homes. This scenario has significantly altered in recent years with the advent of what are known as 'corporate private hospitals'. Several private companies floated by zealous entrepreneurs vie with one another to provide the best medical specialists, equipment and facilities at competitive prices. Some corporates even offer private health-insurance cover to decrease the liability burden of prospective customers. On the whole, health care in the country is becoming a scientifically-managed business enterprise/industry. The fiscal investments in the health sector are beginning to be viewed as positive and mandatory contributions of society to offset huge losses or prohibitive costs of disease and ill health. Almost an identical logic justifies an invitation for higher investment in the rehabilitation sector. An apparent 5 per cent of the handicapped population in the country actually hides more than 20 per cent of the incapacitated population. This is on the assumption that there are at least five members on an average in the family who are equally affected, either as a parent or sibling of the handicapped person. No civil society can afford the neglect of such vast human resources by curtailing fiscal investments in this sector or by leaving it for non-handicapped sections to bear the yoke. It is not a far cry to visualize extension of rehabilitation services in the same vein as the health sector. If the contemporary disability-rehabilitation sector in the country pulls itself out of the prevailing enmeshment of its self-created attitudinal incarceration accompanied with archaic notions of alms giving, public pity, sympathy and charity, there would be a more active and self-determined course to charter for its future. Even before services for persons with disabilities identifies itself as a distinct corporate entity, there is a need to invite an attitude of corporate culture in prevailing establishments. In the existing scenario, there is already evidence of the seeds being sown for such a culture in the country.

## Corporate Culture in Disability Rehabilitation

Many companies are beginning to seek to be perceived as upstanding corporate citizens. Clichés like 'caring for the environment', 'caring for the uncared' and 'community development' have already been abused to such an extent that they have almost become 'meaningless' buzzwords. While some initial skepticism in this matter seems justified in the light of increased pressure of competition, the fact remains that many companies are going ahead to garner goodwill for themselves, either through community welfare activities or by sponsoring social events.

A share of the 'Miss World 1997' collections were reportedly earmarked for spastic children. The Times of India Group recently sponsored the 'Times Hero Award' for a person who saved the lives of dozens of children caught under river waters as a speeding bus turned turtle on a bridge over the Yamuna. The same group gave away a share of their earnings over two weeks from the sale of classified advertising space to a voluntary organization in the service of health and education for children. The Tata Group spent close to Rs 243 crore on various social welfare activities in 1996–97, an increase of 36 per cent over the previous year. After sensing the need to facilitate community development efforts of the 85 Tata Enterprises spread across the country, the Group decided to channel all their activities into one central institution called the Tata Council for Community Initiatives. But community development is not the only way in which companies are nurturing community networks. The trend towards sponsoring events focused on personalities needing funds to enhance their capabilities is on the rise. Most companies sponsor events with an eye on the publicity generated, hoping that it would rub off on the image of their brands. Pepsi, for example, is unlikely to sponsor any event that does not have the 'youth' element in it. The Reliance Group sponsors an art show to bring together a multitude of artists under the theme of 'harmony'. It is no coincidence that Reliance's top-of-the-line furnishing range has the same trade name.

The need for corporate sponsorship and community development can be looked upon as a pragmatic and long-term strategy. To be recognized as an outstanding corporate citizen is a title that the company can flaunt, an edge it can claim psychologically over others. The benefits that arise from this can have a positive snow-balling effect on future and existing employees, consumers and the company's image in a global scenario. In an increasingly competitive environment, talent is keen to be associated with a company that is seen as more respectable in the public eye. For existing employees, it sends messages of trust and helps retention by making a person rethink a decision to quit the place. It establishes credibility and subliminally creates a sense of trust in the minds of the customers. It becomes generally believed that such companies will not indulge in underhand trade practices. Despite these noble measures, there is an urgent need to translate these ideas of welfare and charity into gestures and make them a part of the ethos of the company. Mere lip service will not suffice. It is not adequate to write a fat cheque for a cause and then absolve oneself of all responsibility.

## Boosting Corporate Philanthropy

Industry bigwigs can look for an active role in creating job opportunities for the disabled in the country. Of the about 70 lakh employable disabled in India, only 1 lakh have been provided jobs in the past 40 years. These figures show a deep-rooted apathy towards extending benefits of economic growth to citizens with disabilities. During the International Year of the Disabled (1981), about 12,500 persons with disabilities were found various jobs across the country. Thereafter, the annual placement figures plummeted by more than half to touch 5,800 in the mid-1980s, dropping further to 4,000 per annum since 1991. Clearly, the provision for reservation of 3 per cent jobs in government and public sector has not been sufficient to induce an increase in the recruitment levels of the disabled. What make the matter worse is the appalling inertia of the private sector towards employing persons with disabilities in the country.

There is not an infrequent scepticism as to whether the industry stands to gain by providing employment opportunities for the disabled. In India, no effort has been made to remove the misconception that employing the disabled is expensive or that it hampers production/efficiency. A handful of Indian companies like Telco, Tisco, Eicher Motors and HMT, who have all employed disabled persons, have found them to be motivated, committed and disciplined workers. The Titan factory at Hosur (Tamil Nadu) has 169 disabled persons who comprise 5.22 per cent of the total blue-collar workforce. In high-precision electronic industries, where the tasks are repetitive, workers with disabilities have been found to be less prone to distraction than their non-disabled peers. At Eicher's factory in Faridabad, disabled workers display maximum sensitivity to the Total Quality Management (TQM) programme espoused by the company. It is high time that the corporate sector and disability professionals co-ordinate to identify and categorize jobs that can be performed by persons with different types of disabilities. If necessary, lessons can be learnt from the experience of foreign companies like General Motors, Volvo and Yamaha, and which have a significant number of disabled employees on their rolls. The Confederation of Indian Industries (CII) has an invaluable agenda in all of this for future social action. The special employment exchanges across the country need to play a more active role in this co-ordination between the disability sector and employment generation (Hanumantharao et al., 1994).

One must make sure that community development remains a living corporate value. Focussing on human development through all community initiatives and integrating social development with environment management is a must if community initiative has to work. Further, companies with a negative reputation cannot use community initiatives as a whitewashing exercise in a bid to spruce up their image. The donation of a large sum or sponsoring events for the needy does not automatically ensure a clean image for a company. If one wants to use it as a marketing tool, then it has to have long-term cohesive elements that will integrate it into the marketing strategy and not be just a one-off event. In such instances, short-term tactics are bound to backfire. Even though the industry is becoming increasingly aware of the need for community development activities, disability is still not its focus.

## Role of Government and State

While a discourse on possible collaboration and cohabitation between the cause of the disabled and corporate business culture may seem refreshingly new and promising, at the same time one must not turn a blind eye to the existing realities. In a country where unregistered organizations claiming to take up cudgels for the cause of the disabled thrive in plenty, it may appear far-fetched to speak of a 'corporate culture' or 'rehabilitation service industry'. Needless to say, these matters demand immediate concern. We must think of ways or means for formulating, amending or empowering existing bodies/authorities to oversee, monitor and control the various activities of existing services. It is appreciable that the government has belatedly realized the futility of heavy investments in infrastructure building. In fact, it is a welcome step to disinvest in government-owned services for disabled. Rather, it may take up an active role as a guide, supervisor or monitor to check and control the activities and programmes of voluntary organizations in service of the disabled. The government can help create or equip existing bodies like registrar of societies, Rehabilitation Council of India, national institutes or others with suitable amendments in this direction. Indeed, the registrar of societies is partly empowered to do so. Recently, the Persons With Disabilities (Equal) Opportunities, Protection of Rights and Full Participation Act (1995) envisages an authority to take up responsibilities like certification or ratings of organizations in service of the disabled. It is yet to be seen if these proposals will actually be put into practice. There can be limits on the number of projects awarded to a voluntary organization, and central ministries can take care of miscreants aiding and abetting ephemeral mushrooming of government-aided voluntary organizations. In short, the government or its agencies need only to play the role of a protector, not a policeman; charioteer, not a cop; and driver, not a detective, over the organizations working for the disabled in the country.

## Need for a Separate Ministry

It is heartening to note that several constructive changes are occurring in the area of disability rehabilitation in the country. Several policies are being framed, laws being passed, fresh central- or state-level programmes being drawn up, new schemes being implemented and additional benefits and concessions being provided for persons with disabilities. All these government initiatives are being carried out by several ministries including the Ministry of

Social Justice and Empowerment, Ministry of Rural and Urban Development, Ministry of Human Resource Development, Ministry of Health and Family Welfare, Ministry of Labour and Employment, Ministry of Information and Broadcasting, etc. Some of the programmes are being carried out independently while others require active co-ordination between various ministries. A lot of confusion prevails between the activities of each ministry and its departments. There is more often than not duplication of work by different departments. It has been the experience of this author to have participated in rural camps for identification of the disabled in the same rural area three or four times since they were conducted on different dates by different departments of different ministries!

The Government of India included 'disability' as one of the subjects to be dealt with under 'social welfare' only in 1985. The Ministry of Social Welfare was constituted only on 25 September 1985. The other subjects included under this Ministry was welfare of scheduled castes, scheduled tribes, socially and educationally backward classes and linguistic minorities, social defense relating to victims of alcoholism, drug addiction and juvenile delinquency, welfare of the prisoners, welfare of aged and matters related to administration of *Wakfs*. One could imagine the importance given to the welfare of the disabled in a Ministry with such a lengthy agenda! The Ministry was renamed as the Ministry of Social Justice and Empowerment in May 1998. The subject of animal welfare was added to the list in September 1998. The subject of tribal welfare was removed and put under charge of an independent ministry as an apolitical readjustment in October 1999. There was no national programme for the disabled till 1985. What happened for a few years immediately after 1985 were a few ad hoc plans and schemes. Many of them have since then been scrapped or modified beyond their original recognition. Further, most of those original welfare plans and schemes are left in the hands of state governments to implement and the central government retains only a minor role in the disbursement of grants-in-aid subject to their verification or recommendation from respective state governments.

Budget allocations for the Ministry of Welfare have been sparse in terms of the national budget. With so many sections under the Ministry vying for their share of the pie, the outlay for the disability sector is a pittance with leftover and shop-worn funds. A straight lift of the same attitude that one would have for charities in the home budget. Out of the total budget allocation of Rs 1,843.57 crore to the Ministry of Social Justice and Empowerment in the national budget (1999–2000), a meagre amount of Rs 177.33 crore (9 per cent of the total) was allocated to the disability sector. The per capita expenditure for disabled persons was reported to be Rs 14 per head. Obviously, one does not budget how much money one is going to put up in charities for the year in one's home budget. You give money away from your purse (if you get the impulse to do so) the moment you see a disabled beggar on the street!

An analysis of figures during the Ninth Five-Year Plan period (1997–2002) (Table 6.5) shows only marginal increases in budgetary allocations ranging from 12.64 to 32.97 per cent under schemes, activities or programmes of the Ministry of Social Justice and Empowerment for the disability sector. Further, it must be clarified that the table only presents the financial outlay and not the actual expenses under the heads given thereof. The actual expenses may be even lesser. For example, the proposed outlay for the establishment of the National Institute for Multiple Disabilities, Chennai, is still pending.

**Table 6.5**

**Budget Outlay for Various Schemes/Programmes for the Disabled of the Ministry of Social Justice and Empowerment under the Ninth Five-Year Plan (1997–2002)**

(figures in crores)

| No. | Scheme/Programme | 1997–98 | 1998–99 | 1999–2000 | 2000–2001 | 2001–2 | Total |
|-----|------------------|---------|---------|-----------|-----------|--------|-------|
| 1.  | NIVH | 2.00 | 2.00 | 2.50 | 2.25 | 2.50 | 11.25 |
| 2.  | NIOH | 1.75 | 1.75 | 2.50 | 2.25 | 2.50 | 10.75 |
| 3.  | NIHH | 1.90 | 1.90 | 2.90 | 2.63 | 2.90 | 12.23 |
| 4.  | NIMH | 2.40 | 2.40 | 3.30 | 2.97 | 3.30 | 14.37 |
| 5.  | NIRTAR | 1.96 | 1.96 | 3.71 | 3.60 | 4.00 | 15.23 |
| 6.  | IPH | 0.60 | 0.60 | 1.50 | 1.35 | 1.50 | 5.55 |
| 7.  | NIMD(*) | 1.50 | 1.50 | 0.50 | 1.00 | 1.00 | 5.50 |
| 8.  | ALIMCO | 3.00 | 3.00 | 6.35 | 6.75 | 6.00 | 25.10 |
| 9.  | ADIP Scheme | 15.00 | 25.00 | 30.00 | 28.70 | 47.28 | 145.98 |
| 10. | Promoting Voluntary Action | 27.00 | 46.00 | 62.29 | 55.00 | 65.00 | 255.29 |
| 11. | S&T Project | 0.90 | 1.00 | 1.00 | 1.00 | 3.00 | 6.90 |
| 12. | Special Employment | 0.20 | 0.20 | 1.45 | 1.60 | 1.60 | 5.05 |
| 13. | ISIC | 2.00 | 3.00 | 7.00 | 2.25 | 2.25 | 16.50 |
| 14. | RCI | 0.93 | 3.00 | 15.50 | 7.00 | 3.00 | 29.43 |
| 15. | National Trust | 1.25 | 1.25 | 10.00 | 44.00 | 42.00 | 98.50 |
| 16. | NHFDC | 28.00 | 28.00 | 20.00 | 12.00 | 13.00 | 101.00 |
| 17. | Commissioner of Disabilities | 1.00 | 1.00 | 0.50 | 1.00 | 1.00 | 4.50 |
| 18. | NPRPD | 0.05 | 15.00 | 5.00 | 43.00 | 43.61 | 106.66 |
| 19. | Implementation of PWD Act | 15.00 | 2.98 | 3.50 | 11.75 | 13.75 | 46.98 |
|     | Total | 106.44 | 141.54 | 179.50 | 230.10 | 259.19 | 916.77 |
|     | Percentage Increase (**) | Base | 32.97 | 26.82 | 28.19 | 12.64 | |

**Notes:** (*) National Institute for Multiple Disabilities: not started as yet; (**) against the preceding year.

At this junction, it would be relevant to consider the proposals for the Tenth Five-Year Plan period (2002–2007) as recommended by the steering committee in the field of Social Welfare and Working Group on Empowering the Disabled. The Working Group has recommended a staggering outlay of Rs 2,977 crore (excluding Rs 1,202 crore meant for the NPRPD to be placed in the state sector); a phenomenal 212 per cent increase over the outlay during the Ninth Five-Year Plan (1997–2002)! The steering committee recommends a total outlay of Rs 1,375.20 crore (excluding outlays for NPRPD); which is itself a 44 per cent increase over the outlay during the preceding five-year plan (1997–2002). While these recommendations augur well for the cause of disability sectors in the country, it remains to be seen how the priorities of government are sustained on the ground over the next decade (Table 6.6).

It has been defended that 5 per cent of the population of disabled is a small number in the country to receive higher priorities than what has been accorded. One must acknowledge that there is and can be politics of epidemiology here as well. We have already seen the difficulties in making a correct epidemiological estimate on the prevalence of disabilities in the country. The prevalence percentage quoted in official statistics may be a gross underestimation.

## Alternative Models for Education

Of the 230 million children in India, nearly 40 per cent do not go to school. They are employed for paltry wages that subsidise the family income. Correlate this observation with the fact

---

**Table 6.6**

**Some Important Strategies and Recommendations Given under the Tenth Five-Year Plan Period (2002–2007) by the Steering Committee in the Field of Social Welfare and Working Group on Empowering the Disabled**

1. Disability Sub-plan: To ensure better allocation, there must be disability sub-plan by, or under, different central departments or ministries to earmark funds for activities concerning persons with disabilities in its area of operation.
2. Convergence between Ministries, State Governments and NGOs: All activities or programmes for persons with disabilities must be carried out in close co-ordination between various service-providing agencies in the community.
3. College of Rehabilitation Sciences: The proposed college is to provide comprehensive training in special education and rehabilitation for a highly specialized cadre of specialists.
4. National Programme of Vocational Training and Employment (NPVTE): On the lines of the NPRPD, it is proposed to initiate a NPVTE by including continuous identification of new self-wage employment opportunities for persons with disabilities, skill development, employment-linked vocational rehabilitation training, marketing supports, etc.
5. National Institute for Multiple Disabilities (NIMD): The proposal to establish a NIMD is being procrastinated over since the past five years even though seedling allocations have been made in the Union budget. Likewise, there is a recommendation to merge all the national institutes under one umbrella scheme to bring about synergy and co-ordination in their activities.
6. Design and Development of an Interactive Website on Disability-impairments: It is recommended that a government-sponsored interactive website be launched for providing information on various aspects of disability-impairments.
7. Strengthening Existing NPRPD: There is a proposal to expand and strengthen the NPRPD by earmarking financial outlays exclusively in order to extend coverage across more districts throughout the country.
8. Role of NGOs: While continuing to patronize or assist NGOs, their activities are to be strictly monitored and evaluated in order to ensure the spread of quality services for persons with disabilities across the country.

---

that about 10 per cent of Indian children below 14 years of age have some kind of impairment or disability. The absolute number comes to a staggering 30 million, which mandates the effective role for education in a specialized context. The conventional models of schooling may not suffice, especially for children with lower levels of intelligence, learning disorders, autistic disturbances, conduct problems, multiple handicaps, etc. These children have great problems in coping with regular schools, curriculum and teaching strategies.

There is a need for exploring alternative models for their education including provision for special schools, open schools, home schools, activity centres, sports/music schools, etc. A special case for consideration is especially children with learning disabilities. They are designated as learning disabled because they are unable to swim along the tide of normal curriculum or education. To continue and force them to take up the same conventional curriculum (albeit with some nominal concessions like exemption from a second language, scribe facility or extra examination time) is a euphemism for expression of mistrust against experimenting with alternative models for their education.

The National Open School (NOS) is a welcome alternative to formal education. It is specially suited for the needs of certain categories like school dropouts, girls, mentally handicapped, learning disabled, autistic or such other children. It offers courses which are nominally equivalent to seventh grade, secondary and higher secondary levels or courses. It's programme of open basic education (OBE) for universal elementary education (UEE) is available at three levels, viz., preparatory (equivalent to grade III), primary (equivalent to grade V) and elementary (equivalent to grade VIII) respectively. A list of special accredited institutions for education of disabled under NOS has been identified. However, the NOS is yet to formulate activity based non-formal courses suitable for home-school models of education which may be most suitable for children with disabilities and impairments.

## Legal Vacuum

The first legislative endeavour related to the field of mental health, though not directly linked with the disability sector, could be identified as the Lunatic Asylums Act (1858). The Act was intended to curb private trade in lunacy and wrongful commitment (Varma, 1953). The Act made no distinction between the 'idiot' (old term for mental disability) and a 'person of unsound mind' (legal term for mental illness). The *darogah* of a police station was under obligation to arrest wandering and dangerous lunatics and get them admitted into recognized asylums. While the task of ordering and commitment was allocated to the judicial authorities, the diagnosis of lunacy was seen as a medical function. The Indian Lunacy Act (1912)—another British legacy—came later to safeguard the rights and privileges of persons with both mental illnesses as well as disabilities. This Act also did not differentiate between mental disability and mental illness. In recent times, with pressure from internal, as well as international, mental-health lobbyists and activists, the new Mental Health Act (1987) came to be passed. This Bill safeguards interests, rights and privileges of persons with mental illness. The persons with mental handicaps are excluded. They are left without any legal framework to safeguard their rights, privileges or sanctions.

Marriage of, or with, mentally handicapped persons is still legally considered null and void. They have no marital rights. Spouses can claim divorce or contract a second marriage if it is proved that their partners are mentally retarded. Mentally handicapped persons cannot inherit property directly from their parents or ancestors since it is claimed that they are of 'unsound mind'. The mentally retarded cannot stand for an election or even vote in an election. No labour laws protect their minimum wages, timings of work or working conditions. No wonder many mentally handicapped adults continue to be exploited in all realms of their life—marriage, inheritance, labour and personal independence.

Recently, there was a controversy over the carrying out of hysterectomies (operation for removal of the uterus) for females with mental handicaps on the pretext that the measure could save the girls from the danger of unwanted pregnancies or from the stigma of unwed motherhood. Though the intentions of the protagonists in favour of these practices are unquestionable, these actions raise several issues pertaining to who should decide on the sexual rights of the adult handicapped. Are adults with mental handicap empowered in the first place to make or take their own decisions? Are they provided with healthy and correct sex education? Are they given opportunities for positive social interactions with members of the opposite sex? Without making provisions for any positive growth of these social skills, it is prematurely understood by protagonists that the mentally handicapped are incapable of personal decisions—therefore others deciding on their behalf is the only just and rightful course of action! A mentally handicapped person cannot testify in the court of law. They cannot stand witness since they are of 'unsound mind'. Cases are withdrawn, culprits are acquitted and criminals go scot-free since the key witness or accused was a person with mental retardation—someone whose testimony does not have any value in the court of law.

The passing of the Persons With Disabilities (Equal) Opportunities, Protection of Rights and Full Participation Act (1995) raised a lot of hope in the minds of people as a landmark legislation for the welfare of the disabled in the country. It took more than a year for the MSJE to frame and notify rules to enable implementation of the Act. It took another year to create and put in place the infrastructure as stipulated under the Act. Even seven years after the passing of the Act, there is much to be desired about the implementation process. This tardiness could be attributed, among other things, to the priorities of the Ministry. The multiplicity of subjects dealt with by the Ministry could also be another factor adding to this delay in action for benefit of the disabled. Thus, there is every justification in the demand for a separate Ministry of Disability Welfare as is the case with some advanced counties like Japan, China, the United Kingdom, the United States, etc., as well as some state governments within the country (such as Andhra Pradesh).

## Human Rights Movement

The 'Human Rights Movement' against social problems and issues like gender bias, child rights or the like has also impacted recent trends in disability sectors. The clamour for legislation specifically for persons with disabilities has been a matter for public discussion, declamation and debate since the International Year of the Disabled in 1981. The momentum has picked up since the adoption of a resolution by the General Assembly of the United Nations in its Report of Third Committee, which declared the Universal Rights of Mentally Retarded Persons. Thereafter, the Economic and Social Commissions for Asia and the Pacific convened a meeting at Beijing from 1–5 December 1992 to launch the Asian and Pacific Decade of Disabled Persons (1993–2002). Since India is a signatory to these international bodies and conventions, it has had to take stock of the prevailing legislation for the disabled in the country. Further, some domestic lobbies have also been seeking better deals for persons with disabilities within the country. However, it must be admitted that the pressure from domestic lobbyists has been poorly co-ordinated taking into account the gigantic problem at hand.

## Afflictions in the Voluntary Sector

While it is self-flattering to eulogize the seminal role played by voluntary organizations over the past few decades in the services of the disabled in the country, one must not turn a blind eye to several ills that can be remedied. Even now, many voluntary organizations thrive on the stark sentimentalism of well-meaning philanthropists. Many voluntary organizations are organized on humanitarian concerns by social activists. Most of them are raised on religious zeal and rank sentimentalism with an eye for doing 'good' for the 'unfortunately disabled'. Their services are looked upon as an act of service to God. Even today, quite a few voluntary agencies serve the handicapped on such premises and are manned/supervised by missionaries of different religious faiths or by retired senior citizens with a fervour to spend the last days of their life for a 'noble cause'.

Even if the emotional foundations of such voluntary work are commendable and qualify them to initiate services for handicapped persons, the scientific temper required to sustain quality services by marketing their 'cause' in public is sadly lacking. Further, specific decisions that seem rational from a narrow perspective for individuals or small organizations are at the same time lacking in any overall plan, perspective or purpose for the whole system of service delivery for handicapped persons in the country. The disability rehabilitation sector in India urgently requires professionalism from diverse fields of management, marketing, costing, auditing, human resource development, etc. Professional marketing executives are needed to highlight and advocate enough to raise funds for a cause. Costing and auditing professionals need to scrutinize budget inflows and outflows with their rigours of financial analysis. Manpower capital versus return on investment needs to be scientifically calculated. Cost benefit analyses of fiscal or human resource investments and services accrued need to be studied. Performance audit on asset-utilization ratios as a product of fixed assets and number of beneficiaries per financial year, operational costs per unit of services rendered, debt equity burden ratios as quotient of debt/equity and total number of beneficiaries, etc., can be successfully adapted. Such objective and calculated quantitative indices of human resource utilization is possible even in so-called 'not for profits' service delivery organizations for the handicapped (Venkatesan, 2002c).

## Professionalism in Voluntary Sector

Voluntarism in the rehabilitation industry is yet to come of age in India. Professional interactions, both within and between voluntary agencies, are far from being mutually co-operative or co-ordinated. Each agency works in isolation to aggrandize its own self-image than in common endeavour to promote the cause of handicap welfare. Many NGOs in the contemporary scene are individual-centred and not 'cause'-centred. It is the unique strength of character and influence of a few isolated individuals that raise institutions up. Even though these institutions project an overt guise of having a team of governing body members/trustees; in actuality, one encounters the idolization or even unabashed hero worship of an individual in place of the cause for which such institutions exist.

## Consortium of Voluntary Organizations

A grave repercussion of the prevailing confusion within as well as between voluntary organizations working for the cause of disabled persons in India is that their activities are poorly connected or co-ordinated. There exists an inequitable distribution of voluntarism across the length and breadth of the country. There are either regions or urban conglomerations wherein, within a given circumscribed geographical area, one encounters several agencies duplicating the same activities; or there are areas where there is hardly any voluntary activity visible for persons with disability. This is an avoidable wastage of precious time, money and human resources in a sector in which demand for services outstrips their supply. There is an urgent need to network the activities and programmes of all voluntary organizations in different regions so that one does not reinvent the fire and the wheel. The formation of a consortium of non-governmental organizations with appropriate government mandate, supervision, in-service organizational training avenues, accrediting standards or procedures, etc., would go a long way in lending credibility to the efforts of these institutions.

## Encourage Consumer-based Self-help Movements

Self-help consumer movements appear to hold great promise for the future of disability rehabilitation in our country. They have the potential to become strong pressure groups, points or advocacy nodes to fight for the cause of disabled persons. In due course, they could even become watchdogs that challenge professional behaviour and also signal a death knell for pseudo-philanthropic activities or enterprises by increasing their consumer controls and consciousness. However, this necessitates enablement and empowerment of parents, caregivers or the disabled themselves on their rights, privileges and prerogatives as enshrined in the laws of the land.

A system of third-party sponsors to meet their expenses must also be invoked. Overt competition between self-help groups and voluntary organizations is beginning to appear. Another deviation is that the care industry is shifting from in-patient to ambulatory or itinerant services. The eventual shape that this movement is likely to take in the future is difficult to forecast. The present scenario demonstrates considerable uncertainty. No specific prognostic indicators are now available. More research is required to increase understanding of these changes into a perspective than can improve the rehabilitation care system in the country.

In recognition of the trials and tribulations experienced by parents or caregivers of handicapped children, The National Trust for Welfare of Persons with Autism, Cerebral Palsy, Mental Retardation and Multiple Disabilities Act (1999) has come into existence. The problems of urban parents or two working parents are doubled wherein they are left to fathom the rough seas of co-existence with severe or multiple handicaps in their households. These areas require a new initiative towards social security which ensures that the quality of life in such families are ameliorated. Therefore, it is apt that the Trust has been created as a statutory body to ensure financial as well as other caregiving exercises to these children when their parents or primary family members are unavailable. The objectives of the Trust are guardianship, foster care, mobilization of resources to strengthen the family and community, provision of legal aid and to receive and own properties bequeathed by parents to maintain their handicapped children after their demise.

## Invitation for Research on Organizational Issues

The scientific study of service delivery systems (SDS) in the field of disability rehabilitation is a relatively unstudied pathway for professionals in our country. The field holds promise for a new framework to understand the changing scenario of SDS in our society. There are hardly any studies reported in this direction. In a comprehensive bibliographical search of over a 100 journals published during past 60 years, it was found that there were no more than three theoretical articles related to organizational issues of disability rehabilitation in the country (Venkatesan and Vepuri, 1995). There is a need to develop broad theoretical perspectives or clarify inter-organizational linkages and networks that make up SDS for the disabled in India. An urgent need is to carry out informative case studies to document success/failures of the system, to trace inconsistencies/irrationalities within or in-between organizational sectors. Such intense case studies need to map out relations between various aspects of SDS for the handicapped.

Traditionally, students of business schools and management institutes have perforce concentrated their research and dissertations only on productive organizations. It is useful to distinguish between productive versus service organizations. Products are tangible things we can carry with us. Services are intangible and perishable and are consumed in the process of their production. The person being served often participates in the production process. In product systems, there is little contact between the producers and consumers of the product as much is left to distribution and retailing. On the other hand, human contact is almost the essence of many service systems. Conversion of raw materials to physical products may involve a multitude of inter-related steps. But the processing in service systems is usually simple, involving only a few steps. Demand for products as well as services vary considerably over time. In a sense, variability is higher for the latter. The markets served by productive systems can be regional, national or even international. Conversely, since services cannot be shipped to distant places, they can serve only local markets.

Even though theoretical distinctions are made out between products and services as two differing goals of delivering organizations, in actuality, the differences are likely to be less clear than are made out to be. Even productive systems invariably involve some measure of service, and vice versa. For example, an automobile (product) industry has to back up with after-sales service. Likewise a rehabilitation service for the disabled may be supplemented with dispensing of orthotics or prosthesis (products). Thus, it is valid to think of organizational systems as lying along a continuum of product and service deliveries. Disability rehabilitation service centres may not be producing tangible products that may be stored for later consumption. Their output may be in the form of services like health care, education, advice, guidance, advocacy, etc. The cost and quality of such services, speed and output parameters like a cured patient, informed client, amelioration in their quality of life, etc., can also be quantified by students and researchers of management studies.

Historical analysis of the course and content of organizations must be an inherent ingredient of such case studies. The challenge for researchers would be then to combine these case studies into a comparative and comprehensive analysis to pinpoint lacunae in fundamental co-ordinating mechanisms and identify factors that facilitate rationality in relations within SDS. As it appears, there is no overarching theoretical framework available to integrate the specific findings into a coherent model of organizational systems. An important goal for the next decade would be to produce an integrated study on organizational design that optimizes productivity of services. Another plan of action would be to conduct large-scale surveys of organizations. But such exercises are likely to be expensive and can be ill afforded by our country. Other indirect ways are to conduct systematic and intensive interviews with key informants, establish citizen monitoring councils, consumer forums, extrapolate data on demand versus need for services, etc. Such evaluation should consider the acceptability, accessibility as well as awareness aspects on or about services for persons with disabilities.

For quite some time, the field of disability rehabilitation has been stiflingly ensconced in traditional search and research for appropriate nomenclature, prevalence, etiology, characteristics and clinical/community management of persons with disabilities and impairments. Such customary investigations by social scientists are routinely in demand for circulation in professional literature. However, the time has arrived when professionals rise above such traditional preoccupations, and introspect into the nature or impact of their own skilled interventions with affected populations at organizational levels rather than at individual levels.

# Glossary

**Absurdities in Pictures.** Refers to pictures that depict illogical, silly or meaningless stimuli. For example, a dog with the hind legs of a horse.

**Academic Skills Disorder.** (See Learning Disability.)

**ACPC-DD.** Acronym for 'Activity Checklist for Preschool Children with Developmental Disabilities'. It is a standardized behaviour assessment tool to elicit information on the current level of what a child 'can do' or 'cannot do' in preparation for developing a remediation programme.

**Alternative Sequencing.** Sequencing refers to the arrangement of stimuli in a particular order, such as, arranging number cards from one to five. Alternative sequencing, a higher and more difficult task, involves arrangement of stimuli in a particular order, such as, beads according to red-blue-red-blue-red-blue patterns.

**Amputation.** Refers to loss of limbs (either part of whole) due to trauma, accident or disease.

**Antecedent.** Refers to what happens immediately before the occurrence of a problem behaviour targeted for remediation.

**Articulation Disorder.** (See Phonological Disorder.)

**Asperger's Disorder.** A type of Pervasive Developmental Disorder close to Autistic Disorder but not sharing its delays in language development, and cognitive or developmental delays.

**Athetosis.** A type of cerebral palsy with fluctuating muscle tone and jerky movements of limbs.

**'At Risk' Child.** Refers to children with no existing/current handicaps, but having a strong disposition for developing one or another disability in due course of time.

**Attention.** A psychological process of selection of stimuli from an array that impinge on an individual at any given point of time.

**Attention Deficit and Hyperactivity Disorders.** Characterized by short attention span, impulsivity and over-activity in behaviour.

**Autistic Disorder.** A type of Pervasive Developmental Disorder characterized by typical qualitative abnormalities in reciprocal social interactions and patterns of communication, and by a restricted, stereotyped and repetitive repertoire of interests and activities.

**Autistic Play.** Playing alone or all by oneself in spite of playmates being around.

**BASIC-MR.** Acronym for 'Behaviour' Assessment Scales for Indian Children with Mental Retardation'. It is a standardized behaviour assessment tool to elicit information on the current level of what a mentally retarded school-aged child 'can do' or 'cannot do' in preparation for later developing a remediation programme.

**Behaviour.** Observable or measurable actions of human beings.

**Behaviour Problems.** Actions that are harmful to self or others, interfere in the teaching or learning process, are age-inappropriate or socially deviant and cause immense stress on caregivers.

**Behavioural Objectives.** (See Short-term Goals.)

**Central Auditory Disorder.** Hearing loss due to lesions in the central auditory system with damage to the auditory nerve rather than the external and/or middle ear.

**Cerebral Palsy.** A non-progressive neurological disorder of muscle co-ordination and control.

**Chaining.** A teaching procedure of leading a child along a sequence of steps either in the forward or backward direction towards a behavioural teaching objective.

**Childhood Disintegrative Disorder.** A type of Pervasive Developmental Disorder characterized by an initial course of normal development, followed by a significant loss of previously acquired skills.

**Cognitive.** Refers to the domain under ACPC-DD comprising of activities like clock reading, telling the time, telling the days of week, identification of money, etc.

**Competitive Play.** Involves formal rules and active competition between players, either indoors or outdoors, such as, chess, cricket, etc.

**Conductive Hearing Loss.** When transmission of sound is affected in the outer or middle ear.

**Consequence.** Refers to what happens immediately after the occurrence of a problem behaviour targeted for remediation.

**Cube Assembly.** Involves a series of activities to be performed by the child using one-inch cubes. Cubes are used to stack towers (level 1), make bridges (level 2), trains (level 3) and staircases (level 4).

**Cylindrical Grasp.** Refers to the type of grasp used for holding a bottle or a pipe.

**Deformity.** Refers to an abnormal position assumed by any part of the body that is not passively correctable.

**Developmental Disability.** Refers to a mixed group of children 'at risk' and/or those with permanently handicapping conditions, especially during preschool years of life. They include kids with disabilities like blindness, deafness, locomotor, mental handicaps, learning handicaps, specific speech delays, multiple handicaps, autistic disorders, attention deficit and over-activity disorders, etc.

**Diagnostic Hunting.** A seemingly endless search by parents or caregivers who have not reconciled to the diagnosis of their child with a disability or disease.

**Diplegia.** A type of cerebral palsy wherein both legs rather than the upper limbs are affected.

**Disability.** Usually a consequence of impairment, it is the functional inability of an individual to perform any activity in the manner or within the range considered 'normal' for any human being.

**Disease.** Represents a professional understanding of pathophysiological processes constituting certain signs and symptoms in conjunction with their aetiology and pathology.

**Disorder.** Represents the conjunction of a syndrome with its clinical course.

**Double Hemiplegia.** A type of cerebral palsy wherein both hands rather than the legs are affected.

**Dyspraxia.** Inability to produce correctly sequenced co-ordinated motor movements when presented with a demonstration or oral request.

**Encopresis.** Disorder involving repeated passage of faeces in inappropriate places and times (such as in clothing or on the floor).

**Enuresis.** Disorder involving repeated passage of urine in inappropriate places and times (such as in clothing or on the floor).

**Exploratory Play.** A tendency to show curiosity/eagerness to explore or handle toys and/or pets.

**Expressive Language Disorder.** Characterized by expressive language abilities far below a child's current chronological/mental-age expectations.

**Extinction.** (See Time Out.)

**Fading.** A process of gradual decrease in active assistance by the teacher and increase of independence during behavioural performance by the learner.

**Fine Motor.** Refers to strength, co-ordination and control over smaller groups of muscular activities like grasping, folding, screwing or unscrewing lids of bottles, inserting coins into piggy box, etc.

**Functional Commands.** Refers to comprehension and performance of simple or direct commands like 'Come!', 'Go!', 'Sit!', 'Stand!', 'Give!', 'Take!', etc.

**Generalization.** Application of learning to real life situations or settings.

**Grasp.** Refers to the pattern or position in which an object is held. Different objects require different actions and strength for holding, picking, inserting, transporting, and releasing. There are many types of grasp, like cylindrical grasp, spherical grasp, hook grasp, opponent grasp, palm grasp, pincer grasp, tripod grasp, lateral grasp, etc.

**Gross Motor.** Refers to strength, co-ordination and control over large groups of music activities like walking, running, jumping, skipping, climbing, throwing, etc.

**Handicap.** Is a disadvantage resulting from, or a consequence of, impairment or as well as disability.

**Heller's Syndrome.** (See Childhood Disintegrative Disorder.)

**Hemiplegia.** A type of cerebral palsy wherein only one side of body is affected.

**Home-based Training Programme.** A form of service delivery wherein parents and caregivers are trained to handle their children with developmental disabilities in home settings.

**Hook Grasp.** Refers to the type of grasp used for holding bucket, bag, suitcase, etc.

**Illness.** Refers to parents/family recognition, labelling and experience of a disease as abnormal or as departure from wellness.

**Imitation.** (See Modelling.)

**Impairment.** Any visible structural/anatomical loss of physical or sense organs in an individual.

**Isolated Play.** Playing alone or all by oneself resulting from refusal of or non-acceptance in social play owing to a child's behaviour problems.

**Kyphoscoliosis.** Abnormal curvature of spine both forwards and sideways.

**Kyphosis.** Hunchback or sharply localized forward angulation of spine resulting in an appearance of a lump.

**Lateral Grasp.** Refers to the type of grasp used for holding objects like a deck of playing cards.

**Learning Disability.** Refers to children who show a slowness or incapacity in dealing with one or more academic subjects like reading, writing, spelling and/or arithmetic in the absence of any sensory loss, organic pathology, poor schooling, lack of intelligence, mental illness and/or retardation.

**Learning Handicap.** (See Learning Disability.)

**Long-term Goals.** Statements expressing provisional expectations of caregivers in home-based programmes about their child over the coming three months.

**Lordosis.** Inward curvature of spine.

**Minimal Brain Dysfunction.** An old term for Learning Disability.

**Mixed Hearing Loss.** Combination of sensory and conductive hearing loss with damage to the ear and bone conduction pathways, even though the latter may be the better of the two.

**Modelling.** A procedure of teaching or learning by observation.

**Monoplegia.** A type of cerebral palsy wherein a single limb is affected.

**Multiple Handicaps.** A condition wherein the child has two or more disabilities concurrently.

**Muscle Overflow.** (See Synkinesis.)

**Muscular Dystrophy.** An inherited disorder characterized by progressive muscle deterioration after an initial phase of normal development till about three years.

**Non-participant Play.** Passive observation of others at play. This includes: (*i*) onlooker play and (*ii*) spectator play.

**Normative Approach.** An approach to psychological assessment which involves comparative evaluation of individual children with others who are supposedly like them.

**Object Permanence.** Refers to the child's ability to comprehend that an object continues to exist despite it being hidden from his or her view.

**Onlooker Play.** Passive observation of others at play without comprehending the rules of observed play.

**Opponent Grasp.** Refers to the type of grasp involving opposition between the tip of the forefinger and the thumb, and used for holding objects like a glass tumbler, paper weight, inkpot, etc.

**Palm Grasp.** Refers to the type of grasp used for holding writing instruments like pen, pencil or paint brush at a primitive level.

**Parallel Play.** Playing alone or all by oneself in companionship of available or proximate playmates.

**Pervasive Developmental Disorders.** Represent certain types of psychological disorders characterized by severe and ubiquitous impairment in several areas of child development including reciprocal social and communication skills.

**Pes Cavus.** Claw foot.

**Pes Planus.** Flat foot.

**Phobia.** Anxiety- or fear-evoking circumscribed situations or objects outside an individual which are not currently dangerous and are yet perceived as so.

**Phonological Disorder.** Characterized by failure to use developmentally appropriate expressive-speech sounds for the age or dialect.

**Physical or Locomotor Handicap.** Results from the impairment of limbs or extremities and involves an inability to execute distinctive activities associated with moving the self or other objects from place to place.

**Pica.** A feeding or eating disorder characterized by persistent eating of non-edible or non-nutritive substances.

**Pincer Grasp.** Refers to the type of grasp used for picking or holding very small objects like peanuts, pebbles and needles using the tip of the thumb and the index finger.

**Poliomyelitis.** A result of a neuro-tropic virus affecting the anterior horn cells in the brain stem and spinal cord of the central nervous system from the faecal matter of infected persons.

**Preacademics.** Refers to the domain under ACPC-DD consisting of activities like pre-reading, pre-writing and pre-arithmetic.

**Pre-arithmetic.** Under pre-arithmetic, there are activities like rote recitation of numbers, reading or writing numbers serially, counting and giving away objects, etc.

**Pre-reading.** Under pre-reading, there are activities like comprehension of pictures, arrangement of story pictures, etc.

**Pre-rule Kindergarten Play.** Refers to a type of play seen in toddlers where they either play alone or in a group, but not governed by any elaborate rules and regulations during the said activity. For example, sliding, tunnelling, pat-a-cake, etc.

**Pre-writing.** Under pre-writing, there are activities like scribbling, colouring, joining dots, imitation of simple geometric shapes, etc.

**Primary Colours.** Refers to the colours red, blue and green.

**Primary Rewards.** Edibles with reward value.

**Primary Shapes.** Refers to shapes like circle, square and triangle.

**Problem Behaviours.** (See Behaviour Problems.)

**Procrastination.** Refers to the child's ability to comprehend and delay gratification of needs or postpone wish gratification over a period of time.

**Prompting.** A teaching procedure of giving active assistance, guidance, instruction or help as a child learns specific sub-sets of a target behaviour.

**Psychological Assessment.** A process of systematic collection, organization and interpretation of information about a person and the prediction of that person's behaviour in new situations.

**Psychometric Approach.** (See Normative Approach.)

**Reflexes.** Spontaneous stimulus-response patterns of reactions.

**Regurgitation.** (See Rumination.)

**Rehabilitation.** Refers to the process of identifying the available potential of a given person with disability and providing opportunities and training to optimize these capacities for the near-normalized living of the individual in society.

**Reinforcements.** (See Rewards.)

**Relational Play.** Ability to relate two or more objects as going together during play situations, such as bat and ball, pen and paper, spoon and cup, etc.

**Retts Disorder.** A type of Pervasive Developmental Disorder similar to Autistic Disorder, but invariably diagnosed only in females, with a typical pattern of head-growth retardation, loss of previously-acquired hand skills, appearance of poorly co-ordinated gait/trunk movements and only transient loss of social engagement early in the course of this disorder.

**Rewards.** Pleasurable events or things which happen after a behaviour and which help that behaviour to occur again and again.

**Rumination.** A feeding or eating disorder characterized by persistent ejection of ingested food and rechewing it for ingestion.

**Scoliosis.** Lateral deviation of the backbone.

**Segregated Play.** Playing alone or all by oneself resulting from refusal or non-acceptance in social play by peers.

**Sensory-neural Hearing Loss.** When the nerve cells of the cochlea or acoustic nerve (cranial nerve eight) are damaged.

**Sensory.** Refers to the domain under ACPC-DD comprising of activities to strengthen skills related to sight, hearing, smell, touch, taste and movement senses.

**Sequential Instructions.** Refers to comprehension of three ore more instructions one after another in a sequence, such as, 'Close the door, put on the fan and then go to bed!'.

**Shaping.** A teaching procedure of giving rewards in successive steps for sub-sets of behaviour approximated correctly towards a teaching objective.

**Short-term Goals.** Statements expressing provisional expectations of caregivers about their child for immediate teaching objectives in a home-based training programme.

**Sibling Rivalry.** An unusual degree of competition for attention from parents, negative feelings, overt hostility, strong reluctance to share, lack of positive regard, paucity of friendly interactions, physical trauma or maliciousness towards a sibling.

**Single-step Instructions.** Refers to comprehension of single instructions like 'Open the door!', 'Close your month!', 'Bring me that pen!', 'Throw the ball!', etc.

**Social Rewards.** Verbal praise or actions depicting appreciation with reward value.

**Solitary Play.** Playing alone or all by oneself. This includes: (*i*) autistic play, (*ii*) parallel play, (*iii*) segregated play, and (*iv*) isolated play.

**Spasticity.** Refers to high muscle tone and tight/stiff muscles with rigid type of movements.

**Spectator Play.** Passive observation of others at play with comprehension of the rules of observed play.

**Spherical Grasp.** A type of grasp used for holding round objects like ball, lemon or apple.

**Spina Bifida.** A congenital disorder occurring within the first week of conception owing to a failure of the neural tube to close due to a virus or some harmful agents.

**Stammering.** (See Stuttering.)

**Stuttering.** Disturbance in normal fluency and time patterning of speech that is inappropriate for the individual's age.

**Symbolic or Dramatic Play.** A type of play seen in young children where they act out a concept as perceived by the performer. It contains rule-based play without lines or with few props. It includes: (*i*) pretentious play: pretending to eat with spoon, drink milk from a cup, going to sleep, etc., (*ii*) representational play: using surrogates to represent objects or situations in play, such as, leaves for money, wooden block as a car, etc., and (*iii*) enactive play: role-playing entire sequences of behaviour of various persons/situations around, such as playing a teacher, father, bus driver, etc.

**Synkinesis.** Manifests itself as unintended muscle movements.

**Tali pes.** Club foot.

**Task Analysis.** The procedure of teaching children in small and simple steps.

**Time Out.** A behavioural procedure of correcting problem behaviours in a child by removing the child from a rewarding situation or removing the rewarding situation from the child.

**Tokens.** Items with no inherent value, yet desired by some as having reward value since they have been assigned such a value under a specific set of circumstances.

**Toy-pet Play.** Use of toys or pets during play.

**Triplegia.** A type of cerebral palsy in which three limbs are affected.

**Tripod Grasp.** Refers to the type of grasp used for holding writing instruments like pen, pencil or paint brush at normal adult level.

**Turn Talking.** Refers to the ability to wait for one's turn in a play situation or group activity.

**Two Unrelated Commands.** Refers to comprehension of two related set of actions for instructions like 'Close the door and bring me that book', 'Keep the bag in the cupboard and remove your shoes!', etc. Do not prompt the child during or at the end of performing the first part of the instruction.

**Understands 'All Gone'.** Refers to child's comprehension of experiences related to hiding of objects from his or her line of vision—that he or she is being misled.

# Bibliography

**American Association of Mental Deficiency.** (2002). *Definiton of Mental Handicap: 2002*. New York: American Association of Mental Deficiency.

**American Psychological Association.** (1974). *Standards for Educational and Psychological Tests*. New York: American Psychological Association.

**Arya, S., Peshawaria, R., Naidu, S.** and **Venkatesan, S.** (1990). *The Problem Behavior Checklist*. Secunderabad: National Institute for the Mentally Handicapped.

**Baer, D.M., Wolf, M.M.** and **Risley, T.** (1969). 'Some Current Dimensions of Applied Behavior Analysis'. *Journal of Applied Behavior Analysis*, 1: 91–97.

**Becker, W.C.** and **Engleman, S.** (1976). *Teaching and Evaluation of Instruction*. Chicago: Science Research Associates.

**Bharatraj, J.** (1983). *Manual on Developmental Screening Test*. Mysore: Padmashree Publishers.

**Bock, E.F.** (1975). *The Minnesota Developmental Programming System*. Minnesota: Academic.

**Chowdhry, S.** (1995). *Child Welfare/Development*. New Delhi: Atmaram.

**Cornelius, D.J.K.** and **Rukmini, J.** (1998). *Assessment of Vocational Readiness*. Chennai: Navjyothi Trust.

**Desai, A.N.** (1995). *Helping the Handicapped: Problems and Prospects*. New Delhi: Ashish.

**Dhanda, A.** (2000). *Legal Order and Mental Disorder*. New Delhi: Sage Publications.

**Fiske, D.W.** and **Pearson, P.B.** (1970). 'Theory and Techniques of Personality Development'. *Annual Review of Psychology*, 21: 41–86.

**Gandhi, J.S.** and **Agarwal, K.G.** (1969). 'Attitude of Public towards Mental Retardation'. *Indian Journal of Mental Retardation*, 2(1): 21–25.

**Glaser, R.** (1963). 'Instructional Technology and Measurement of Learning Outcomes'. *American Psychologist*, 18: 519–21.

**Glaser, R.** and **Nitko, A.J.** (1971). 'Measurement in Learning and Instruction'. In R.L. Thorndike (ed.), *Educational measurement*. Washington, D.C.: American Council on Education.

**Grossman, G.** (1972). *Manual on Terminology and Classification on Mental Retardation*. Washington, D.C.: American Association of Mental Deficiency.

**Halpern, A.S.** and **Fuhrer, M.J.** (1984). *Introduction to Functional Assessment in Rehabilitation*. Baltimore: Paul B. Brooks.

**Hammill, D.D.** (1987). 'Assessing Students in the Schools'. In D.D. Hammill (ed.), *Assessing the Abilities and Instructional Needs of Students*. Texas: Pro-Ed.

**Hanumantharao, P., Venkatesan, S.** and **Vepuri, V.G.D.** (1993). 'Community Based Rehabilitation Services for People with Disabilities: An Experimental Study'. *International Journal of Rehabilitation Research*, 16: 245–50.

———. (1994). 'Employment Opportunities for Mentally Handicapped Individuals in Rural Areas: A Proposed Model'. *Journal of Indian Academy of Applied Psychology*, 20(2): 131–37.

**Hawkins, R.P.** (1979). 'The Functions of Assessment: Implications for Selection and Development of Devices for Assessing Repertoires in Clinical Emotional and Other Settings'. *Journal of Applied Behavior Analysis*, 1: 97–106.

**Howell, K.W., Kaplan, J.S.** and **O'Connell, C.Y.** (1979). *Evaluating Exceptional Children*. Columbus: Charles E. Merrill.

**Jeffree, D.M., Mc Conkey, R.** and **Hewson, S.** (1977). *Let Me Play*. London: Souvenir.

**Jeyachandran, P.** and **Vimala, K.** (1983). *The Madras Developmental Programming System* (III edn.). Chennai: Vijay Human Services.

**Jeyachandran, P.** and **Vimala, K.** (2000). *The Madras Developmental Programming System* (VI edn.). Chennai: Vijay Human Services.

**Jones, H.G.** (1970). 'Principles of Psychological Assessment'. In P. Mittler (ed.), *The Psychological Assessment of Mental and Physical Handicaps*. London: Tavistock.

**Kamat, V.V.** (1967). *Measuring Intelligence of Indian Children*. Bombay: Oxford University Press.

**Karoly, P.** (1981). 'Self-management of Problems in Children'. In E.J. Mash and L.G. Terdall (eds), *Behavior Assessment of Childhood Disorders*. New York: John Wiley.

**Kiernan, C.** (1987). 'Criterion Referenced Tests'. In J. Hogg and N.V. Raynes (eds), *Assessment in Mental Handicap*. London: Croom-Helm.

**Kohli, T.** (1986). Portage Basic Training Course for Early Stimulation at Pre-school Children in India. New Delhi: UNICEF.

**Kurani, J., Miranda, S.N., Shane, P.A.** and **Shroff, G.S.** (1999). *Assessment cum Curriculum Guidelines for Vocational Training in School and Rehabilitation Centers*. Mumbai: Jai Vakeel

**Lansdown, R.** (1985). *Child Development Made Simple*. London: William Heinmann.

**Mager, R.F.** (1962). *Preparing Instructional Objectives*. Belmont: Pearson.

**Malin, A.J.** (1961). *Manual for Vineland Social Maturity Scale, Nagpur Adaptation*. Nagpur: Child Guidance Clinic.

**Mash, E.J.** and **Terdall, L.G.** (1976). *Behavior Therapy Assessment: Diagnosis, Design and Evaluation*. New York: Springer.

**Melin, L., Sjoden, P.O.** and **James, J.E.** (1983). 'Neurological Impairment'. In M. Hersen, V.B.U. Hasselt and J.L. Matson (eds.), *Behavior Therapy for the Development and Physically Disabled*. London: Academic Press.

**Murthy, R.S., Wig, N.N.** and **Dhir, A.** (1980). 'Rural Community Attitudes to Mental Retardation'. *Child Psychiatry Quarterly*, 13: 81–88.

**Narasimhan, M.C.** and **Mukherjee, A.K.** (1995). *Disability: A Continuing Challenge*. New Delhi: Wiley Eastern.

**National Sample Survey Organization.** (1991a). A Report on Disabled Persons: Forty-seventh Round (July–December 1991). New Delhi: Department of Statistics: Government of India.

_____. (1991b). A Report on Delayed Mental Development among Indian Children: Forty-seventh Round (July–December 1991). New Delhi: Department of Statistics: Government of India.

**National Trust for Welfare of Persons with Autism, Cerebral Palsy, Mental Retardation and Multiple Disabilities Act.** (1999). New Delhi: Ministry of Law, Justice and Company Affairs, Government of India (Website: http://disabilities.org.in/legal/nationaltrustact 1999.html).

**O'Leary, K.D.** (1979). Behavioral Assessment. *Behavioral Assessment*, 1: 31–36.

**Pandey, R.S.** and **Advani, L.** (1996). Perspectives in Disability and Rehabilitation. Delhi: Vikas.

**Peshawaria, R., Menon, D.K.** and **Reddi, S.** (1991). *Play Activities for Young Children with Special Needs*. Secunderabad: National Institute for the Mentally Handicapped.

**Peshawaria, R.** and **Venkatesan, S.** (1992a). *Behavior Assessment Scales for Indian Children with Mental Retardation*. Secunderabad: National Institute for the Mentally Handicapped.

_____. (1992b). *Behavioral Approaches to Teaching Children with Mental Retardation: A Manual for Teachers*. Secunderabad: National Institute for the Mentally Handicapped.

**Peshawaria, R., Venkatesan, S.** and **Menon, D.K.** (1988). 'Consumer Demand of Services by Parents of Mentally Handicapped Individuals'. *Indian Journal of Disability and Rehabilitation*, July–December: 43–57.

_____. (1990). 'Behavior Problems in Mentally Handicapped Persons: An Analysis of Parent Needs. *Indian Journal of Clinical Psychology*, 17: 63–70.

**Peshawaria, R., Venkatesan, S., Mohapatra, B.** and **Menon, D.K.** (1990). 'Teachers' Perception of Problem Behaviors among Mentally Handicapped Persons in Special School Settings'. *Indian Journal of Disability and Rehabilitation*, January–June: 23–30.

**Piaget, J.** (1962). *Play, Dreams and Imitation in Childhood*. New York: Norton.

**Popham, W.J.** (1973). *Criterion Referenced Instruction*. Belmont: Pearson.

**Ramdas, G.** and **Mishra, R.R.** (1987). 'Rural Attitude towards the Disabled'. *Indian Journal of Disability and Rehabilitation*, 1: 49–53.

**Salvia, J.** and **Ysseldyke, J.E.** (1988). *Assessment in Special and Remedial Education*. Boston: Houghton Mifflin.

**Shroff, G.S., Merchant, V.J., Adhikari, H.** and **Kurani, J.** (1989). *Pro-forma on Developmental Data and Academics*. Mumbai: Jai Vakeel.

**Singh, A.K.** (1986). *Tests, Measurements and Research Methods in Behavioral Sciences*. New Delhi: Tata McGraw-Hill.

**Skinner, B.F.** (1953). *Science and Human Behavior*. New York: Mac Millan.

**Sundberg, N.D.** and **Taylor, L.E.** (1962). *Clinical Psychology*. New York: Appleton Century Crofts.

**Thorndike, R.L.** and **Hagen, E.P.** (1977). *Measurement and Evaluation in Psychology and Education*. New Delhi: Wiley Eastern.

**Ullman, L.P.** and **Krasner, L.** (1965). *Case Studies in Behavior Modification*. New York: Holt, Rinehart & Winston.

**Varma, L.P.** (1953). 'History of Psychiatry in India and Pakistan'. *Indian Journal of Neurology & Psychiatry*, 4(1 and 2): 26–53; 4(3 and 4): 138–64.

**Venkatesan, S.** (1991). 'Psychological Assessment of Individuals with Mental Retardation: Some Perspectives and Problems'. *The Creative Psychologist*, 3(2): 65–75.

————. (1993). 'Disciplining Children: Some Problems and Issues'. *Journal of Indian Education*, July: 7–11.

————. (1994a). 'Development of Curriculum for Preschool Education: Some Psychological Considerations. *Journal of Indian Education*, November: 1–9.

————. (1994b). 'Recent Trends and Issues in Behavioral Assessment of Individuals with Mental Handicap in India'. *The Creative Psychologist*, 6(1 and 2): 1–7.

————. (2000). 'Play Activities in Children with Mental Retardation'. *Indian Journal of Clinical Psychology*, 27(1): 124–28.

————. (2001). Parental Opinion on Prevailing Practices in Preschool Education'. *Journal of Indian Education*, February: 57–63.

————. (2002a). 'Extension and Validation of Gessells Drawing Test of Intelligence in a Group of Children with Communication Handicaps'. *Indian Journal of Clinical Psychology*.

————. (2002b). 'Reappraisal of Bombay-Karnatak Version of Binet-Kamat Intelligence Scales (1964)'. *Indian Journal of Clinical Psychology*, 29(1): 72–78.

————. (2002c). Building Bridges: Fiscal Analysis of Not for Profits for Disabled in India. Unpublished Dissertation. Mysore: All India Institute of Speech and Hearing.

**Venkatesan, S.** and **Choudhury, S.** (1995). 'Psychological Assessment of Rural Children with Mental Handicaps in India: Some Problems and Issues'. *The Creative Psychologist*, 7(1 and 2): 1–9.

**Venkatesan, S.** and **Das, A.K.** (1994). 'Reported Burden on Family Members in Receiving/Implementing Home Based Training Programs for Children with Mental Handicaps'. *Journal of Psychological Researches*, 38(1 and 2): 39–45.

**Venkatesan, S., Hanumantharao, P., Ravi, C.** and **Anuja, K.R.** (1994). 'Exposure of Mentally Handicapped Children to School Settings'. *Disabilities & Impairments*, 8(1): 21–22.

**Venkatesan, S., Peshawaria, R.** and **Anuradha, M.P.** (1996). 'Reward Preferences in Parents/Caregivers of Children with Mental Handicaps'. *Indian Journal of Applied Psychology*, 33(1): 11–17.

**Venkatesan, S.** and **Rao, P.M.** (1990). 'Validity of Parental Estimates against Actual Test Estimates in Mentally Handicapped Individuals'. *The Creative Psychologist*, 2(2): 71–75.

**Venkatesan, S.** and **Reddy, K.R.** (1990). 'Idiometric Approaches to Functional Assessment in Mentally Handicapped Adults: Report of a Pilot Study'. *Indian Journal of Clinical Psychology*, 17: 21–27.

————. (1991). 'Validation of an Idiometrically Based Functional Assessment Battery for Mentally Handicapped Adults: Report of a Pilot Study'. *Indian Journal of Clinical Psychology*, 18: 31–34.

**Venkatesan, S.** and **Reddy, K.R.** (1992). 'Sensitivity of an Idiometrically Based Functional Assessment Battery to Changes in Neuro-psychological Functions in Adults with Mental Handicap'. *The Creative Psychologist,* 4(2): 7–11.

**Venkatesan, S.** and **Vepuri, V.G.D.** (1993a). 'Parental Perception of Causes and Management for Problem Behaviors in Individuals with Mental Handicap'. *Disabilities & Impairments,* 7(2): 29–37.

**Venkatesan, S.** and **Vepuri, V.G.D.** (1993b). 'Content Errors in Prearithmetic Performance of Children with Specific Arithmetic Retardation'. *Journal of Psychological Researches,* 37(1 and 2): 46–51.

————. (1995). *Mental Retardation in India: A Bibliography.* New Delhi: Concept Publishers.

**Wahler, R.G.** (1976). 'Deviant Child Behavior in the Family: Developmental Speculations and Behavior Change Strategies'. In H. Lertenberg (ed.), *Handbook of Behavior Modification & Behavior Therapy.* New York: Englewood Cliffs

**Witt, J.C., Elliot, S.N., Gresham, F.M.** and **Kramer, J.J.** (1989). *Assessment of Special Children: Tests and the Problem Solving Processes.* Illinois: Scott Foresman.

**World Health Organization.** (1980). *International Classification of Impairments, Disabilities & Handicaps.* Geneva: WHO.

————. (1992). *International Classification of Diseases* (Tenth Revision). Geneva: WHO.

————. (2002). *International Classification of Impairments, Activities & Participation.* Geneva: WHO.

————. (2003). *Beta-2 Draft: Short Version.* Geneva: WHO.

# Index

# About the Author

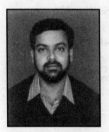

**S. Venkatesan** is Reader in the Department of Clinical Psychology, All India Institute of Speech and Hearing, Mysore, Karnataka. He was earlier a faculty member at the National Institute for the Mentally Handicapped (NIMH), Secunderabad, and subsequently Officer-in-Charge at NIMH's Regional Centre, Patna, Bihar.

Dr Venkatesan has previously published eight books (in English and Telugu) including *Behavioral Approaches in Teaching Mentally Handicapped Children: A Manual for Teachers; Managing Problem Behaviors in Children;* and *Mental Retardation In India: A Bibliography.* A Fellow of the Society for Advanced Studies in Medical Studies, New Delhi, he was conferred the N.N. Sen Memorial Award for the Best Research Paper by the Indian Association of Clinical Psychologists in January 2002.

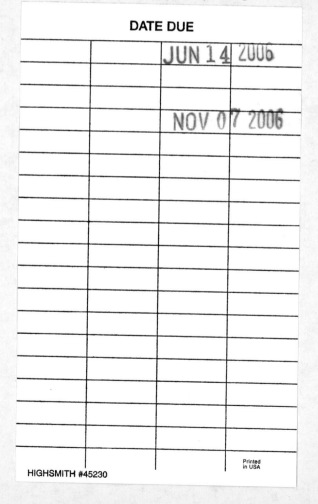